D1123794

NATURE'S MEDICINES

NEW UPDATED EDITION!

NATURE'S MEDICINES

FROM ASTHMA TO WEIGHT GAIN, FROM COLDS TO HIGH CHOLESTEROL— THE MOST POWERFUL ALL-NATURAL CURES

UNLEASH THE HEALING POTENTIAL OF
vitamins * minerals * herbs
amino acids * plant nutrients

By Gale Maleskey and the editors of **Prevention** magazine

© 2011 by Rodale, Inc.

Printed in the United States of America
Rodale Inc. makes every effort to use acid-free ♾, recycled paper ♲.

Book design by Kara Plikaitis

Library of Congress Cataloging-in-Publication Data

Maleskey, Gale.
    Nature's medicines: from asthma to weight gain, from colds to high cholesterol: the most powerful all-natural cures/by Gale Maleskey, and the Editors of Prevention.
        p.   cm.
    Originally published: 1999.
    Includes index.
    ISBN 978–1–60961–077–7 hardcover
    1. Naturopathy. I. Prevention (Firm: Emmaus, Pa.) II. Title.
RZ440.M34   2011
615.5'35—dc23   2011015768

    4   6   8   10   9   7   5   hardcover

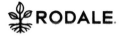

We inspire and enable people to improve their lives and the world around them.
For more of our products visit **prevention.com** or call 800-848-4735

contents

3: *Fighting Disease with Supplements*

Index   625

introduction

health rewards from Mother Nature

Sometimes, the keys to good health come in very small packages.

Many of those packages are sitting, right now, on the shelves of your nearest drugstore, supermarket, or health food store. That's where you'll find supplements that scientists, nutritionists, and doctors have distilled from nature's storehouse of healing remedies.

Some of these supplements—truly, nature's medicines—are derived from fruits and vegetables. Others come from minerals—yes, the same minerals that make up stone and soil. Still others are highly concentrated versions of many herbs that have been used for centuries in healing teas, tinctures, and tonics.

Alongside the nutritional and herbal supplements, however, you'll also find substances so unusual that they almost seem bizarre—from bee pollen and brewer's yeast to shark cartilage and fish oil. Even some living, beneficial organisms have their place among nature's medicines.

Faced with so many choices, how do you know which of these natural supplements are right for you?

That's where this book comes in.

In this updated edition of *Nature's Medicines,* you'll find out exactly how and when to take these supplements to improve and maintain your health. You'll discover how they can protect you from disease, keep your immune system powered up, and help you maintain sturdy, strong bones. Some will free you from aches and pains; others can help relieve heartburn or indigestion. Nature's medicines can even help your blood carry all of the necessary nutrients to your cells.

The benefits don't stop there. In these pages, you'll discover how to keep your skin healthy and flexible and free of itching, rashes, and infections. You'll learn how to restore worn-out tissue; fight cancer; and help your liver, kidneys, and bladder do the cleanup chores that they're supposed to do. You'll find out which supplements can help keep your heart healthy, your arteries clean, and your lungs clear.

In this book, you have a complete, authoritative guide to the most effective supplements that are currently available. You'll find specific, sound advice from many experts, including medical doctors, researchers, and a wide range of naturopaths, herbalists, and other practitioners of alternative medicine.

Look in Part 1 to learn how nature's medicines were first discovered and how to choose from among the many vitamins, minerals, herbs, and other supplements that are available today. Then turn to Part 2 for an A-to-Z guide to the healing powers of the world's most effective natural medicines. In Part 3, you can look up your specific health concerns to find out which of the powerful healing supplements can help protect you or speed your recovery from disease.

There are many ways to use this wealth of information. Want the most up-to-date and reliable evidence about leading supplements? You'll find that in Parts 1 and 2. Want to know which remedies are most highly recommended by leading experts for specific health concerns? Turn to Part 3 for authoritative answers, plus advice on appropriate dosages.

On every page, you'll learn how nature's medicines go hand in hand with other health measures, such as a nutritious diet and stress-relieving, immunity-boosting exercise. By combining these strategies, you can provide the best all-around health care for yourself and your family.

At the same time, however, it's important to know which of nature's medicines might not be appropriate. Before taking any supplement, you should note the cautions that are described in the Supplement Snapshots in Part 2. If you are pregnant, nursing, or have a chronic illness, be sure to consult a medical doctor or other qualified health-care practitioner before using any of the supplements described in this book. If you are taking prescription medication or treatments (such as chemo, radiation, or physical therapy), always talk to your doctor about possible interactions or side effects before taking supplements. Also, do not give these supplements to children.

1

what you
need to know
about
supplements

vitamins
and minerals

essential ingredients for a healthy body

Hippocrates got it right in one sentence: "Let food be thy medicine."

It took an additional 2,000 years of observation, plus a century of modern scientific research, to find out why food has the healing powers that Hippocrates ascribed to it—and the details are still being worked out.

Take vitamins, for instance. Ancient Greek and Egyptian physicians prescribed "liver juice" for night blindness. They had no way of knowing that their prescription contained a remarkable amount of vitamin A. It wasn't until 1930, in fact, that Swiss researchers determined the chemical structure of vitamin A and its precursor, beta-carotene. We now know that people who don't get enough vitamin A can experience night blindness, an early symptom of deficiency.

The discovery of vitamin C followed a parallel route. By 1601, some astute observers had noted that consuming citrus fruits prevented scurvy, a disease that wiped out countless crews of sailors who lived on salted meat and dried biscuits while at sea. It took two more centuries before British navy ships were required to carry rations of lime or lemon juice, and even then, the advocates of this practice had no idea why these tart fruits helped prevent the dreaded sailors' disease. It wasn't until more than 100 years later that vitamin C was finally isolated.

As vitamin C revealed the power of vitamins, iron was the telltale clue to the potential of minerals. "Metals of heaven"—iron-rich meteorites—were used therapeutically by the ancient civilizations of the eastern Mediterranean. The oldest surviving manuscript, the Ebers Papyrus, details two iron-rich remedies. In 1932, iron deficiency was officially recognized as the cause of chlorosis, a type of anemia found in teenage girls, and we were also well into the 20th century before scientists proved that iron is a component of hemoglobin, a protein in red blood cells. Now it's universally recognized that we all need iron to help rebuild blood.

What Makes a Mighty Multi?

Scan the shelves of your local pharmacy, and you're likely to see a multitude of multivitamin/mineral supplements. Obviously, each contains a wide variety of vitamins and minerals, and if you carefully compare labels, you'll find that some brands have a little more of this, while others have a little more of that. Beyond shaking the bottles, checking the prices, and comparing labels, how should you look for a multi?

No matter what the state of your health, it's smart to take a supplement that contains 100 percent of the Daily Value (DV) for most essential vitamins and minerals. The trouble is, none of the multis contains 100 percent of what you need. If you eat a healthful diet, you'll get many of the vitamins and minerals that you'll find in a multi, but many diets come up short on the following nutrients, experts say. You can get them by taking a multi along with a few individual supplements. Here are the suggested amounts.

Daily Multivitamin/Mineral Supplement

- Vitamin A/beta-carotene: 5,000 international units (mixed carotenoids)
- Vitamin B_6: 2 milligrams
- Vitamin D: 600 to 800 international units
- Folic acid: 400 micrograms
- Chromium: 200 micrograms

Small Stuff, Big Action

The scientific definition of a vitamin is "an organic compound, not a lipid or amino acid, required in very small amounts for essential functions in the body." Anything that's organic—from mulch and tree trunks to toenails and earlobes—contains the element carbon, the same element that's found in every vitamin. Lipids (fats) and amino acids are also organic, but they are not vitamins.

The customary means of getting vitamins into our bodies is to eat plants or animals that make or store these compounds. Plants use sunlight, air, water, and nutrients from the soil to synthesize folate in their leaves. Some plants and animals make their own vitamin C. Vitamins can also be synthesized from organic compounds in a laboratory. Thus, when you buy

- Copper: 2 milligrams
- Magnesium: 350 milligrams
- Selenium: At least 100 micrograms
- Zinc: 15 milligrams

As for iron, unless you have iron-deficiency anemia, look for a supplement that doesn't include it. You probably don't need extra iron, and studies have linked high iron levels with increased risk of heart attack and atherosclerosis (hardening of the arteries). Some premenopausal women, however, may need extra iron to compensate for menstrual blood loss.

Additional Supplements

You won't find the optimal dose of the following nutrients in most multis, so buy these supplements separately.

- Vitamin C: 250-milligram tablets. The optimal dose is 500 milligrams a day, but you'll absorb more if you take two doses spaced 12 hours apart.
- Vitamin E: 100 to 400 international units (mixed tocopherols, and ideally, mixed tocotrienols) once a day.
- Calcium: 500 to 1,000 milligrams once a day.
- Vitamin D: 800 international units.

a vitamin supplement, you might be getting compounds that have been put together by plants and animals or you might be getting identical, look-alike compounds that have been assembled in a laboratory.

Minerals are inorganic, but these, too, are available from organic sources. Plants absorb minerals from the ground, and animals get them from the plants they eat, so the root source of all minerals is the Earth.

By definition, anything officially labeled a "vitamin" is in some way absolutely necessary to human health. "If a substance found in food has a defined biochemical function in the human body, it is considered essential," says Forrest Nielsen, PhD, director of the USDA Human Nutrition Research Center in Grand Forks, North Dakota. It may take many years of research, however, before scientists know whether a component is essential, he adds.

Where Phytos Finish
in the Nutrient Race

When it comes to stocking your body with nutrients, the essentials are just that—essential. They include protein, carbohydrates, fats, vitamins, minerals, and water.

Then there are the phytonutrients. Phyto means "plant," so phytonutrients are simply nutrients derived from plants. Phytonutrients may promote good health, but unlike vitamins, they have not been found to be essential, says Cyndi Thomson, PhD, RD, clinical nutrition research specialist at the University of Arizona Cancer Prevention Center in Tucson.

Then where does that leave our green vegetables? Weren't we all told to eat our peas and broccoli or we'd wither and fade away?

Despite what you were told, or even what you told your kids, "you will not die if you do not eat broccoli—but you may not be as healthy, either," Dr. Thomson says. In fact, there's only one class of phytonutrients, the carotenoids, that has been shown to have vitamin activity. The beta-carotene that you get from carrots and some other fruits and vegetables is changed

Essential nutrients may be parts of hormones. The trace mineral iodine, for instance, is needed to manufacture thyroxine, the thyroid gland's major hormone. Vitamin D is a steroid hormone. Nutrients may also be needed to break down food for energy, as many of the B vitamins are.

Nutrients can also break down wastes that are subsequently eliminated from the body. The trace mineral manganese serves this role, converting the toxic ammonia that we form in our bodies into urea, which is excreted in urine.

Some nutrients appear to be essential even though their biochemical functions have yet to be defined, Dr. Nielsen says. Chromium, nickel, and boron are examples. Arsenic, a substance that we label a poison, is one of the possibly essential nutrients under investigation. We know we need trace amounts of it, although we're not sure exactly why.

It's likely that more nutrients will make the "essential" list as research continues. "There are a lot of gray areas left to explore," says Gerald Combs Jr., PhD, professor of nutrition at Cornell University in Ithaca, New York. He cites omega-3 fatty acids and the amino acid carnitine as two examples. "Now we realize that omega-3 fatty acids are required for by your body into different compounds, one of which is much-needed vitamin A.

So even though you can survive without vegetables, you do need them. While it's true that some phytonutrients are available as nutritional supplements, no matter how "complete" the supplements are, they're bound to leave out many of the phytos that are found in fruits and vegetables. Not only that, but the mixture of these nutrients that you get naturally from carrots, blueberries, broccoli, and other plant foods provides some benefits that generally can't be duplicated by a laboratory-produced pill.

You're better off supplementing your diet with a wide range of fresh fruits and vegetables. Especially good sources of the phytonutrients that will help you thrive are berries, garlic, dark leafy greens, deep yellow and orange fruits and vegetables, grape juice, tomatoes, and yes, broccoli and other cruciferous vegetables, such as cabbage and kale.

neurological development and eye development in infants," says Dr. Combs. "Some experts also think that carnitine may be required for infants under some circumstances."

As we develop better technology, we can scrutinize the additional properties of vitamins and minerals even more closely, Dr. Combs adds. "We can measure things we couldn't even conceive of earlier." Within the last four decades, for example, the ability to measure zinc has improved tremendously. "Twenty-five years ago, we thought there were five or six zinc-containing enzymes because that's all we could measure," Dr. Combs observes. "Now we know there are more than 300, simply because we can detect tinier and tinier amounts."

Getting Your DVs

Although each of us has somewhat different requirements for vitamins and minerals, we all need a certain basic supply of nutrients. Based on research, experts have drawn up a set of nutrition guidelines that are universally used as a standard of measurement by the federal government.

The nutrition information that you'll find on any packaged food—and on most bottles of vitamins and minerals—is based on those guidelines.

Wherever you see the abbreviation DV, it stands for Daily Value. The DV column on a label lists the percentages of the DV for vitamins or minerals in a serving of a food or a single dose of a supplement, based on an intake of 2,000 calories a day. The DV for vitamin C, for instance, is 60 milligrams, so a supplement containing 60 milligrams has 100 percent of the DV. The label of a supplement containing 30 milligrams of vitamin C would indicate that it has 50 percent of the DV.

Since each of us has different needs, your vitamin C requirement might be higher than the DV if you're older, if your immune system needs some boosting, or if you're recovering from an infection. Smokers, for instance, have an enhanced risk of many diseases, so the recommended dose for them is 100 milligrams—more than 160 percent of the DV that applies to most nonsmokers. (Many experts, however, consider even 100 milligrams an inadequate dose for smokers.)

Age differences, sex differences, and stage of life can also affect your nutrient needs, meaning that your actual daily requirements for vitamins and minerals may vary from the DV for many reasons. For both men and women, vitamin and mineral requirements are likely to change somewhat with age, and very active or athletic people are likely to need more than those who are less active. All of these factors have an impact on individual nutrient requirements.

Some of these differences are readily apparent. Consider the needs of infants. Per pound of body weight, nutrient needs are highest when an infant is growing rapidly, as it does during the first year of life, says Kathryn Kolasa, PhD, professor of nutrition education at East Carolina University School of Medicine in Greenville, North Carolina. Nutrient needs are also high during teenage growth spurts, usually from ages 12 to 20 for boys and 10 to 18 for girls.

A Little Something Extra

To help us get our DVs of vitamins and minerals, as well as meet other basic nutritional requirements, nutrients are routinely added to foods that many of us eat nearly every day. When this is done, the foods are called fortified or enriched. This program, regulated by the federal government, has been highly successful in helping to eliminate severe nutritional deficiencies.

In the United States, iodine has been added to salt since 1930. Before then, in areas where people had little or no iodine in their food supplies, it was fairly common to see the medical condition called goiter. An enlargement of the thyroid gland, goiter is a direct result of iodine deficiency, says Paul Lachance, PhD, professor and executive director of the Nutraceuticals Institute at Rutgers University in New Brunswick, New Jersey.

Slightly less than ½ teaspoon of iodized salt a day provides enough iodine to prevent goiter. Noniodized salt, such as kosher salt, is still available, but manufacturers are required by law to offer the iodized version as well. People are so used to buying iodized salt that goiter problems have been virtually eliminated, but people who use sea salt or "gourmet" salts may not be getting enough iodine since those salts aren't fortified.

Vitamin D is another cause célèbre of the government's nutrition program. Since the 1940s, vitamin D has routinely been added to milk to help prevent childhood rickets, a disease that causes bones to become deformed or soften. This fortification program has helped to reduce the incidence of childhood rickets in the United States, Dr. Lachance says. Researchers now think we may need even more D, as people seem to benefit from attaining blood levels that are higher than the traditional "low-normal" range of 20 ng/ml.

Vitamin A is also added to milk, particularly reduced-fat, low-fat, and fat-free milk. In the 1940s, when this vitamin was found to improve immune response and correct some vision problems in children and women, the government began requiring that it be added. Whole milk naturally contains some vitamin A—about one-third of the DV in a quart—but extra vitamin A is sometimes added. Most powdered milk contains vitamin A, along with vitamin D.

Since 1942, white flour, cornmeal, and polished (white) rice have been enriched with three B-complex vitamins—thiamin, riboflavin, and niacin—and with iron. In 1998, folic acid was added to the list of required fortifications. Whole-wheat flour is not enriched because it naturally contains these and other nutrients, although in smaller amounts than those added through enrichment.

Even with this fortification program, we can't take all of these nutrients for granted, Dr. Lachance says. While fortification has made serious deficiencies much less likely to develop, iron deficiency is still common in the United States, he says. It's also likely that you're not getting enough vitamin D if you don't drink much milk, since other foods don't offer much. In fact, people consuming adequate vitamin D through milk can still be vitamin D–deficient during the winter months.

Deficiency Detection

When someone is deficient in an essential nutrient, symptoms are sure to crop up after a while. Health problems ensue. Fatigue, muscle weakness, irritability, reduced resistance to infection, poor healing, and slowed growth are common to many vitamin and mineral deficiencies.

Despite these well-known signs, the detective work isn't easy. Anemia, for example, is a condition that's characterized by many of the symptoms of overall nutrient deficiencies—particularly fatigue and muscle weakness. It occurs when there's a reduction in the number of red blood cells, but there are many possible causes of that reduction. In some people, anemia is caused by iron deficiency. Others may display symptoms of other kinds of anemia because they're short on vitamins A, B_6, B_{12}, C, and E, or folate, riboflavin, or copper. Sometimes looking at red blood cells (or bone marrow cells, where red blood cells originate) under a microscope gives a clue to what type of anemia a person has.

In other cases, initial symptoms are more distinct or tend to show up first in a certain area of the body. If a wound takes longer than usual to stop bleeding, for instance, that slow clotting time might indicate a vitamin K deficiency, or someone may develop poor night vision, a tip-off for vitamin A deficiency. These days, a suspected vitamin or mineral deficiency can usually be confirmed with tests that measure blood levels of the nutrient or that test a particular enzyme or cell function associated with the nutrient, Dr. Nielsen says.

There are some nutrients that we can take for granted, however. We get lots of them every day in our diets. These include sodium, phosphorus, sulfur, and chloride.

Adequate versus Optimal

Over the years, as researchers have explored the effects of different amounts of vitamins and minerals, a new approach has emerged. In the past, they tried to determine the minimum necessary amounts of nutrients that were needed to prevent deficiencies and thereby prevent the health problems caused by deficiencies. Today, scientists are paying greater attention to the amounts of nutrients needed for optimal nutrition.

"We're asking different questions than we used to," Dr. Combs says. "For the last 100 years, since the first vitamin, thiamin, was discovered, the questions have been, 'Do you need this vitamin? Will it keep you alive? Will it prevent a deficiency disease, such as scurvy or beriberi?' Now that those diseases are pretty much gone from our society, we are looking at other health problems related to diet."

Among the leading problems related to nutrition, Dr. Combs points out, are cancer, heart disease, and certain kinds of diabetes. "Thus, we are asking different questions to determine whether there may be benefits at higher levels [of vitamin consumption]," he says.

Some of the vitamins studied in this regard include the antioxidants, such as vitamins E and C; vitamin D; chromium; and various B vitamins. But as we learned from vitamin E, studied in clinical trials for its apparent ability to help prevent heart disease, answers aren't as easy to find as we would like them to be. "In population studies, groups taking vitamin E supplements clearly had a lower risk of heart disease," Dr. Combs says. "However, these people possibly had other healthier behaviors than those who didn't take supplements, so it still needs to be determined if this big reduction in heart disease can indeed be directly attributed to vitamin E." Researchers continue to try and find out how much prevention vitamin E actually offers to those who are at risk for heart attack, or even whether the kind of vitamin E used in studies—most often dl- or d-alpha-tocopherol—provides less heart protection than the eight forms of vitamin E found naturally in foods.

Supplement-Making Made Simple

How are vitamin and mineral supplements made, tested, packaged, and sold? How do you know if you're getting what the label says?

Vitamins, whether synthetic or "natural," are processed in huge, modern plants. There are a dozen or so large companies worldwide that produce most vitamins so that hundreds of companies can purchase them as ingredients for vitamin pills.

Each vitamin is produced through a unique series of steps. Vitamin C, for instance, can be made from natural-source dextrose, a type of sugar.

Sustenance from Sunbeams— And Other Sources

Most of our nutrients come from food, but there are notable exceptions. Given enough exposure to the sun's ultraviolet rays, our bodies convert one kind of fat in our skin to vitamin D. Sunlight has traditionally been considered health-reviving for that reason.

Getting adequate vitamin D helps prevent crippling bone deformities like rickets, which began to appear more than 200 years ago as northern European countries became industrialized. With more people living in cities and more cities darkened by an overhang of smoke from industrial production, sunlight was fighting a losing battle with man-made interferences.

A Polish doctor named Sniadecki first made the connection between the need for sunlight and the bone diseases that appeared to be a slow-moving epidemic in these industrialized areas. He advised parents to take their rickets-ridden children into the country, or to at least carry them into the sunlight as often as possible. He had no idea what healing power was in the rays, but whatever it was, he surmised, these children needed it.

There are also instances in which lifestyle does the doctoring. In countries such as India, people who are strict vegetarians suffer from shortages of vitamin B_{12} in their diets. Some of the lack is made up from an unusual source—bacteria in food. Unappetizing as it seems, certain bacteria

The process involves nine steps. Technically complex, those steps mimic the way animals manufacture the vitamin in their bodies.

Vitamin B_{12}, another vitamin in high demand, requires the use of a particular kind of bacteria that can break down sugar into alcohol. It's no coincidence that the French, who are famous wine producers, are also the world's leading producers of vitamin B_{12}.

Making vitamin E, on the other hand, is a very different process. This vitamin is oil-soluble, which means that it's dissolved and carried in a medium of vegetable oil. The natural-source vitamin E must be isolated from soybean oil, while the synthetic form is synthesized by a chemical process.

Once isolated, each vitamin can be run through a series of chemical analyses, called assays, to make sure that it is pure and has the right chemical structure. Manufacturers of any vitamin made in the United synthesize vitamin B_{12}. Our bodies need only a tiny amount of this vitamin, and bacteria make enough to compensate.

Some forms of yeast, which is actually a living fungus, also synthesize B_{12}. Since this is especially true of brewer's yeast, a strict vegetarian who drinks beer may have a ready source of this vitamin, says Gerald Combs Jr., PhD, professor of nutrition at Cornell University in Ithaca, New York. (Of course, the average beer contains only 0.06 microgram of B_{12}, so even if vegetarians have an occasional cold one, they must take supplements to get the Daily Value of 6 micrograms.)

Extra minerals can also be obtained in some unusual ways. Take iron, for instance. The iron in cast-iron pots or skillets is actually transferred to food when we cook with those utensils. Although the transfer might seem insignificant, it can increase the iron content of foods by two to six times.

The skins of fruits and vegetables, especially root vegetables like carrots and potatoes, are also good mineral "supplements" because trace minerals are concentrated in the pores of the skins. True, you need to wash these foods before eating them to remove unwanted bacteria and pesticides, but you'll still get some minerals once you start munching.

States or imported for use do these appraisals voluntarily. Some do these assays faithfully, while others do them seldom or not at all. It's one of the "loopholes" in the nutritional supplements laws that forces the industry to police itself and that makes smart consumers stick with well-regarded brands or see a health care professional for recommended brands.

All vitamins sold in the United States are supposed to meet the manufacturing quality standards set by the US Pharmacopeia (USP), a scientific, standard-setting organization for the drug industry. Even if the vitamins are made in China, for example, they should meet USP manufacturing standards to be sold here, says Frank Girardi, director of market services at Roche Vitamins in Parsippany, New Jersey. Unfortunately, these standards aren't often enforced through inspections or restrictions, at least not outside the United States.

Keep or Toss?

Vitamins can be an investment—and the best way to protect that investment is to store supplements in a cool, dry place.

But what's considered a cool, dry place?

The bathroom's out because the steamy shower jacks up the humidity, and the cupboard above the stove is out because it gets hot up there. You have a lot of other choices, though.

"Keep them in a spot that's not exposed to direct sunlight, excess humidity, or heat," says V. Srini Srinivasan, PhD, senior scientist with the US Pharmacopeia, a private standard-setting organization for the drug industry. For most people, a kitchen cupboard fits that bill, as long as it's well away from the stove.

To find out how long a supplement is likely to remain effective, check the expiration date on the bottle before you buy it. The label might carry a code such as 010112, which means that the expiration date is January 1, 2012. An expiration date may be two to four years from the date of manufacture, depending on what's in the supplement.

Minerals are a different story. Unlike most vitamins, minerals are obtained from natural sources, and that often means mining. Sent to manufacturing laboratories, the minerals go through a purification process. Then they're usually combined with some other ingredient to make them stable, nontoxic, and more absorbable.

Sabinsa, a company in Piscataway, New Jersey, makes a product called selenomethionine. At the heart of that supplement is the mineral selenium. Sabinsa buys selenium from producers around the world and purifies it. Then the manufacturer uses a chemical process to bond the pure selenium with methionine, an amino acid. The purpose of this process is to make selenium more available to the body.

Many companies worldwide prepare minerals for use in multivitamin/ mineral supplements. Most handle only one or two types of minerals, though, so a supplement manufacturer that offers many kinds of minerals may purchase them from a wide range of suppliers.

Mineral product manufacturers also use the USP standards of testing. Since the companies that do the formulations are buying batches of vitamins and minerals from hundreds of different suppliers around the world,

Experts say it's best not to buy or use expired supplements because of reduced potency. As long as a product is properly stored, though, it's guaranteed to meet the potency listed on the label up to the expiration date. After that, the product begins to degrade, and its potency slowly drops.

You'll lengthen the life of your supplements if you store them in the refrigerator or freezer. If you do, though, don't leave the cap off after you take them, since moisture will condense inside the bottle. Recap the bottle quickly and return it to the refrigerator or freezer.

Some additional tips: Always keep bottles tightly closed, and don't leave supplements inside a hot car. It's also important to keep them out of the reach of children. Even though they're not as poisonous as many household products, an overdose can be dangerous or even fatal. Discard any product that begins to look or smell strange. It might have become contaminated by mold, bacteria, or other harmful organisms.

testing is important. An incoming batch that was previously tested may be tested again by a reputable company upon arrival at the manufacturer to make sure that it meets certain specifications.

The first step is to "culture" the batch to see if any unwanted bacteria or yeast starts to grow. After that, individual ingredients are weighed out, mixed together, sampled and tested again, and put into tablets or capsules. Finally, they are bottled and placed on store shelves.

Natural versus Synthetic

Looking at this vast and profitable manufacturing process, you may begin to wonder whether the selected, purified nutrients that end up in supplements are really very natural at all.

Of course, food is the most obvious natural source of vitamins and the Earth is the most natural source of minerals, but the vitamins and minerals in supplements are several times removed from their original sources. While some manufacturers isolate vitamin E from soybean oil and derive vitamin C from acerola berries, unless they are specifically labeled as "whole food" supplements, most vitamins aren't made that way these days.

Although some people think "natural" means "better," there's a practical reason for synthetic vitamins: The laboratory process is much more efficient and less expensive than isolating these nutrients from foods. Also keep in mind that even vitamins labeled "natural" undergo several steps in processing before they arrive in their final form.

Still, most experts agree that, in general, it's best to take vitamins that are biochemically identical to the forms found in foods. That's because some synthetic forms, like dl-alpha-tocopherol, may actually interfere with the biological activity of natural forms.

With minerals, the question of natural versus synthetic never comes up. Since minerals are elements, they can only be purified—not created—in the lab. If they aren't mined from the ground, they're separated from other natural sources. Calcium, for instance, is derived from limestone, oyster shells, eggshells, or naturally occurring beds of calcium carbonate.

What is synthetic in the case of mineral supplements is the way the minerals are combined to make them less toxic and easier for our bodies to absorb. Chromium picolinate, for instance, is a patented form of chromium that's been combined with picolinic acid. In this form, the metal chromium is easier to absorb, Dr. Nielsen says. Many minerals are chelated, or combined with an amino acid, to make them more absorbable so you can take less and still get the same nutritional benefits.

Meeting Special Needs

In the Supplement Snapshots in Part 2 of this book, you'll find the DV listed for each of the vitamins and minerals discussed. Keep in mind, though, that as we've mentioned, your specific needs may exceed the recommended DV, depending on your sex, age, and various health factors.

Pregnant women need twice as much iron as nonpregnant women, and their requirements for vitamin D and folic acid are more than double. Expectant mothers also need much more of vitamins C and E, as well as all of the B vitamins. Among minerals, extra calcium is critical for pregnant women, and more zinc and magnesium are also required.

If a woman nurses her baby, requirements for some nutrients during the first 6 months of nursing soar even higher than the levels required during pregnancy, Dr. Kolasa says. This is true for vitamins A, C, and E

Do Dinosaurs Have What You Need?

If you have children, it's possible that you have some vitamins around that are grape-flavored and resemble prehistoric cartoon characters. Dinosaur-shaped vitamins are fine for the kids, but will they do you any good?

It's perfectly okay to take one or two each day, says Cathy Kapica, PhD, RD, assistant professor of nutrition and clinical dietetics at Finch University of Health Sciences/The Chicago Medical School in North Chicago. In fact, "if you have trouble swallowing, chewable vitamins are a reasonable way to supplement," she says. Liquid vitamins are also available, she notes.

Most chewables will not provide adequate nutrition for an adult. You'll want to read labels to compare what you'd get in a children's vitamin to what you'd get in an adult multivitamin. This will vary by brand. If you're looking for high amounts of antioxidant nutrients, for instance, you won't find them in dinosaur-shaped, multicolored chewables. Even if you have a dinosaur as a supplement appetizer now and then, you're better off with adult-size supplements for adult-size doses, Dr. Kapica advises. Some brands even have chewables, liquids, and powders for grown-ups.

and most of the B vitamins, along with magnesium, zinc, and selenium. "That's why women are advised to continue taking their prenatal vitamins until they wean their babies," she says.

Women also have an increased need for iron during their childbearing years because they normally lose iron every month during menstruation. If you're a woman whose menstrual flow is heavy and you often feel tired, you should probably see your doctor about an iron supplement, says Dr. Kolasa.

The iron requirements for men are generally less than those for women because men normally have larger iron stores. Men don't lose much iron unless they have chronic internal bleeding, such as from a bleeding ulcer. Since high iron stores have been associated with an increased risk for conditions such as heart disease and cancer, men are usually advised not to take supplemental iron unless they have been tested for deficiency and advised by a doctor, Dr. Kolasa says.

Safety with Supplements

Like prescription and over-the-counter drugs, any kind of supplement needs to be taken responsibly, says Mark Stengler, ND, a naturopathic doctor and author of *The Natural Physician: Your Health Guide for Common Ailments.* Before you start taking any supplements that are new to you, heed the following suggestions from Dr. Stengler.

• To avoid or minimize any side effects, start with a lower dosage than the one stated on the label, then gradually increase the dosage until you reach recommended levels.

• Consult a knowledgeable physician or health practitioner before using any new supplements. Certain vitamins, herbs, and dietary supplements can be toxic in higher doses.

• If you are pregnant or nursing, avoid all supplements unless they have been prescribed or approved by your doctor. Also, check with your physician before using supplements if you are taking prescription medication. People who are taking anticoagulant (blood-thinning) medications, for example, should not take high doses of vitamin E, fish oil, or a number of other supplements that thin the blood.

The need for some nutrients—such as the B vitamins, which are used to help metabolize food—is based on calorie intake. These nutrient requirements are higher for men, who usually eat more calories each day, than they are for women. The differences are slight, however. People who eat lots of "empty calories," such as soft drinks and other sugary foods, are likely to need more B vitamins and magnesium because it takes a lot of these nutrients in order to break down these low-quality foods for energy.

Calcium is often singled out as a nutrient that's needed more by women in menopause than by premenopausal women, but men also need it, Dr. Kolasa points out. "Men get osteoporosis, too," she says. Vitamin D also plays a crucial role in preventing osteoporosis after menopause.

Increasing Your Supplements as You Age

Research by the FDA shows that we need a higher maintenance dose of certain nutrients as we age, says Robert Russell, MD, associate director of the Jean Mayer USDA Human Nutrition Research Center on Aging at Tufts University in Boston.

"It's simple," Dr. Russell says. "Older people are eating less food. They are less active." Since we're more sedentary when we're older, we're likely to eat less—and that means that we probably don't get enough nutrients.

Contrary to popular belief, Dr. Russell says, most older people can absorb most nutrients just as well as younger people can. In fact, their ability to absorb vitamin A appears to increase, which means that they have to be careful not to overdo it with this potentially toxic nutrient.

There are exceptions. Absorption of one form of vitamin B_{12} can be a problem for up to one-third of older people. They don't need larger amounts of it, but they need to take it in the form that their bodies can use, says Dr. Russell. That form, methylcobalamin, can be found in fortified food products or in supplements, which is why a lot of senior multi formulas have it.

Older people also have trouble with vitamin D. "Their skin doesn't manufacture it as well as it did when they were younger, so they need to get more from foods or supplements," Dr. Russell says. Some experts are recommending amounts as high as 4,000 IU a day, but it's best to get your blood levels checked to determine the dosage that will work best for you.

Riboflavin, too, can be a problem for older people, Dr. Russell notes. Since many seniors have smaller appetites, they often get less riboflavin than they should in their diets. To adjust the balance, you'd have to consume several servings of dairy products each day, he says. He recommends at least 1.3 milligrams of riboflavin a day for men over 50 and at least 1.1 milligrams for women.

Vitamin B_6 requirements also seem to be higher among seniors. About one-third of older people show signs of deficiency, Dr. Russell says. He recommends that men over 50 get 1.7 milligrams and women take 1.5 milligrams.

Older people might also benefit from getting more than the DV of thiamin, especially if they drink alcohol, Dr. Russell says. In one study, when women who got an average of less than 1 milligram a day of thiamin were given supplements of 10 milligrams a day, they reported sleeping better and having better appetites. They also reported that they felt more cheerful.

Studies also indicate that it might be helpful for older people to get more of the antioxidant nutrients, specifically vitamins C and E and selenium.

Rather than focusing on large amounts of just one antioxidant, such as vitamin E, though, it's best to take a mix of antioxidants in smaller amounts. That way, you'll get a variety of antioxidant activity that targets many parts of your body.

As for minerals, the DVs are usually adequate for older people. In fact, the DVs for some minerals, such as chromium and magnesium, may even be set too high, Dr. Russell says. If many older people don't get the recommended amounts, it could be because they aren't eating the foods that supply these needed nutrients.

How Do You Know When Enough Is Enough?

If you take in more supplements than your body can handle, what was beneficial at a lower dose becomes potentially toxic, says Henry Lukaski, PhD, research leader for mineral nutrient functions at the USDA research center in North Dakota.

In the Supplement Snapshots in Part 2, you'll find information about cautions and side effects to help ensure that you take safe and reasonable doses. This advice comes from doctors and researchers, based on studies and observations.

When scientists talk about the toxicity of a vitamin or mineral, they are referring to the concentration at which it becomes harmful—the point at which it begins to act more like a poison than a medicine.

Each vitamin and mineral with known toxicity has its own unique symptoms. If you get way too much of the trace mineral selenium, for instance (as once happened to people who took an improperly made dietary supplement), you might lose your hair and fingernails and develop a garlicky odor. If you take too much vitamin A, as people who are self-treating for acne sometimes do, you'll develop a headache, vomiting, hair loss, and dry mucous membranes.

If you take vitamins and minerals within their safe ranges, you'll get the benefits rather than the toxic effects. For each vitamin and mineral, however, the range is different, according to John Hathcock, PhD, director of nutrition and regulatory science for the Council for Responsible Nutrition in Washington, DC. The DV for vitamin A, for instance, is 5,000 IU, but toxic effects have been reported at amounts above 10,000 IU.

With other nutrients, the range of safety is so broad that toxicity has never been reported. Chromium appears to be safe even at more than 1,000 micrograms, which is more than eight times its DV of 120 micrograms.

Memory Joggers:
How to Remember to Take 'Em

One man put the bottle in his shoe. "He could remember to take his pills in the evening, but he could never remember in the morning," says Joyce Cramer, a medical researcher in psychiatry at West Haven–Yale Veterans Affairs Medical Center in Connecticut and an authority on drug-taking behavior. He had one pair of sneakers that he wore every day, "so he put his pill bottle in there."

Sound silly? "It worked for him," Cramer says. "And if it works for you, do it. It's just like car keys. Some people put them in their pocket, some hang them by the door—whatever it takes to remember to take them when you leave the house."

If you've been forgetting to take your daily supplements and you want some easy memory joggers, you might want to try one or both of the following tactics.

• Use a daily chore as a cue. Using a habit as a reminder can go a long way, but if it's going to work, you have to get it established. The cue needs to be something that you do at a regular time every day, like drinking a morning cup of juice. If you always take a vitamin after drinking your juice, your mind will cue you, "Oops, I forgot something" if you neglect to do it.

• If you take a number of different supplements, visit a drugstore and get a plastic pill organizer. A typical kind has a row of seven boxes, and some have separate compartments for up to four doses a day. If you can't remember whether you've taken a supplement, just snap open the right box and have a look. You can tell at a glance which pills you missed. Plus, this method ensures that you don't take two doses when you should take only one. If you like beepers and gadgets, you can even get a pill box that has a programmable timer on top. Ask your pharmacist for more information.

Vitamin C has no reported adverse effects at doses of 1,000 milligrams and, except for causing occasional bouts of diarrhea, seems to be safe at any amount. Vitamin B_{12} does not appear to have any toxic effects, says Dr. Hathcock. "For most vitamins and minerals, the amounts that are safe and beneficial are far below the amounts that are toxic," he concludes.

Pushing the Limits

Given the careful guidelines that scientists have established, it may seem odd that some doctors prescribe doses that are much higher than what is usually considered safe. This is a considered risk, because large amounts—even amounts that could be toxic—may be needed to treat a particular condition.

If you're taking large, therapeutic doses of a vitamin or mineral for a long period of time, you need to be careful, says Dr. Hathcock. These large doses can have damaging effects on organs or tissues. The occasional liver-damaging side effects of large doses of niacin (nicotinic acid)—prescribed to reduce cholesterol—are well-documented, he notes. (Don't take more than 35 milligrams per day without a physician's supervision.) So are the nerve-damaging effects of huge doses of vitamin B_6. (Don't take more than 100 milligrams per day without a physician's supervision.)

In addition, there are limits that are simply unknown. No one knows the potential side effects of many vitamins and minerals when taken in large doses over the long term. While we know that large amounts of calcium can impair absorption of other minerals such as zinc and manganese, for example, what are the other possible side effects? A total calcium intake of 2,500 milligrams is safe, but we don't know what levels might cause long-term problems, says Dr. Hathcock.

Your best bet is to work with a doctor who's knowledgeable in nutrition. Confirm with your doctor that the amount of each nutrient you're taking is within a safe range. Don't take extra multivitamin/mineral pills to get more of one nutrient. Take single supplements of individual nutrients if necessary, says Dr. Hathcock. And be careful when you take several combination supplements. Add up the nutrients in each to make sure you are not going over the safe limit of any single nutrient.

Doctors advise that you not mix different multinutrient pills unless you've confirmed that the totals are within a safe range. If you have been diagnosed with a chronic health condition or you take prescription drugs regularly and want to use any of the remedies mentioned in this book, talk with your health-care practitioner first. Women who are pregnant or nursing or who are trying to become pregnant should always consult their doctors before using any home remedy, including vitamins and herbs. Also, if you have kidney, liver, or heart problems, it's best to check with your doctor before you take anything other than a standard multivitamin/ mineral supplement that offers the DV of most nutrients.

Food in a Pill?

Why bother with real food if you can just pop a pill that provides all the nourishment you need? That's what the Jetsons did for breakfast in the cartoon series set in an imaginary 21st century, and they had more than enough energy.

If you're really into pill popping, it's true that you can get all the known essential nutrients from vitamin and mineral pills. You can also buy protein and carbohydrate powders and capsules of essential fatty acids. In fact, some people who are unable to eat food live on liquid versions of the same; it's called parenteral nutrition.

You won't want to live on synthetic food alone if you have a choice, though, says Scott Smith, PhD, research nutritionist for NASA at the Johnson Space Center in Houston. "The engineers would be happy if we could get to that point, but not the astronauts or the medical staff."

Why? For the astronauts, shared meals of real food provide a major psychological benefit, Dr. Smith says. "On long flights especially, with very few things that look like home, food reminds them of something they had back on Earth," he explains. The same sorts of foods that you may have found reassuring as a kid—such as pudding, for instance—provide some psychological comfort in outer space.

In addition to psychological benefits, real food also provides some distinct nutritional advantages over pills and powders. Your digestive system is accustomed to handling real food. It needs bulk. Even aromas and appearance play a role by stimulating your appetite and prompting some food-processing enzymes to jump into action, initiating the process of breaking down foods for absorption into the body. Real food also offers a sense of fullness and satiety that pills and powders just can't provide, Dr. Smith says.

That's why even astronauts dine on meals that are as close to real food as they can get. The usual space shuttle fare is reconstituted freeze-dried, packaged food similar to the lightweight stuff that back-packers sometimes eat. These foods can provide all the energy, vitamins, and minerals the astronauts need.

In addition, astronauts may take along vitamin and/or mineral supplements if they like, Dr. Smith says. On longer missions, supplements may be required to compensate for potential deficiencies.

Within individual chapters, you'll find dosage recommendations, contraindications, potential side effects, and other essential information about specific supplements. This information is based on advice from health-care professionals who have worked extensively with supplements and on guidelines from authoritative references. Remember, a remedy is most effective when used properly.

Watching the Clock

Is there a best—or worst—time to take a supplement? If you can benefit from taking a specific supplement at a certain time or in a certain manner, you'll find that advice in Part 2. Meanwhile, here's some general information that can help you decide when to take your supplements.

When it comes to taking a multivitamin, your best bet is to keep it simple. "Just take the darn thing every day, and don't worry about where or when or with what," says Paul Saltman, PhD, professor of biology at the University of California at San Diego.

That said, most people take multivitamins with meals, and that's just fine, Dr. Saltman says. Digestive juices that flow when you eat help you digest the ingredients in the pill, too. There are some elements in foods, such as fiber, that interfere somewhat with nutrient absorption, but unless you have serious gastrointestinal problems, you'll still absorb plenty.

Here are some additional ways to optimize vitamin and mineral absorption.

• Take fat-soluble vitamins—E, D, A, and K—with a meal that contains a teaspoon or so of fat to aid absorption, says Dr. Saltman.

• Take these fat-soluble vitamins in small doses throughout the day rather than in one large dose. If you take a large, one-a-day dose, more of the vitamin is likely to be stored rather than utilized, he says.

• If you are taking a therapeutic amount of a water-soluble vitamin such as vitamin C, it's also best to divide the dose into three or more smaller doses, according to Dr. Saltman. This way, you absorb more of the vitamin, plus your blood levels of the vitamin will stay more steady throughout the day than if you take one large dose.

• Avoid taking minerals with meals that are mostly fiber, such as a high-fiber breakfast cereal, he says. As good as it is for you, fiber impairs mineral absorption.

• Minerals are also better absorbed in divided doses, says Richard Wood, PhD, associate professor at Tufts University School of Nutrition. If you're taking 750 milligrams a day of calcium, for instance, you might want to try dividing it into three 250-milligram doses taken at midmorning, midafternoon, and before bed.

Minerals can compete for absorption as well. If you are taking a supplement containing many minerals, dividing it into three doses will increase absorption of all minerals.

In the next two parts of this book, you'll find everything that you need to know about vitamins and minerals. If you want details on a specific vitamin or mineral and how it works in your body, you can read about it in Part 2. Along with each vitamin or mineral that's included, you'll also find specific information—what it's recommended for, the DV, cautions about its use, and other details. If you have a particular health problem, turn to Part 3 for details on the vitamins and minerals that show promise for that condition.

botanical medicines and herbals

our green allies in health and healing

Every culture on Earth has used plants to cure disease, ease pain, and heal the ills and discomforts of the human body. Herbal medicine undoubtedly predates written history. We can assume that at the same time that human beings were learning which plants were good to eat and which were poison, they also were discovering which plants could heal them.

People first started to keep records of herbal medicine some 5,000 to 7,000 years ago in China and Mesopotamia. Much later, in AD 78, a Greek physician named Dioscorides described some 700 healing plants in a comprehensive work called *De Materia Medica*. For several centuries afterward, this was the foundation text for practitioners of herbal medicine throughout Europe.

The New World added new pages to the growing book of herbal cures. When Europeans stepped ashore in North America, they found Native Americans who had a flourishing apothecary that drew on healing plants of the forests and prairies. As white settlers pushed farther into the interior, many turned to Native American plants and herbal practices when they needed frontier treatments for illness and infection.

Native American herbs were still used by North American doctors throughout the 19th century and well into the 20th. Entrepreneurial pharmacists drew on Native American lore when they started marketing patent medicines. They would grind up some of the traditional ingredients and include them in cures for a wide range of ailments.

Today, the search continues for plants with healing properties. Ethnobotanists, who study how botanical medicines are used in other cultures, continue to study plants from places as remote as South American rain forests. Even drug companies have gotten into the act, hoping through exploration and experimentation to discover sources of new chemicals for the development of possible drugs.

In other words, herbal healing is nothing new.

What Is an Herb?

Simply put, a healing herb, or a botanical medicine, is a plant, so the range of potential sources of medicines is just as diverse as the plant kingdom itself. Botanicals range from the towering, rock-hard lapacho tree of the Brazilian rain forests, which has an inner bark that helps cure fungal infections, to the lowly, common feverfew, a weed found in roadside ditches that does a remarkable job of preventing migraine headaches.

Discovering that a plant or part of a plant has healing properties is only part of the challenge, however. Anyone who prescribes or uses herbs and other botanicals also would like to know how these plants can deliver the most healing benefit to our bodies. During the several millennia that humans have known about herbal healing, practitioners have used botanicals in a wide range of forms, from teas and tinctures to poultices and compresses—and today, as capsules and other supplements.

When medicines are derived from healing plants, they're called phytomedicines, botanicals, or herbal supplements. The terms are interchangeable, and all refer to medicines derived solely from plant material. Today, these botanicals are widely distributed. Many are available in drugstores, health food stores, grocery stores, and even department stores. Others may be provided by naturopathic doctors, practitioners of traditional Chinese medicine, or practitioners of alternative medicine who use herbs as important elements in their healing regimens.

In Parts 2 and 3 of this book, you'll find details about what these herbal supplements can do for you, the most effective ways to use them for particular health conditions, and specific cautions that you'll want to observe. Before you turn there, though, it's helpful to know something about herbal supplements in general and why some are considered far more effective than others.

Isolating Medicinal Properties

Many of the medicines that we consider pharmaceuticals actually come from plant sources. It was in the early 1800s that scientists first began to isolate and extract healing compounds from plants. Poppies yielded morphine, the narcotic that can help to dispel pain but can also be addictive. From willow bark comes aspirin, perhaps the most universal of all pain relievers. Quinine, widely used to prevent and control malaria, comes from a plant species called cinchona. A wildflower, foxglove, yields digitalis, which is used as a medication for a wide range of heart problems. Taxol, an extract from the bark of the yew tree, is used as an anticancer drug.

Concentrating an active ingredient that's derived from a plant—or synthesizing that chemical in the lab—has its advantages. Drugs allow doctors to deliver a powerful dose of medicine that's intended to cure a specific ailment. The concentrated active ingredient delivers a well-aimed punch.

When ingredients are intensely concentrated in a small package, however, taking large doses can have unwanted effects. "Whenever you use an isolated ingredient, you're increasing the likelihood of side effects," says Eran Ben-Arye, MD, a researcher at the natural medicine research unit at Hadassah University Hospital in Jerusalem. "That's one reason that you might want to try an herb," he says. "Herbs are not so concentrated and are almost always milder on your system."

Another reason is that you may not need the powerful punch of a pharmaceutical. A tea of valerian, passionflower, and hops, for instance, may be all you need to help you fall asleep—and help you avoid an expensive sleeping pill habit. Or a tincture of echinacea and goldenseal may be enough to knock out an upper respiratory infection and avoid GI-disrupting antibiotics.

Making a Comeback

Botanical medicines are making a comeback in America. Before the 1940s, many doctors were still prescribing phytomedicines for health problems, but that all changed with the advent of antibiotics during World War II. Considered "wonder drugs" because of their remarkable ability to fight bacterial infections, antibiotics spawned a whole new generation of pharmaceuticals specifically targeted to mow down bacteria. Plant-based medicines quickly fell out of favor.

"People were looking for magic bullets," says Steven Dentali, PhD, a natural products chemist with Dentali Associates in Troutdale, Oregon, and a member of the advisory board of the American Botanical Council. "When we adopted these new medicines, we left behind herbs and a way of healing that had served many people well for a long time. Herbs just weren't in vogue anymore."

Choosing an Herbal Supplement

They're sold under many brands, with a wide range of information on their labels. So what should you look for when you're choosing an herbal supplement? Here are some tips.

Buy the standardized extract. If you can find the supplement you want in the form of a standardized extract, it's your best assurance that the product contains a measured amount of a particular ingredient that's thought to be the active ingredient in the herb.

"A standardized extract gives you some guarantee that what's supposed to be in the product is probably in there. It's a good quality marker," says Alison Lee, MD, a pain-management specialist and medical director of Barefoot Doctors, an alternative medicine practice in Ann Arbor, Michigan.

Remember, though, that a standardized extract contains many other beneficial substances besides the "primary" ingredient listed on the label.

Check the botanical name. Look for the genus and species names on the product label to make sure you're getting the right herb. (You'll find the correct Latin names of recommended herbs in the Supplement Snapshots in Part 2.) That's important because a common name can sometimes refer to two or three different herbs. Ginseng, for instance, is a common name, but each of three bottles of ginseng might contain a different species of the herb, and each species has different properties.

Check expiration dates. Herbal products age rapidly when exposed to light and heat. Buy the freshest supplements you can find, says Steven Dentali, PhD, a natural products chemist at Dentali Associates, in Troutdale, Oregon, and a member of the advisory board of the American Botanical Council.

Keep it cool. Herbs generally stay potent longer if they're kept cool, says Dr. Dentali. Store them in the refrigerator.

Buy from the big guys. Large companies like Nature's Way, the Eclectic Institute, and Enzymatic Therapy have established reputations for quality control, says Andrew Weil, MD, director of the Center for Integrative Medicine at the University of Arizona, in Tucson, and author of *Eight Weeks to Optimum Health*. Without federal regulation of herbal products, you have to rely on the manufacturer for quality control. Look for GMP-certified companies. (GMP means "Good Manufacturing Practices.")

This was true only in the United States, however. In Europe, healing herbs continued to be recommended, prescribed, and used by mainstream medical doctors. European private companies, sometimes with government support, extended their research into plant-based medicines. In central Asia and China, where herbal traditions date back thousands of years, it was virtually unthinkable for plant medicines to be neglected as they had been in the United States. In these Asian countries, scientific methods of investigation continue side by side with traditional medicine. Hospitals and research institutions frequently analyze and find scientific evidence to support the use of many herbal cures, Dr. Dentali says.

As was almost inevitable, researchers and doctors in the United States are now looking more closely at phytomedicines, says William Page-Echols, DO, an assistant clinical professor of family medicine who teaches alternative medicine at the Michigan State University College of Osteopathic Medicine in East Lansing. People hear about herbal alternatives, and naturally they ask their doctors whether these herbs are effective.

People want medicines that are less invasive, easier on their systems, and readily available. They're learning that herbs offer another way of healing, a way to help the body help itself, says Dr. Page-Echols.

Saw palmetto, for example, is said to help shrink an enlarged prostate. "I have patients who come in and ask me about saw palmetto," says Dr. Page-Echols. "They've heard about it in the media or from other men who have the same problem."

Also, people who have had less-than-satisfactory experiences with conventional medications are likely to consider an herbal alternative. If you have insomnia, for instance, an MD might immediately prescribe a pharmaceutical sleeping pill. As many people have discovered, though, a sleeping pill is less than magic. While it may put you to sleep at night, you may find that you wake up the next morning feeling hungover and spaced-out.

In the search for alternatives, you might turn to valerian, passionflower, or hops, the phytomedicines used for insomnia. Many people who have used these botanicals report that they relieve anxiety or "take the edge off" enough to allow an easier transition to sleep and an awakening free of the typical side effects of pharmaceuticals. "A gentle herbal remedy may be much better," says Woodson Merrell, MD, a specialist in alternative and complementary medicine and assistant clinical professor of medicine at the Columbia University College of Physicians and Surgeons in New York City.

Food, Spirit, and Magic

Native Americans introduced several important phytomedicines to Western medicine, including cinchona, sarsaparilla, coca, black cohosh, sassafras, witch hazel, capsicum, goldenseal, and echinacea.

When Europeans first encountered the healing traditions of Native Americans, their perception was shaped by an entrenched attitude toward healing medicines. To the Europeans, herbs were medicines that you took when you were sick—and that was all. To Native Americans, herbs represented not only food and medicine but also spirit and magic, says David Winston, a professional member of the American Herbalists Guild and a practicing herbalist in Washington, New Jersey.

"North American Indians saw plants as living beings," says Winston. "They were used with great respect. Plants had life and power."

Religious and mystical overtones pervaded Indian herbal traditions. While the average Native American probably knew 100 to 200 useful plants, a medicine man or shaman might be learned in using some 800 plants, says Winston.

"Sometimes, there was a certain allure or quality associated with Native American medicine," says Winston. Frontier physicians who practiced native medicine often advertised themselves as Indian doctors. Hucksters of patent medicines boasted that their elixirs contained Indian herbs with wondrous healing properties. In fact, the *Pharmacopoeia of the United States of America,* first published in 1820, contained more than 200 indigenous drugs. Most of these were the plants originally used by Native Americans.

There's another appeal, as well. "Herbs fit in with self-healing and prevention," says Dr. Merrell. "That's one reason that you're seeing them out in the marketplace in such quantity."

A Regulatory Purgatory

Currently, herbal medicines sold in the United States are in limbo between regulation and free-market distribution. Since they are classified as dietary supplements, not drugs, they can be purchased without a prescription.

This policy raises doubts in the minds of many health practitioners. In Europe, where phytomedicines are common, people are accustomed to having herbs prescribed by doctors. In the United States, however, you can just walk into a health food store and buy them in quantity. Why should there be such a discrepancy in the way they're distributed?

"Just because they are readily available or advertised as so-called natural products does not mean that they are completely safe and free of side effects," warns Dr. Ben-Arye. "You really should treat herbs like drugs. They shouldn't be used indiscriminately or taken for fun."

The quality of the products is another concern. The US government does not hold supplement manufacturers to the same standards as drug companies. The potency and quality of herbal products vary greatly. You can't always be sure you're getting the real thing. "Many of the products are overpriced and ineffective. Also, there's a great deal of promotion about health benefits by these companies that is pure baloney," says Andrew Weil, MD, director of the Center for Integrative Medicine at the University of Arizona, in Tucson, and author of *Eight Weeks to Optimum Health.*

By law, manufacturers of herbal supplements aren't allowed to make specific health claims for their products, Dr. Weil says. They can instead make general statements about an herb's effect on the body's structure and function. Thus, a supplement label will not say "prevents atherosclerosis" or "relieves arthritis." Instead, the label is likely to say that it is "good for circulation" or "good for joint health."

Despite these limitations, there's a rich tradition and a long history of anecdotal evidence as well as a growing body of scientific references to support the use of herbs for overall, general good health and for specific health problems. Just because the landscape is confusing doesn't mean that you should ignore what you can find. It does mean, however, that if you're going to use herbs, it will help to have the guidance of a book like this one. Or you may want to go a step further and consult with a health practitioner who has experience with herbal medicines.

If you do consult an experienced practitioner, you have a number of choices. One is to find a certified herbalist who is a member of the American Herbalists Guild. Or you might want to see a licensed naturopathic doctor, who will integrate the use of herbs with other healing techniques. A doctor of traditional Chinese medicine will also prescribe herbs. Some chiropractors and some physicians—both MDs and DOs—have taken the time to learn about phytomedicines. In addition, you may find some pharmacists who are quite knowledgeable.

Unfortunately, it's impossible to say which practitioners are fully qualified to prescribe herbal medicines. Just as there are no set standards for botanicals, we have no government or professional organizations that oversee the standards of practitioners.

Word-of-mouth recommendations and professional reputations are important. In gathering the information on herbal supplements that you find in this book, we turned to herbalists and practitioners who are recommended by their peers or who have made significant contributions to the research on the subject. In addition, we have asked the opinions of many medical doctors and well-qualified naturopathic doctors who observe practical results in their daily practices. As you read about herbal supplements in Parts 2 and 3, you'll find dosages and cautions that have been recommended by these experts. You'll also learn how to take these supplements for maximum effect and discover how other supplements can boost or reinforce their healing power.

Thinking about Herbs

Whether you visit an herbal practitioner or choose to self-medicate, there are two ways to consider herbal supplements.

One view is that botanicals are simply substitutes for drugs. If you have a tension headache, for instance, you want instant relief, so you reach for an over-the-counter pharmaceutical like aspirin, ibuprofen, or acetaminophen. If these are no longer effective or have undesirable side effects, you might consider taking an herbal supplement instead. In a case like that, you're really looking for a one-to-one substitute—an herb to relieve a symptom instead of a drug to relieve a symptom.

Looking for quick, targeted relief is a mindset of Western medicine. The model is allopathic, which simply means trying to substitute a new, benign condition (no headache) for a condition that's causing a lot of discomfort (oh, that aching head). In the allopathic model of medicine, when you have a symptom or a disease, you expect to find some treatment that will produce a different effect and relieve whatever ails you as soon as possible.

Sometimes, the treatment addresses the underlying cause. If so, that treatment might get rid of the pain or discomfort and also keep it from

Look to Germany

In Germany, people seeking herbal medicines have access to nearly 700 plant-based remedies, and the cost of many of them is covered by health insurance. In fact, some 70 percent of German physicians routinely prescribe phytomedicines. Drugstores carry them, and pharmacists are knowledgeable about their many uses.

Germany has undertaken the most comprehensive science-based investigation of herbs of any Western country. In 1978, the German government established Commission E to evaluate herbal medicines and write a series of monographs, or scholarly works, on them. A team of physicians, toxicologists, pharmacologists, and other specialists set out to produce the most comprehensive study ever attempted.

The commission's series of monographs covers some 400 herbs. For each herbal medicine, Commission E sets certain guidelines for dosage and uses. Unlike the Food and Drug Administration in the United States, which uses a requirement of "absolute certainty" before licensing a drug, Commission E uses a criterion of "reasonable certainty" to determine if an herb is effective. To arrive at its conclusions, the commission took scientific studies into account, but it also considered historical use, anecdotal evidence, and information from field studies as well as other sources.

coming back again. But what happens if you just treat the symptom without eliminating the cause? A tension headache is a good example of that. Aspirin or ibuprofen might beat the pain and help you get through the rest of the day, but they do nothing to prevent the headache from recurring a day or a week later.

Herbalists and naturopathic doctors tend to look beyond the allopathic model for just that reason. Why not address what's causing those headaches, they ask, on the chance that they can be prevented in the future? Symptoms are important clues to an underlying imbalance. A skilled herbalist can use botanicals to treat hormone imbalances, stress, or allergies that cause a headache, not just provide anti-inflammatories that subdue the immediate pain. Yes, herbs can be used for particular problems, but they also provide nourishment for the whole body.

"Herbs can help the body achieve a healthier condition so it can better protect and heal itself," says Jennifer Brett, ND, a naturopathic doctor at the Wilton Naturopathic Center in Stratford, Connecticut. "It's really a nutritive or positive cure viewpoint."

The second view of using herbs is a more holistic model, meaning that the body is viewed as a whole, rather than as a set of isolated parts. Instead of seeing a headache as an isolated problem that begins somewhere above your shoulders, as the allopathic practitioner would, a holistic practitioner wonders what's happening all over. Is digestion a contributing factor? Mood? Lifestyle factors? Posture? In the view of the holistic practitioner, if we understand how other body factors contribute to the problem, we can better address the causes.

In many cultures, it's not unusual to consume different healing herbs at different times of the year to keep the whole body healthier and prevent disease. When winter comes on, the Chinese often add astragalus to their soups and stews as a way to boost their immune systems and fight off seasonal colds and flu. Unlike antibiotics, astragalus fights both bacterial and viral infections. People living on the Indian subcontinent use red pepper, curry, and garlic on their food all year round, not just as spices but also as medicines to aid digestion, improve liver health, and lower cholesterol, Dr. Brett says.

Balms and Cures

Of course, herbs wouldn't be your first choice if you had an acute-care situation, such as a heart attack, pneumonia, or a broken leg. In these cases, it's best to get yourself to the hospital, says Dr. Brett.

Herbal supplements are well-suited for preventing illness, building up the body's defenses, and easing the symptoms of long-term conditions such as heart disease, diabetes, migraines, and asthma. They can also make a big difference if you have problems that often elude solutions like insomnia, anxiety, depression, or lack of energy, she adds.

Unlike synthetic drugs designed to cure specific ills, herbs tend to have a wide range of applications. In fact, the very terms *drug* and *medicine* are inappropriate descriptions of what they actually do. Many herbalists use other terms, such as *tonic* and *adaptogen*. Tonic herbs restore, nourish, and support individual organs or the entire body. Adaptogens help restore balance in the body, particularly helping it to adapt to stress, be it physical, environmental, or emotional.

An adaptogen can make adjustments on the plus or the minus side. Let's say you're feeling run-down and sluggish, or just the opposite—stressed-out and wired. Although the symptoms seem totally different, the cause may be the same—adrenal glands that are not working optimally, says Dr. Brett. Maybe your adrenal glands are overactive, producing more hormones than they should, or perhaps they're not producing enough. Either way, an adaptogen might help.

By taking an adaptogenic herb that supports adrenal health, you can restore the balance of the adrenals and normalize function, says Dr. Brett. "An adaptogen really shunts in wherever it is needed. It just helps your body do what it should be doing."

Subtle Healing

In most instances, you'll find the work of herbs to be subtle and gentle, says Dr. Dentali. Sometimes, you really need to pay attention to notice whether they're working. Also, if they're causing a side effect, that might not be readily apparent.

Feverfew, for example, has been very successful in limiting migraines, but it may take weeks before the herb has an effect. If you start taking it, your headaches may ease so gradually that it may seem as if the herb has nothing to do with the relief you're getting. The cause-and-effect relationship isn't entirely clear.

"If you are going to self-medicate, you really need to pay attention, and even take notes on your condition. That way, you can better tell if the herb is working," says Dr. Dentali.

Stanley W. Beyrle, ND, a naturopathic doctor at the Kansas Clinic of Traditional Medicine in Wichita, says that after 18 years of practicing herbal medicine, he tends to prescribe much lower dosages than he once did. "A little bit can be enough. What you're looking to do is nudge the body in one direction or another so it can take care of itself," he says. "You don't want to overdo it."

Timing is also a factor. Like medication, herbs should only be used for the time you need them. There are really very few herbs that you should be taking long-term unless it's to address a chronic condition, says Alison Lee, MD, a pain-management specialist and medical director of Barefoot Doctors, an alternative medicine practice in Ann Arbor, Michigan.

From Plant to Shelf: How Your Herbal Supplements Make It From the Wild to Your Bottle

The way herbal supplements are made these days is a far cry from the traditional hunter-gatherer methods of yore. As with any complex manufacturing operation, supplement makers require a steady stream of raw materials, and there are many checkpoints for quality control throughout the process.

When you step inside the doors of Herbalist and Alchemist, an herbal medicine manufacturer in Washington, New Jersey, the complexity of the operation is immediately apparent. In the factory, which employs 13 people, technicians make herbal tinctures in a processing room that's the picture of scrupulous hygiene. People wear gowns, goggles, hair and beard nets, and rubber gloves. Some have respirators. In an area that resembles a very neat, well-organized chemistry lab, there are checklists and formulas, glass beakers, electronic scales, and a computer that assigns lot numbers and expiration dates to bottled products.

Herbs come from a wide range of sources. Nearby herb farms in New Jersey supply plants that are native to the region. Kava kava is imported from Hawaii and Vancouver. Botanical brokers on the West Coast link small farmers and organic growers to this hub of manufacturing activity in New Jersey. Other brokers represent the people who gather plants from fields and forests in the Carolinas.

All the herbs used by Herbalist and Alchemist are grown organically and gathered responsibly, according to Beth Lambert, the company's chief executive officer. Once delivered to the facility, the herb is ground, measured, and placed in 5-gallon glass jars with a solution of ethanol and distilled water. The solution, called a menstruum, extracts the healing chemical compounds from the plant material. Most plants soak in the menstruum for about 2 weeks. A technician then strains and presses out the plant material. What's left behind is tincture, a colored liquid with a strange but earthy odor of alcohol and plants.

Depending on the herb, the manufacturing process can be more complicated. Herbs may be cooked or percolated in the menstruum.

Plants are sometimes shredded when wet. Processing times can be shortened or extended. Sometimes, several tinctures are mixed together in herbal combinations developed by David Winston, the company's founder.

The company makes only tinctures, even though they may be higher-priced than other popular forms of the herb, such as capsules or teas. "We only make tinctures because we believe that once the active ingredients are extracted by the menstruum, the medicines are more easily assimilated into the body," Lambert says.

Despite the high-tech trappings, the sampling and selection of ingredients is a subjective process based upon the instincts and experiences of the people who scan the raw material and maintain quality control. The key people in that selection process are Winston and Betzy Bancroft, both herbalists who are professional members of the American Herbalists Guild.

"We do our own grinding," says Bancroft. "We want our herbs as whole as possible because they stay fresher longer that way."

She and Winston subject every shipment to a detailed examination. It's the first hurdle that the product must pass before it can be approved by the two certified herbalists. They use sight, smell, taste, and feel to evaluate whether the raw materials pass muster. If a shipment of ginger arrives, Winston will taste it to make sure the plant meets his criteria for gingerols, the active ingredients that give ginger its pungent taste.

As for the rest of the process, the strict hygiene and quality-control practices are self-imposed rather than required by law, according to Lambert. She thinks that these careful processes will someday be required of everyone. The labeling of their products also follows strict guidelines. "We can trace a bottle of our tincture at a health food store right back to the herb supplier," she says.

Begun in 1982, the company sells most products wholesale to medical doctors, naturopathic doctors, homeopaths, herbalists, chiropractors, and health food stores.

A Few Studies, a Lot of Tradition

Determining the effectiveness of an herb is difficult. Many people who are enthusiastic about herbal remedies and who strongly believe in alternative medicine may experience a so-called placebo effect when they take herbs. Yes, they feel better, but no one knows whether they feel better because the herb is causing some kind of change in the body or because the positive messages about herbs are changing how they feel. Both count, of course. Any remedy that makes you feel better is worth taking, as long as it has no harmful side effects. In the interest of scientific curiosity, though, we'd all like to know how these things work and whether they can help everyone.

Some herbs, like hawthorn, garlic, and ginkgo, have quite a bit of scientific research behind them. Others, such as cat's claw, have little. If you take cat's claw, you're relying on anecdotal evidence and tradition—sometimes going back centuries.

Why aren't there more studies of herbal medicines? For one thing, testing a phytomedicine is difficult and expensive. In the United States, the Food and Drug Administration (FDA) relies on drug companies to finance research and development. If a drug wins approval from the FDA, the economic rewards can be enormous. Along with a patent for the medicine, the company gets exclusive rights to sell the drug to the public before it becomes public domain, explains Dr. Dentali.

Phytomedicines can't be patented. Hawthorn, echinacea, and thousands of other herbs belong to everyone, and the supplements derived from them are universally available. Without the expectation of a high-profit license to pay the costs of exhaustive research, drug companies have little incentive to make the exorbitant investment required to get FDA approval.

The other barrier to herb testing is the sheer volume of active ingredients that would have to be tested. The classic method of understanding the active compounds in a plant or drug is to isolate each chemical and test it for medicinal properties, using first cell-based, then animal, and finally human studies to supply evidence, says Dr. Dentali. That type of isolation and testing, applied to the scores of active ingredients in an herb, turns into a prohibitively expensive and time-consuming task. It may also be fruitless. Many scientists believe that the chemicals in healing herbs frequently act together. By singling out the "active" ones, they say, we'll neglect all the other ingredients that make herbs different from drugs.

That's why herbalists say that herbs are meant to be taken as a whole, including all of their chemical constituents, known and unknown, and they don't recommend extracting the active ingredients so that they become plant-derived chemicals that act independently. You might say that an herbal treatment is like the sound produced by an orchestra. Each instrument plays a separate part, but you don't get the orchestral sound until they're all playing together.

Dosage Dilemma

The lack of "scientific evidence" and research studies supporting the effectiveness of herbal preparations in humans has an impact on the medical community. Not many MDs are writing prescriptions for herbs, and that's largely because of the lack of studies, says Jonathan Sporn, MD, an oncologist and associate professor of medicine at the University of Connecticut Health Center in Farmington.

Eating more garlic or taking a garlic supplement is probably good for your heart and circulatory system. It may very well prevent stomach cancer as well, says Dr. Sporn. There are questions, however: How much garlic should a person take? How often? In what form? Doctors who want to answer these questions hear many opinions but few firm recommendations.

"We do know that garlic has some anticancer properties," says Dr. Sporn, "and there's evidence that eating more garlic or taking a garlic supplement may prevent gastrointestinal cancer. That's all that science can tell us right now, though. We can't tell you whether garlic should be generally recommended as an anticancer agent."

Instead, what doctors and herbalists have to rely upon is the clinical experience of herbal practitioners, the folklore of native healers, and centuries of traditional use.

"Up until 5 to 10 years ago, with many of these herbs we only had anecdotal or clinically based evidence—how they've been used in the past or within the doctor's own practice," says Dr. Merrell. "More recently, however, there have been hundreds of well-designed, published studies examining the scientific basis and clinical outcomes to help guide us on the safe and effective use of herbal medicines."

Evaluating herbs is like trying to pin down the benefits that we get from food, observes Dr. Dentali. "Sure, you could attempt exhaustive studies on these herbs, but is that any better than doing exhaustive studies on something like a carrot, so we know what every little chemical in a carrot does for us? What we already know is that carrots are good for you. Moreover, we know that about many of these herbs. Centuries of use by people tell us that." Still, in this modern-day world, even herbs used for centuries face new situations. St. John's wort, for instance, used to treat depression, has fallen out of favor as it becomes apparent that it interacts with many drugs and can also cause severe sun sensitivity. In fact, drug–herb interactions are one of the best reasons to see a health-care practitioner, or at least do some research, before you self-medicate with herbs.

Selecting a Supplement

Considering all the different kinds of herbs and the ways that we use them, what's the best way to take them? Should you eat the plant? Drink it as a tea? Extract its active ingredients? Or take it as a pill or capsule?

In years past, people simply added medicinal herbs to their foods, or they made some kind of brew using the dried and ground-up plant. Today, the large and small companies that distribute herbs have developed many ways to process them for consumption. Squeezing the herb into a pill or capsule certainly makes it convenient to take, but certain decisions are made by the producers when herbs are processed this way.

In an extraction process, it's possible to isolate specific chemicals from the plant. When those chemicals are included at a specific, guaranteed concentration, they're said to be standardized.

If you buy St. John's wort in supplement form, the label may tell you the amount of St. John's wort extract in each capsule. It will also say that the supplement is standardized for a certain percentage of hypericin, which is what some phytochemists think is the most important ingredient in the herb. This is the supplement maker's "guarantee"—without any regulatory verification—that each capsule contains a specific amount of the extract and a specific percentage of a primary ingredient.

Purists may say that the only way to take herbs is in their raw form, but there's a lot to be said for herbal supplements that come as capsules, pills, and liquid tinctures, especially if they're labeled as standardized extracts. The supplements offer convenience, uniform doses, and specific concentrations of certain ingredients.

They're also tasteless, which is sometimes a real plus, especially if you're taking an herb like valerian. When made into a tea, valerian smells and tastes downright obnoxious. Those familiar with its rank odor have dubbed it the gym-sock herb. Taken as a pill, however, it has no taste at all, so you can get the benefits without the challenge.

Putting the Genie in the Bottle

As their name implies, wildcrafted herbs are gathered in the wild. Cultivated herbs, however, ensure a constant supply with more consistent qualities. Nearly all ginseng, echinacea, and ginkgo, to name just three popular herbs, are now farmed as regular crops. Since some herbs, such as echinacea, are becoming scarce in the wild due to overharvesting, you should buy cultivated herbs whenever possible, says Jill Stansbury, ND, assistant professor of botanical medicine and chair of the botanical medicine department at the National College of Naturopathic Medicine in Portland, Oregon.

Whether gathered in the field or in the wild, the herbs are dried before they're packaged. Throughout the growing, harvesting, drying, and packaging processes, reputable manufacturers will take steps to ensure that the final product has consistent, assured qualities. It's important that dried herbs be of consistent quality to yield a potent supplement.

Three kinds of herb supplements are most common. Here's a rundown.

Pills. The ground herb is pressed together and held by a binding substance. Some pills may have an enteric coating, a kind of second skin that's gradually dissolved by enzymes in the intestines. The coating ensures that the pill passes undisturbed through the stomach and starts to dissolve only when it reaches the intestines.

Capsules. These work in much the same way as pills, but they're constructed somewhat differently. The ground herb is inside a gelatin shell, where the ingredients are protected from light, moisture, and exposure to oxygen.

Extracts. These are concentrated preparations made from dried or fresh plant parts. The herb is soaked or cooked in a liquid to concentrate active ingredients or remove unwanted components. If the active ingredient is known or suspected, manufacturers may try to include or concentrate that ingredient in their products. The content of desired constituents is calculated and standardized.

A tincture is a type of liquid extract in which alcohol is used as a solvent to extract active constituents from dried or fresh plant material.

If you have difficulty swallowing pills or capsules, tinctures are a good way to go. You can simply use an eyedropper to put drops of an alcohol-based solution on your tongue, in a cup of tea, or in water.

Glycerites are a type of liquid extract in which active constituents are held in glycerin, a sweet-tasting fatty compound with a syrupy consistency. Glycerin makes herbs taste better, which can help if the raw herb is bitter or has a disagreeable flavor. Glycerites are a good choice if you want to avoid alcohol.

Mostly Mild, Mostly Safe

The mild nature of many herbal supplements makes them relatively safe, but that's not true of every herb. That's why it's important to follow any directions from your health practitioner, as well as the dosage recommendations on the product's label. Don't exceed the dosage, says David Winston, a professional member of the American Herbalists Guild and a practicing herbalist in Washington, New Jersey.

"A lot of folks have this idea that if a little is good, more is better. That's never a good idea, even with herbs," says Winston. "Just because herbs are natural does not necessarily mean that they are harmless."

Also, be cautious if you're already taking other medications. Side effects are possible when you mix pharmaceutical drugs and herbs. If you have concerns about possible side effects or interactions, be sure to consult a health practitioner who has experience with herbs. Also, to guard against potential drug interactions, tell your regular doctor about any herbs that you're taking.

emerging
supplements

exploring the outer boundaries

Walk through the supplement section of your local health food store, supermarket, or drugstore, or shop online, and you'll discover many supplements that don't fit in the categories of either vitamins and minerals or herbal supplements. You'll see strange names like phosphatidylserine and chondroitin sulfate, mysterious abbreviations like DHEA and GABA, large selections of sports supplements, weight-loss aids with eye-catching labels, and sexual enhancement supplements with attention-grabbing names.

How do we classify these other supplements that are neither vitamins, nor minerals, nor herbs?

There are so many different kinds that they defy a single classification. Since all of them are in some stage of being tested, challenged, advertised, and marketed, however, it seems simplest to call them emerging supplements.

Many of the emerging supplements are substances found naturally in the body, such as coenzyme Q_{10}, ribose, or melatonin. So if you make them, why would you want to buy them? When given in higher amounts than your body can create on its own, some of these supplements may improve biochemical functions, such as energy metabolism, sleep, or nerve conduction.

In fact, there is a whole new field called "functional medicine" that focuses on improving physiological function, such as energy metabolism or liver detoxification, to help prevent and treat chronic illnesses such as diabetes, cancer, and heart disease. These functional medical providers use nutritional supplements, including emerging supplements, to improve or enhance things your body already does, such as energy metabolism, fighting off illness, and hormone production.

Natural sources generate other up-and-coming supplements, and because they come from the Earth (like plants), they're not regulated as pharmaceuticals. That said, they're still far removed from the teas and foods we think of as plants. They are refined, highly concentrated, and often reconfigured in laboratories. Take theanine, for instance. This calming amino acid is naturally found in tea, but companies have found a way to isolate and then concentrate the active form of it to sell in supplement form. Curcumin is another example: This cancer-fighting compound is naturally found in the spice turmeric, but in that form it's poorly absorbed. So manufacturers patented a way to increase absorption by 20 times.

It doesn't happen to every supplement, but some that show promise catch the interest of people who are more interested in making a quick buck than they are in healing, says Wes Seigner, a Washington, DC–based attorney specializing in food and dietary supplement laws. "As more suppliers join the market—especially on the Internet or late-night TV—the quality and price of a supplement usually go down," he says. And thanks to the Internet, you can order a supplement from almost any country in the world—and know nothing about its safety or regulation. Although the two enforcement agencies that police this industry, the FDA and the Federal Trade Commission (FTC), can stop a shipment coming into the United States, the likelihood of that happening is pretty low, admits an FDA spokesperson.

It's definitely "buyer beware" out there. Given this uncertainty, why are we so willing to try these emerging supplements—or any supplements, for that matter?

For the most part, it's because we want to be in charge of our own health. "People are taking more control over their own health, and supplements are a way of becoming proactive," says Mark Stengler, ND, a naturopathic doctor and author of *The Natural Physician: Your Health Guide for Common Ailments*. "They realize that preventing disease is the key to good health, and they know that, when it comes to prevention, nutrition and lifestyle are key." Some people and medical professionals also believe that supplements are part of staying healthy, says Stephen DeFelice, MD, founder and chairman of the nonprofit Foundation for Innovation in Medicine in Cranford, New Jersey.

The Roads to Discovery

Sometimes, the discovery of a supplement begins with simple observation and a powerful sense of curiosity. In other cases, a new supplement is found when scientists look closely at existing data.

There are many ways that supplements are discovered. Modern researchers may take clues from ancient medical texts or modern-day folk medicine. They may accidentally stumble across the next big supplement or test a hypothesis based on years of research.

Consider the intriguing case of fish oil. Doctors working in the Arctic in the 1970s observed that the Eskimo people were rarely afflicted with heart disease, despite eating a high-fat diet of whale meat, seal meat, and fish.

Later, researchers in Japan in the early 1980s also noted a low death rate from heart disease in their country. Like the Eskimos, the Japanese people ate a lot of fish. Scientists began to wonder if a diet high in fish was the common link.

On closer examination of the statistics, researchers found that this theory seemed to hold up. In Japan, the lowest death rates from heart disease were found on the island of Okinawa, where fish consumption was about twice as high as in mainland Japan. Another study compared a fishing village where residents ate as much as 250 grams of fish each day with a farming area where people ate about 90 grams of fish each day. Sure enough, the lower incidence of heart disease was in the fishing village.

These early observations led researchers to study whether some aspect of seafood was protective against heart disease. Much of the research zeroed in on omega-3 fatty acids, which were found in fish oils.

Today, research points to the conclusion that the omega-3s in fish oil reduce the risk of heart disease by influencing blood clotting and blood pressure. They may also reduce the risk of irregular heartbeat. Beyond heart health, researchers are now considering how fish oil can help reduce the risk of other conditions, including rheumatoid arthritis, cancer, and other chronic conditions caused by inflammation.

Given these promising findings, it was almost inevitable that supplement makers would begin to manufacture fish oil supplements. In fact, if you check the shelves of almost any drugstore or health food store, you'll find dozens of different brands and concentrations.

Gaining Respect

Nearly every week, it seems, we read about a new supplement that's going to reverse aging, help us sleep better, improve our sex lives, or boost our immune systems.

So how does a supplement move from obscurity to acceptability?

The Strange Case of Red Yeast Rice

Long before we even knew what cholesterol was, there was red yeast rice (RYR). It actually is a red yeast that's grown on rice, and it's been used for centuries in traditional Chinese medicine for heart and circulation problems. It does lower cholesterol. In fact, one of the first cholesterol-lowering drugs, lovastatin, is based on one of the active ingredients in red yeast rice, a compound called monacolin K. The drug company that developed lovastatin was able to get a patent for its efforts, but by law, no patent is permitted for monacolin K because it is considered a natural substance. Still, the two are chemically identical. And that's a problem. Is RYR a natural product? Is it a drug? Is it both?

Gray areas like these have had federal regulators and product manufacturers at odds over what's legal and what's not. In 1999, the FDA ruled that RYR was a drug and ordered it removed from the shelves. That decision was initially overruled by a district court in Utah, but a federal court of appeals later agreed with the FDA that RYR could be regulated. In 2000, the FDA declared that RYR could be sold legally in the United States, but

In a best-case scenario, a major research institution decides to spend the time and money on a supplement that seems promising. (This doesn't happen a lot, but it does happen.) That's what happened with alpha lipoic acid. The supplement was being used in some circles to treat diabetic neuropathy, a painful side effect of diabetes. The treatment drew the interest of the Mayo Clinic in Rochester, Minnesota. Their research showed that this natural product works as well as the most commonly used drug for diabetic neuropathy, without all the side effects.

In other cases, a supplement may have a lifelong researcher–advocate whose persistence finally pays off, as was the case with Peter Langsjoen, MD, and coenzyme Q_{10}. The Tyler, Texas, cardiologist has studied CoQ_{10} for about 30 years, and now there are four major CoQ_{10} research centers in the United States, including the Mayo Clinic and the State University of New York at Stony Brook. "It is gratifying to see some of these new centers doing good work," Dr. Langsjoen says.

But in most cases, a supplement moves slowly from obscurity to acceptability as scientific evidence or clinical use confirms that it works, Dr. DeFelice says. Research that determines a dietary supplement's only if steps were taken during the manufacturing process to remove the lovastatin—presumably eliminating its effectiveness.

Then, in 2007, the FDA found that at least some RYR available in the United States, promoted and sold on the Internet, still contained lovastatin and took further steps to purge the "tainted" products.

Currently, as far as the FDA is concerned, the RYR that you can buy in the United States contains no lovastatin. (In fact, it does, but only that which occurs naturally in the yeast.) It also contains other monacolins that may also lower cholesterol and other cholesterol-lowering ingredients such as sterols and stanols.

But since RYR is still considered a dietary supplement, its formulation and content are still not regulated—and it is very difficult if not impossible to find out what it does contain. That's not much help to consumers, and the manufacturers don't like it, either. "It's kind of like 'Don't ask, don't tell,'" one RYR manufacturer admits. "The law is very awkward in this regard and should be rewritten," adds Dr. DeFelice.

mechanisms of action is helpful in establishing credibility. Research can also use "biomarkers" such as lower blood sugar, lower cholesterol, or lower homocysteine levels to infer that a supplement can help. But the usual "gold standard" of evidence—the randomized, blinded, controlled clinical trial—is not often done with dietary supplements, Dr. DeFelice says. Why? Because these studies cost millions of dollars and can take many years to complete and, unlike in the drug industry, there simply are not billions of dollars to be made in dietary supplements to pay back the millions spent on research. This lack of gold standard research may prevent conventional medical doctors from recommending dietary supplements, but it hasn't slowed consumer interest.

Making Pills with Possibilities

With so much interest in emerging supplements, what does it take for a new discovery to make the grade and win acceptance?

To answer that question is to tell the story of how an emerging supplement, well, emerges.

Although the process may seem mysterious, it's actually a lot like a very big homework assignment. For instance, at Thorne Research, one of the country's biggest makers of professional-grade dietary supplements, scientists in the technical division regularly scour existing research for anything that looks promising. Officers in the company attend conferences where leading researchers in the field present new research findings. Often, the company itself is contacted by smaller research and development firms that are in the process of developing an ingredient that Thorne may want to market. Thorne may work with them to develop standards for the ingredient, says Thorne CEO Paul Jacobson. "There are lots of potential products out there, but for a product to interest us it has to pass a kind of screening test," Jacobson says. "We look for clinical evidence that it works. We like to see at least some clinical work done. We need to know that we can manufacture it to our stringent standards. The ingredients themselves have to be completely clean and pure and hypoallergenic. And, finally, we need to know that when we formulate it according to our standards, the product is still going to work." If a new product, or potential new product, can meet all of those criteria, there's a good chance Thorne, or another large, well-known manufacturer, may want to obtain exclusive rights to it.

Once a company has decided to manufacture a supplement, Jacobson says, the supplement is thoroughly tested to make sure that it contains the right mixture of ingredients and is free of contamination. Samples are run through a laboratory, where an analysis is done to ensure that the product is completely mixed. A state-of-the-art instrument takes an infrared "fingerprint" of a product sample, which is then compared with the verified standard for the product and compared by computer with the other batch samples to ensure complete mixing.

The next step is to get uniform amounts of the mixture into capsules, which are made from gelatin. To make sure that all of the capsules contain the right amount of materials, samples are taken randomly and weighed. If necessary, the machine that makes the capsules is adjusted to make sure that each capsule falls within an acceptable weight range.

All dietary supplements in the United States are required to comply with good manufacturing practices (GMP) standards put out by the FDA. These regulations require that manufacturers, processors, and packagers of dietary supplements take steps to ensure that their products are safe and pure and contain what is listed on the label. Most countries, including the

United States, will only accept for import and sale supplements that have been manufactured to international GMP standards, but this regulation can be hard to enforce.

Your Selection Process

Given all of the companies offering supplements, how do you know which ones are most reliable? How can you be reasonably sure that the product you buy contains what it says it does and is free of contaminants?

Buy brands recommended by a trusted professional, either a nutritionally trained doctor or a health food store owner or store employees with training and a good reputation in the community. Brands such as Thorne Research, Scientific Botanicals, PhytoPharmica, Eclectic, Naturopathic Formulations, Metagenics, Enzymatic Therapy, and Tyler Encapsulations sell mostly to health-care professionals such as doctors, naturopaths, dietitians, and nutritionists, although some are available directly to consumers through compounding pharmacies or direct sales.

Read the label. Look for any potentially allergenic substances such as Red Dye #4. If the product does not clearly state ingredients and their amounts, do not buy it.

Make sure the product has a real address and location. This should be listed on the bottle or, at the least, on the company's Web site. Companies that make cheap, poor-quality, or tainted products are in business simply to make quick money. They will list only a post office box so they can fold quickly if the FDA and FTC come after them. They sometimes reappear later with a different company name and, perhaps, different products.

If you buy products online, stick with reputable companies. Fly-by-night companies are most likely to market their products online.

Ask for proof. The supplement company should be able to provide you with a product analysis of potency and purity, such as from ConsumerLab.com. (This is called a third-party assay.) In addition, check to make sure the product is Good Manufacturing Practices (GMP) certified. This gives you some assurance that the product you choose is free of contaminants such as bacteria, pesticides, and heavy metals.

Get as much background as you can on the company you're buying from. Consider their number of years in the industry and the quality of their educational materials. The company should also be able to tell you where the raw materials for their products come from, such as organic herb farms. Other measurements are the quality of their product analysis and their commitment to research and scientific validation.

Check the FDA's Web site. Visit www.fda.gov/Safety/MedWatch to see if the product you have bought or are thinking about buying has been cited by the FDA for safety issues. For instance, some sexual enhancement supplements have been found to contain sildenafil, the same active ingredient found in Viagra. The stuff works, but it can interact with nitrates found in some prescription drugs and lower blood pressure to dangerous levels. Another product, called Fruta Planta, marketed for weight loss, has been found to contain sibutramine, a controlled substance that was withdrawn from the market in October of 2010 for safety reasons. The product poses a threat to consumers because sibutramine is known to substantially increase blood pressure and/or pulse rate in some people and may prove risky to people with heart disease.

Besides being knowledgeable about labels and manufacturers, of course, you need information about the newest supplements and the claims that have been made for them. In Part 2, you'll find many emerging supplements along with the vitamins, minerals, and botanical medicines that experts prescribe.

2

the powerhouse of nature's medicines

alpha lipoic acid

Alpha lipoic acid was considered a vitamin until scientists realized that our bodies actually make this vital energy-producing coenzyme. Together with a substance called pyrophosphatase, alpha lipoic acid helps produce adenosine triphosphate (ATP), the body's major fuel source. In other words, when you have enough lipoic acid, your body can generate the energy it needs to keep functioning (not just your get-up-and-go energy, but the actual energy your cells need to do their jobs). When you start to run short, the whole energy metabolism process slows down—and your health suffers with it.

Restoring lipoic acid levels to normal helps to restore proper energy metabolism in cells, and that helps cells to survive and can also help stem cells regenerate organs, such as the liver and nerves, says Burt Berkson, MD, PhD, author of *The Alpha Lipoic Acid Breakthrough* and medical director of the Integrative Medical Center of New Mexico.

Alpha lipoic acid has another disease-preventing role. "It activates a group of about 250 antioxidants, all made in the body, that help protect cells from damage," says Bruce Ames, PhD, professor of biochemistry and molecular biology, University of California, Berkeley, and a senior scientist at Children's Hospital Oakland Research Institute. In fact, alpha lipoic acid is one of the best generators of glutathione, a powerful antioxidant that's been linked with protecting the body from aging, heart disease, and cancer. And since alpha lipoic acid has the ability to concentrate in cells' mitochondria, it plays a major role in shielding these tiny energy generators from damage. Animal studies have shown that supplemental alpha lipoic acid can actually make aging mitochondria act like those years younger, which is how it gets its reputation as an antiaging supplement.

Alpha lipoic acid is both water-soluble and fat-soluble, so it can get into more places in the body, Dr. Ames says. "It really can get into any cell, including the brain and nerves and liver cells," he says. It can regenerate both vitamin E, which is fat-soluble, and vitamin C, which is water-soluble. Because it can get anywhere and can be used by any cells, it helps a wide variety of conditions, Dr. Berkson says.

Helpful for People with Diabetes

Some people with diabetes develop nerve damage, called peripheral neuropathy, that can be painful and lead to more serious complications. In Germany, intravenous and oral alpha lipoic acid are prescribed treatments for diabetic neuropathy. In the United States, researchers from the Mayo Clinic in Rochester, Minnesota, found that people with diabetic neuropathy who took alpha lipoic acid had a significant reduction in symptoms such as burning, pain, numbness, and prickling of the feet and legs. Those who took the largest dose of 1,800 milligrams got the most relief, which started around 3 to 5 weeks after starting treatment.

"There appears to be a rather large effect on the pain of diabetic neuropathy with ALA," says Peter Dyck, MD, Mayo Clinic neurologist and

---

SUPPLEMENTSNAPSHOT

▶Alpha Lipoic Acid

May help: Peripheral neuropathy, liver diseases, burning mouth syndrome (if related to diabetic neuropathy,) peripheral artery disease (claudication), insulin sensitivity, cardiac autonomic neuropathy, conditions of energy metabolism disorder such as chronic fatigue syndrome and fibromyalgia, taste and smell disorders (if due to nerve damage), and regulation of certain immune cells called T-lymphocytes.

Good food sources: Red meat, organ meats, spinach, broccoli, potatoes, yams, carrots, beets, and yeast.

Special instructions: Alpha lipoic acid works well with certain other supplements, such as acetyl-l-carnitine and milk thistle. It is used both orally and intravenously.

Cautions and possible side effects: May cause a drop in blood glucose levels. Dosing adjustments for insulin or oral hypoglycemic agents may be necessary. High-dose alpha lipoic acid can quickly cause B vitamin deficiencies and *must* be taken with B complex vitamins to be effective.

peripheral nerve specialist. "The magnitude of the change is considerable. We were surprised by the magnitude and the rapidity of the response." How does it work? In animal models, alpha lipoic acid increases blood flow in nerves, makes the nerves take up glucose better, and increases amounts of antioxidants that our bodies make, including glutathione.

If you have diabetes but don't have neuropathy, you should still consider taking ALA. Researchers think alpha lipoic acid might help to prevent nerve damage if you start taking it early. "It's very safe," says Dr. Dyck. "There have been no known complications."

Along the same lines, alpha lipoic acid seems to help reduce pain in cases of peripheral arterial disease—damage to the smaller arteries in the legs. And alpha lipoic acid may help other types of neuropathy, as well, Dr. Berkson says. In one study, it improved symptoms in people with cardiac autonomic neuropathy, a type of nerve damage that affects the nerves in the heart that control heartbeat.

Alpha lipoic acid has been found to improve insulin resistance and control glucose levels in type 2 diabetes. Patients who took 600 to 1,800 milligrams orally had significant improvement in insulin resistance and glucose effectiveness after 4 weeks. ALA seems to help insulin "signaling"—that is, it helps in the production of biochemicals that transport glucose inside a cell.

Burning Fat for Fuel

ALA also helps with fatty acid oxidation, so it may help the body burn fat for energy. It also seems to reduce appetite by working directly in the hypothalamus, the part of the brain that sends out hunger and satiety signals. It suppresses a hunger-causing enzyme and results in reduced appetite and food intake.

In animal studies, it also helps to reverse some fat-related aspects of heart disease, such as high cholesterol. In one study, animals on a high-fat diet that got supplemental alpha lipoic acid had a 73 percent reduction in total cholesterol, a 75 percent reduction in triglycerides, a 71 percent reduction in harmful LDL cholesterol, all while more than doubling their beneficial HDL.

Researchers have found that alpha lipoic acid actually changes the action of genes that control cholesterol. It cranks up the production of enzymes that act as free radical scavengers, and it lowers production of LDL cholesterol.

Help for Ailing Livers

Fatty liver disease—a problem that used to be common only among alcoholics—has become more common in the rest of the population due to the rise of abdominal obesity. But in animal studies, researchers have shown that ALA causes the liver to store less fat, even when consuming a high-fat diet. Dr. Berkson uses alpha lipoic acid as part of his treatment for many types of liver disease, including chronic hepatitis C and alcohol-induced cirrhosis. In fact, research shows that lipoic acid can be helpful in liver diseases where oxidative stress is a factor, especially if chemical toxins are involved. "The liver has a remarkable capacity to regenerate itself if it is given the support it needs to recover," Dr. Berkson says.

May Help with Stroke and Dementia

Studies in animals, and some human studies from Russia, have shown that ALA can help to reduce brain damage when given to people who are at a high risk of stroke, or intravenously immediately after a stroke. It reduces what is called reperfusion injury, a scenario where oxygen-rich blood causes oxidative damage. There is also preliminary research to suggest that lipoic acid might improve function in people with dementia, but it needs to be taken long-term before improvements are seen.

How to Use Alpha Lipoic Acid

Keep a few things in mind if you decide to take alpha lipoic acid. First of all, not all alpha lipoic acid is created equal. The purest product is made in Germany and other European countries, where it is regulated like a drug. This European-made alpha lipoic acid is bought by companies in the United States who use it to make their own products. So before you buy any alpha lipoic product, find out the source of the alpha lipoic acid in the product, Dr. Berkson says. You will need to call the manufacturer to get this information. And be prepared to shell out a few bucks. "You can pretty much be assured that a cheap product will not contain pharmaceutical-grade alpha lipoic acid, but you are not assured that an expensive one does," he says.

If you're taking ALA simply as an antiaging supplement, about 300 milligrams a day is a good dose, Dr. Ames says. If you're taking it to treat diabetes and peripheral neuropathy, doses of both 600 and 1,200 milligrams daily, in divided doses, have been used effectively. For cardiac autonomic neuropathy in patients with type 2 diabetes, 800 milligrams daily in divided doses is recommended.

Alpha lipoic acid is easily absorbed when taken orally, and once inside cells it is quickly converted to its most potent form, dihydrolipoic acid. Alpha lipoic acid does need to be taken with B vitamins, because it depletes B vitamins. Chemically, it is similar to biotin, one of the Bs. If you take alpha lipoic acid and don't get enough biotin, you may develop a skin rash. Alpha lipoic acid also can quickly deplete thiamin, especially in people who abuse alcohol. "I always give a B-50 complex, which contains 35 milligrams of thiamin, along with alpha lipoic acid," Dr. Berkson says.

amino acids

Thumb through a muscle magazine, and you're likely to see advertisements for amino acid supplements that offer the promise of bigger, stronger muscles.

While complete amino acid supplements, such as whey from milk, offer a good source of lean protein, most of us get more protein than we need. But that doesn't mean that we can't sometimes benefit from getting additional amino acids. They play critical roles in our day-to-day lives and can sometimes be used to help fight or treat health problems.

Amino acids are the building blocks of protein. Twenty of them combine to form the 50,000 to 100,000 different proteins in the body. Nine amino acids are classified as essential because your body is unable to produce them and you must get them by eating foods that supply them. They are histidine, isoleucine, leucine, lysine, methionine, phenylalanine, threonine, tryptophan, and valine. Meat, poultry, fish, eggs, milk, cheese, yogurt, and soy are considered complete proteins because they provide us with all nine aminos.

The other 11 amino acids that scientists have studied are considered nonessential. That doesn't mean that they are unnecessary, only that we don't need to get them from foods because most people's bodies can produce them as needed. Our bodies use the essential amino acids to make the nonessential ones—alanine, arginine, asparagine, aspartic acid, cysteine, glutamic acid, glutamine, glycine, proline, serine, and tyrosine.

Just as your right hand is the mirror image of your left, amino acids occur as mirror image forms. The left-hand forms are known as "l" and the right-hand forms are known as "d." You get l-amino acids from food, since they're part of proteins, and they are the ones that are packaged as supplements. If you look at the label of an amino acid supplement and it doesn't indicate "l" or "d," you can't assume it's the "l" form, however. Choose only supplements that are labeled as the "l" form, says Joanne

Larsen, RD, of Nutritional Data Services in Minneapolis, author of *Edmund's Food Ratings for Dieters.*

Amino Activities

Amino acids play several vital roles in keeping us healthy, says James Heffley, PhD, director of clinical nutrition for the Nutrition Counseling Service in Austin, Texas. Their main function is to build the protein that gives structure to such body components as skin, membranes, muscles, organs, and bones.

SUPPLEMENTSNAPSHOT

▶Amino Acids

May help: Heart disease, high blood pressure, low immunity, indigestion, heartburn, diarrhea, diverticulitis, prostate problems, erectile dysfunction, intermittent claudication, infertility, wound healing, depression, and ADHD.

Good food sources: Meat, poultry, fish, eggs, milk, cheese, yogurt, soy, and quinoa supply all nine essential amino acids; other good sources are beans, peas, seeds, and nuts.

Cautions and possible side effects: Don't take individual amino acids without the supervision of a knowledgeable doctor.

People who have genital herpes should not take arginine because it may increase herpes outbreaks. Also, don't take arginine and lysine at the same time, as they can interfere with each other.

Cysteine in high doses can cause kidney stones in people who have cystinuria, and it can inactivate insulin, so use caution if you have diabetes. Taking cysteine may deplete zinc and copper, so if you plan to use cysteine or n-acetylcysteine for more than a few weeks, take it with a multivitamin/mineral supplement that supplies the Daily Value of these minerals.

Tyrosine and phenylalanine supplements can raise blood pressure to dangerous levels, especially in people taking MAO inhibitors as antidepressants. Do not take phenylalanine if you have phenylketonuria.

Some amino acids also act as neurotransmitters, the chemicals that ferry information from one nerve cell to another, says Dr. Heffley. Others are precursors of neurotransmitters, which means that they're involved in creating the compounds that do the transmitting. Tryptophan, for example, is a precursor of the neurotransmitter serotonin, which in turn is a precursor of melatonin, a hormone that's important in sleep and sensory perception. So, if you don't get enough of the tryptophan that helps produce serotonin, you may end up with a shortage of that neurotransmitter. You may also have some sleep problems because you're short on melatonin.

Amino acids are also the foundation for some hormones, including insulin, and they help vitamins and minerals do their jobs. Taurine, for example, helps transport magnesium and potassium from the bloodstream and into the cells.

Protein and amino acids are so abundant in the foods we eat that very few people in the United States are deficient. If anything, we consume too much protein, says Larsen.

The only people who might be low in a particular amino acid are those with genetic defects that prevent them from making or using certain amino acids, she says. People with a hereditary condition called phenylketonuria, for example, can't metabolize phenylalanine properly. If they get this amino acid in their food, their bodies can't process it, and if the condition is left untreated, mental retardation and poor muscle coordination can result.

Zooming In on Specifics

Amino acid supplements come in many forms. Some are combinations of many different kinds of amino acids, but you can also get individual supplements.

Since most of us don't have an amino acid deficiency, you may wonder why anyone would take supplemental protein at all. Most are trying to get the benefits of extra protein—weight loss and increased muscle mass—without taking in all the calories that come with high-protein foods such as dairy, beans, and meat. But individual amino acid supplements should be used only for a specific reason and only under the supervision of a medical professional who's familiar with amino acids, says J. Alexander Bralley, PhD, director and CEO of Metametrix Clinical Laboratory in Atlanta.

As for the kinds of supplements to take, Dr. Bralley advises doctors and their patients to stick with amino acids labeled "free-form." These types of amino acids are easily absorbed into the bloodstream and don't have to be digested, according to Dr. Bralley.

Here is what some of the specific amino acid supplements might be able to do for you, if taken with a doctor's guidance.

Alanine, glutamic acid, and glycine. Some studies have shown that these three amino acids may help relieve the symptoms of one kind of prostate problem in men. Called benign prostatic hyperplasia (BPH), the problem occurs when the prostate gland swells and presses against one part of the urinary tract—the urethra. BPH is especially prevalent among older men and is characterized by an increased frequency of urination, waking at night to empty the bladder, and a reduced flow of urine. Many amino acids are present in the prostate, but alanine, glutamic acid, and glycine seem to be the ones that can help control BPH symptoms.

Arginine. This nonessential amino acid is involved in nitric oxide production, and it may be this action that makes it helpful to our bodies. Nitric oxide relaxes the muscles of the arterial walls and helps to open up the arteries, says Michael Janson, MD, president of the American College for Advancement in Medicine, based in Laguna Hills, California, and author of *The Vitamin Revolution in Health Care.* That is why it is used to treat erectile dysfunction and to help establish collateral circulation around blocked arteries. Studies suggest that arginine supplements may help with high blood pressure and coronary heart disease. It is also thought to help boost immunity and speed wound healing.

Branched-chain amino acids (BCAAs). This is a group that includes three essential amino acids: leucine, isoleucine, and valine. Branched-chain amino acids are a favorite with bodybuilders and other athletes. Dr. Bralley says they may improve performance and help prevent the muscle breakdown that occurs during endurance training. They are sometimes used to help prevent the muscle wasting that occurs in HIV/AIDS patients, in people confined to bed, and during cancer treatments. BCAAs are found mostly in muscle, and they break down and are used up for energy during prolonged exercise. If there isn't a readily available pool of amino acids to draw upon, the protein synthesis doesn't remake muscle as quickly and efficiently. BCAAs help to boost the muscle-building process. "From what we've seen, branched-chain amino acids do tend to conserve muscle mass," says Dr. Bralley.

Carnitine. Carnitine is an amino acid made in the liver from two other amino acid building blocks—lysine and methionine. It's not one of the 20 amino acids that are used in protein synthesis, says Dr. Bralley, but it helps transport fat into the mitochondria within cells, where fat is burned for energy. Carnitine has been found to lower serum cholesterol and triglycerides, build muscle tissue, and increase stamina. A deficiency may cause muscle weakness, confusion, or angina. A deficiency can also lead to an increase of fats in your bloodstream, especially a harmful type called triglycerides. Your doctor can spot a deficiency of carnitine with a blood or urine test.

Studies have shown that l-carnitine increases exercise capacity in people with some kinds of artery disease and improves muscle function and exercise capacity in people with kidney disease. Acetyl-l-carnitine, a closely related amino acid, has been found to slow memory loss. A third form, d-carnitine, is synthetic and does not have any beneficial effect in the body. There is no reason to take d-carnitine or dl-carnitine.

Cysteine. Cysteine is needed to make another amino acid, taurine, which is anti-inflammatory, says Dr. Bralley. According to studies, cysteine can remove heavy metal toxins from the body, including mercury, cadmium, lead, and arsenic.

In the form of n-acetylcysteine, cysteine has been used to stimulate the synthesis of another amino acid, glutathione. Glutathione has antioxidant properties, so it helps to block free radicals—the free-roaming, unstable molecules that harm cells.

N-acetylcysteine may also help combat the side effects of chemotherapy and radiation therapy as well as help to clear mucus out of the lungs of smokers and cystic fibrosis patients. It is often used by alternative doctors to aid in detoxification.

Glutamine. Under normal circumstances, glutamine is not considered an essential amino acid, but some people do need supplements in certain situations, says Dr. Heffley. Cancer cells like an acidic environment, and glutamine helps to shift the body chemistry in the other direction, creating a less acidic, more alkaline environment. This happens even when cancer is present.

Glutamine has also been used for its calming effects. Once in the body, it's made into gamma-aminobutyric acid (GABA), a neurotransmitter in the central nervous system. But the calming effect is not universal. In fact, Dr. Heffley says that in 1 person in 10, glutamine can act as a stimulant.

That's because it can also be made into glutamic acid, which sends signals that excite the nerves rather than calming them. There's no real danger, however, even if you happen to experience stimulating effects from glutamine, he says. The worst that can happen is a restless night.

Glutamine is also used for wound healing, to repair the small intestine, to boost depressed immunity, and to break addictions to caffeine and other stimulants. It may also help treat diarrhea that's caused by gluten intolerance, Crohn's disease, AIDS, and other conditions, adds Larsen. If you take it for this purpose, you'll know within 3 days if it's working.

Lysine. This essential amino acid can decrease outbreaks of the herpes simplex virus, which is responsible for cold sores and genital herpes. With either kind of outbreak, a lysine supplement can help the infection heal more quickly.

If you're low on lysine, you might end up with a deficiency of carnitine. A lysine deficiency may also lead to calcium loss, which could increase your risk of developing osteoporosis. Lysine deficiencies occur more often in people who do not consume any animal products than in those who do, says Dr. Heffley. The best way to tell if you are lysine deficient is to have your doctor perform a urine or blood test.

Lysine competes with arginine for absorption and use by the body, so if you're taking lysine, you'll get less-than-optimal results from arginine, and vice versa.

Phenylalanine and tyrosine. Phenylalanine is an essential amino acid that is used to make another amino acid, tyrosine. Tyrosine in turn is transformed into three kinds of neurotransmitters, the nerve-related chemicals that help messages travel through your body. Since phenylalanine and tyrosine have an energizing effect, studies suggest that they are useful in treating depression and lethargy.

There's a synthetic form of phenylalanine called d-phenylalanine. It's not used by the body in the same way that the naturally occurring l-form is, but it may be beneficial as a treatment for chronic pain, especially lower back pain and dental pain.

A combined form, called dl-phenylalanine, however, does have some separate benefits. Some studies suggest that it may be useful in treating the chronic pain of osteoarthritis and rheumatoid arthritis, lower back pain, menstrual cramps, and migraine, among other conditions. It's thought that it blocks certain enzymes in the central nervous system that are responsible for breaking down the brain's own painkillers. If it interferes with those enzymes, the theory is that the natural painkillers in your brain will be free to do their work of suppressing pain.

Taurine. This amino acid is important for the normal functioning of the heart, brain, gallbladder, eyes, and vascular system. It's the most abundant free amino acid found in the heart. In Japan, it's widely used to treat heart disease.

astragalus

Chinese folks are as likely as Americans to have soup or stew simmering on the stove top for the evening meal. Unlike beef stew or tomato soup, though, that Chinese broth probably contains a medicinal element—a few sticks or slices of astragalus root to keep away the colds and flu that come with the winter season.

Astragalus is a member of the pea family whose name was derived from an ancient Greek word meaning "anklebone." These bones were once used as dice, and it's thought that the name originated because the rattling seedpods of the Mediterranean variety of the plant sounded like rolling dice.

Western herbalists classify astragalus as a tonic herb, meaning that it helps the body return to a condition of normal functioning. In China, this popular herb is believed to strengthen *chi*, the body's defensive energy that protects against invading pathogens such as bacteria and viruses.

The root is the medicinal part of the plant, a perennial that can grow to about 2 feet tall. There are 2,000 species of astragalus worldwide—400 of them in North America—but the medicinal variety is found only in central and western Asia. Also known as *huang qi*, it was used in China for at least 2,000 years before European botanists wrote about its medicinal qualities in the 1700s.

"For the Chinese, astragalus is really a classic healing herb. It's thought to have a warm tonic action on chi, the protective energy," says Jennifer Brett, ND, a naturopathic doctor at the Wilton Naturopathic Center in Stratford, Connecticut. "A lot of elderly people make it a part of their diets."

Defense, Defense

In Western terms, strengthening chi translates to bolstering the immune system, and astragalus appears to have a positive effect on resistance to diseases and infections, says Dr. Brett. It's like food or nourishment for your immune system, essentially giving it more vitality and "muscle" so it can ward off disease on its own. Some studies in China have shown that it can prevent or shorten the duration of colds.

Chinese doctors usually mix this chi tonic with other herbs, depending on a person's complaint. It's been used to combat shortness of breath, weakness, night sweats, respiratory diseases, lingering diarrhea, uterine and rectal prolapse, boils and sores, and other maladies, but its main use is to make the body's defenses a little tougher, says Dr. Brett.

"It's an herb that helps you cope with the physical and emotional stress that can make you more susceptible to getting sick," she says. "It doesn't so much stimulate the body as tone it."

Arming the Body

Astragalus has been used for centuries in Fu Zheng therapy, an herbal treatment used by practitioners of traditional Chinese medicine to promote or bolster the immune system. In trying to strengthen their patients' natural defense mechanisms, doctors of traditional Chinese medicine have even begun to use Fu Zheng therapy to help treat cancer patients. They use astragalus to boost immune function during and after radiation or chemotherapy treatments.

SUPPLEMENT SNAPSHOT

▶Astragalus

Botanical name: *Astragalus membranaceus;* also known as *huang qi.*

Origin: Medicinal species grows only in Asia.

May help: Low immunity due to disease, including cancer; fibromyalgia; stress; chronic fatigue syndrome; and poor appetite. Has been used in traditional Chinese medicine to treat shortness of breath, weakness, colds and flu, night sweats, respiratory diseases, lingering diarrhea, uterine and rectal prolapse, boils, and sores.

Cautions and possible side effects: Generally regarded as safe, but has not been well studied in the United States. More than 28 grams a day can suppress immunity.

When cancer invades your body, your immune system naturally weakens. In the advanced stages of the disease or after rounds of chemotherapy or radiation—which are lifesaving but very toxic treatments—your immune system can be devastated. Shamelessly opportunistic, a routine cold can turn into a deadly infection.

The effectiveness of astragalus and the Fu Zheng treatment was put to the test in a study of cancer patients undertaken at the MD Anderson Cancer Center in Houston in the early 1980s. After giving a specially prepared astragalus extract to 19 cancer patients and 15 healthy people, doctors found that the treatment restored immune system functioning in the majority of the patients. In some cases, it made the cancer patients' immune systems resemble those of the healthy subjects. The researchers concluded that astragalus contains a potent immune stimulant.

"Those kinds of results really fit with the traditional use of astragalus," says Steven Dentali, PhD, a natural products chemist with Dentali Associates in Troutdale, Oregon, and a member of the advisory board of the American Botanical Council. "It's an herb that supports the immune system."

Down to the Marrow

Astragalus appears to influence the bone marrow, where immune cells are manufactured, says Dr. Dentali. Compounds called polysaccharides seem to stimulate white blood cell production and increase the activity of killer T cells, the body's defenders that hunt down and destroy invaders.

Astragalus also increases the production of interferon, a natural protein that adheres to the surfaces of cells and stimulates production of other proteins that prevent viral infection. In other words, it makes your cells more thick-skinned so viruses have a harder time getting in.

In people with chronic hepatitis, a viral infection, astragalus seems to improve liver function. In animals, astragalus also reduces heart damage from the Coxsackie virus. Astragalus is also thought to dilate blood vessels and help the heart pump more blood, which might be beneficial in angina, congestive heart failure, and after a heart attack.

As a general tonic, Dr. Brett recommends astragalus—usually in combination with other herbs—to people who feel run-down or stressed, have poor appetites, or can't shake colds. "It's an energy tonic that can do a lot to increase your stamina," she says.

Astragalus can also be useful if you're making a lot of trips to the bathroom at night. Dr. Brett sometimes recommends it for its diuretic effect. It can temporarily increase urination and clean out the urinary tract, she notes, so if you take it well before bedtime, the diuretic effect kicks in before the lights go out. "The astragalus tends to normalize urination so you don't have to get up so often," she explains.

In health food stores, you'll probably find bins of sliced and whole root, sometimes labeled as huang-qi. Either form is good for a tea. You can also take a tincture or capsule. Look for a product that contains astragalus root extract standardized to contain 40 percent polysaccharides. Dosages vary with the form of astragalus you are using. A usual dosage of standardized extract is 250 to 500 milligrams, three or four times a day; a usual dosage of powdered root is 500 to 1,000 milligrams, three or four times per day. Follow the label directions or work with a knowledgeable doctor for best results.

vitamin B₆

Make up a list of health problems that each vitamin or mineral is supposed to help, and there's a good chance that the list for vitamin B_6 will be the longest. This essential B vitamin has been recommended for everything from kidney stones and morning sickness to diabetes and PMS.

While it may actually help some of these conditions, there's just not enough scientific evidence yet to nail down many of its benefits, says James Leklem, PhD, professor of nutrition and food management at Oregon State University in Corvallis.

Like other vitamins and minerals, B_6 works with enzymes, the chemical spark plugs that start reactions in the body. It is an essential part of more than 100 enzymes that are involved in the production of energy and protein. B_6 has to be on hand when your body breaks down stored sugar for energy, when it creates the building blocks that will become protein, and when it makes the brain and nervous system of a developing fetus. Research also suggests that B_6 can help reduce the risk of heart disease and complications of diabetes.

Generating Energy

If we eat more food than we need for immediate energy, some of the excess calories are converted to a form of glucose (blood sugar) called glycogen, which is stored in the liver and muscles. When blood sugar drops, glycogen is broken down into glucose and used for fuel. The enzyme that does this requires B_6.

People start to use glycogen for energy if they've been exercising for an hour or longer or if they're dieting to lose weight. "But you'd have to be extremely deficient in vitamin B_6 to have a problem breaking down glycogen," Dr. Leklem says. "Most people just don't have this problem."

Vitamin B_6 also helps link the molecules that make up certain amino acids, Dr. Leklem explains. Strung together like pearls, amino acids are the "bits" that make proteins. So B_6 indirectly aids protein production in the body.

This vitamin also helps link the molecules of nucleic acids, which make up our cells' genetic material. Low B_6 levels can slow down amino acid or nucleic acid production enough to lead to impaired immunity. In extreme cases, the deficiency can lead to a rare condition called sideroblastic anemia, Dr. Leklem says.

Good for the Heart and Brain

Our bodies need vitamin B_6, along with vitamin B_{12} and folic acid, to be able to break down a potentially toxic amino acid by-product called homocysteine. "High levels of homocysteine have been associated with

SUPPLEMENTSNAPSHOT

▶Vitamin B₆

Also known as: Pyridoxine.

Daily Value: 2 milligrams.

May help: Morning sickness, PMS, menstrual problems, depression, canker sores, peripheral neuropathy (sometimes diagnosed as carpal tunnel syndrome), endometriosis, diabetes, angina, heart disease, HIV, and kidney stones. With vitamins B_{12} and folic acid, can also lower blood levels of homocysteine to reduce risk of heart attack and prevent intermittent claudication, phlebitis, Alzheimer's disease, angina, and high blood pressure.

Good food sources: Chicken, fish, pork, and eggs. Spinach, broccoli, tomato juice, bananas, watermelon, acorn squash, and fortified cereals are good vegetarian sources.

Who's at risk for deficiency: Alcoholics, elderly people with poor diets, people taking drugs that interfere with B_6 absorption, and people with intestinal absorption problems.

Special instructions: If you're supplementing with 50 milligrams or more, take in divided doses two or three times a day.

Cautions and possible side effects: Doses of 200 milligrams a day or more for several months may cause nerve damage.

increased risk of heart disease and stroke," says Alan Gaby, MD, a specialist in nutrition and preventive medicine in Pikesville, Maryland. Compared with B_{12} and folic acid, however, B_6 seems to play a lesser role, according to Dr. Gaby. "Only about 15 percent of people with high homocysteine levels respond to B_6," he says.

A study from the Harvard School of Public Health showed that women who got at least 3 milligrams a day of B_6 had half the risk of having heart attacks as did women who got 1.5 milligrams. This is still more than a woman's average daily intake of B_6, which is about 1.2 milligrams.

Vitamin B_6 also helps out neurotransmitters, the chemicals that our nervous systems produce in order to send out messages. It is needed to make an impressive array of neurotransmitters that help to activate and speed up communication among nerve cells. These include serotonin, taurine, dopamine, norepinephrine, and histamine.

"Unfortunately, there's not much research to tell us what all this may mean in terms of actual mental performance," Dr. Gaby says. But there is some. Higher blood concentrations of B_6 were associated with better performance on two tests of memory in a study by researchers at Tufts University in Boston.

Helping Hormones and Blood Sugar

Vitamin B_6 plays a role in maintaining normal hormone balance. When B_6 levels are low, hormones may have a stronger-than-normal action on specific cells or organs, Dr. Leklem says. In animals, the vitamin inhibits the way a hormone hooks up or binds within a cell, which is a step in the cell's activation. "In humans, however, we don't know for sure how it works," Dr. Leklem says.

Still, B_6 is known to help regulate a number of specific hormones, including estrogen, progesterone, androgens (male hormones), and glucocorticoid (a stress hormone.) This may be one reason why the vitamin sometimes seems to be an effective treatment for PMS and morning sickness, says Dr. Leklem.

For different reasons, vitamin B_6 may also be able to help people who have diabetes. One result of this disease is that blood sugar has the ability to stick to proteins, a process called glycosylation. "It's fairly well accepted that glycosylation of proteins is one of the things that causes the complications of diabetes, such as kidney and nerve damage and cataracts," Dr. Gaby says.

In a study at Yale University, researchers found that people with diabetes got some benefits from taking a B_6 supplement because of its apparent effect on glycosylation. When they took 50 milligrams of B_6 three times a day for 6 weeks, the participants had significant drops in the glycosylation of hemoglobin, a protein found in red blood cells.

Vitamin B_6 deficiency has been linked to glucose intolerance, a condition in which blood sugar rises sharply after eating. It has also been implicated in impaired secretion of insulin and glucagon, both hormones that are essential in regulating blood sugar levels.

Blood levels of B_6 are low in 20 to 25 percent of people with diabetes, and in some, levels fall abruptly when they are given sugar, Dr. Leklem says. "We don't know why this happens, but we do know that there are several good reasons that people with diabetes should make sure they are getting enough B_6. Preventing diabetes-related organ damage is apparently one of them." Vitamin B_6, along with thiamin, also can help reduce the nerve damage in feet and hands, called peripheral neuropathy, that plagues so many people with uncontrolled diabetes.

Interactions with Others

Vitamin B_6 interacts with magnesium, an essential mineral used in more than 300 biochemical reactions in the body. In some cases, both the vitamin and the mineral are needed to activate the enzymes that start biochemical reactions such as breaking down sugar for energy. Some research also suggests that B_6 depends on magnesium to help it get inside cells, where it can do its work. "One thing we do know is that an extremely low intake of magnesium will compromise the body's ability to use B_6 properly," Dr. Leklem says.

The vitamin also interacts with oxalate, a by-product of metabolism that plays an important role in the formation of kidney stones. Some people who develop kidney stones have a genetic abnormality that leads to a buildup of oxalate, and high concentrations in the kidneys cause it to form stones. Taking B_6 at doses of 10 to 50 milligrams a day can help, Dr. Gaby says. "And taking magnesium along with the B_6 is warranted," he adds. In his view, the magnesium helps prevent oxalate from crystallizing into stones. Your doctor should determine whether taking B_6 and magnesium would be beneficial if you've been diagnosed with kidney stones.

The Bottom Line

The more protein you eat, the more vitamin B_6 you need, because this vitamin assists in protein metabolism. Some protein-rich foods contain good amounts of B_6, but you can't count on all of those foods to be super suppliers. Good sources include meats, fish, poultry, shellfish, legumes, fruits, egg yolks, whole grains, and leafy green vegetables. Dairy products, on the other hand, are relatively poor sources, and processed lunch meats like sliced ham or turkey lose 50 to 70 percent of their B_6 in processing.

Alcoholics are most likely to be deficient, because alcohol actually promotes the destruction of B_6 and its loss from the body. If you're elderly and don't eat well for any reason, you're more likely than a younger person to have a deficiency. Others who might have a problem are people with absorption problems such as celiac disease and those who take drugs that interfere with the body's use of B_6.

More than 40 drugs can compromise absorption, including isoniazid (Laniazid, Nydrazid), a tuberculosis drug, and penicillamine (Cuprimine, Depen), used to treat Wilson's disease and rheumatoid arthritis and to prevent kidney stones. "Birth control pills used to be on the list of possible B_6 antagonists, but low-estrogen pills don't cause this problem," Dr. Leklem says. Some environmental chemicals may also hinder the body's ability to use B_6, Dr. Gaby says.

People who are short on B_6 are likely to be weak and irritable and have trouble sleeping. They may also develop depression, impaired glucose tolerance, convulsions, cracking of the lips and tongue, and skin problems such as seborrhea or eczema.

vitamin B₁₂

Imagine having a disease that will very likely kill you—unless you can somehow choke down ⅔ pound of raw liver a day. Awful? Yes. But that was once the cure offered to people with pernicious anemia.

The researchers who discovered this cure won the Nobel Prize for medicine in 1934. It wasn't until 1948 that researchers isolated from raw liver the small red crystals of the nutrient that we now call vitamin B_{12}.

Unless you're a vegan (strict vegetarian), pernicious anemia is not often due to a lack of this essential vitamin. It's actually a problem with absorption. B_{12} differs from other vitamins in that before it can be absorbed into the cells lining the intestines, it has to hook up with a protein (called *intrinsic factor*) that is secreted as part of the stomach's digestive juices.

Some people, especially when they're older and on low-protein diets, don't make enough intrinsic factor to absorb all the B_{12} they need. Since intrinsic factor is provided by the body, not by food, when the body doesn't make enough, we can be at risk for B_{12}-related health risks.

Only about 1 percent of people develop the classic symptoms of B_{12} deficiency—anemia and nerve damage. About 30 percent of older people show signs of deficiency when their blood is tested, says Robert Allen, MD, professor of medicine and biochemistry and director of hematology at the University of Colorado Health Sciences Center in Denver.

Even a low-level deficiency can have negative health effects. People may have depression, forgetfulness, trouble walking, and even incontinence. Sometimes, though, these are problems of old age rather than symptoms of vitamin deficiency. That's why proper testing is so important.

B₁₂ Basics

This vitamin is essential to every cell in your body. It must be on hand for DNA synthesis, the process by which your body makes the genetic material that comprises the cell nucleus. Vitamin B$_{12}$ is far more than a cheerleader in this process. It rolls up its sleeves and goes to work, helping to make the nucleic acids that are strung together like pearls to form DNA, the genetic e-mail system. It also helps make RNA, the copy of DNA that's sent along to each cell.

When cells are rapidly dividing, as they do during growth and development, more B$_{12}$ is needed for this process, according to John Pinto, PhD, associate professor of biochemistry at Weill Cornell Medical College in New York City and director of the nutrition research laboratory at Memorial Sloan-Kettering Cancer Center, both in New York City. Extra B$_{12}$ is also necessary in areas where cells normally have rapid turnover, such as the intestines and the blood, he says.

SUPPLEMENT SNAPSHOT

▶Vitamin B$_{12}$

Also known as: Cobalamin, cyanocobalamin, hydroxocobalamin, and methylcobalamin.

Daily Value: 6 micrograms.

May help: Pernicious anemia and nerve problems related to B$_{12}$ deficiency; sometimes used for shingles, multiple sclerosis, canker sores, diabetes, depression, age-related cognitive problems, chronic fatigue syndrome, and to help delay the progression of HIV to AIDS. With vitamins B$_6$ and folic acid, can lower blood levels of homocysteine to reduce risk of heart attack and prevent intermittent claudication, phlebitis, Alzheimer's disease, angina, and high blood pressure.

Good food sources: Cooked oysters and clams and all meats.

Who's at risk for deficiency: People age 60 or older who have a condition that causes low stomach acid, people with problems related to intrinsic factor, people with Crohn's disease, strict vegetarians, and breastfed babies of strict vegetarians.

Special instructions: People with B$_{12}$ deficiencies might not be able to rely on oral supplements and should see a doctor, who may recommend B$_{12}$ injections as well as other supplementation.

Cautions and possible side effects: Generally regarded as safe.

When B_{12} is in short supply, DNA and RNA synthesis slows, and cells can no longer divide and multiply. This can show up in several ways. In the blood, it can mean anemia—a shortage of red blood cells—since the cells in the bone marrow that make red blood cells normally crank them out at the rate of at least 200 million a minute. In the intestines, it can mean absorption problems that create a domino effect, accelerating nutrient deficiencies as cells are deprived of the supplies that are delivered like groceries by the red blood cells.

In some places in the body, such as the cervix and intestines, a shortage of vitamin B_{12} can begin to interfere with cell growth; the resulting cell abnormalities can lead to cancer. Your ability to fight infection may slow down because your body can't crank out enough infection-fighting white blood cells. In fact, one study showed that people with HIV, the virus that causes AIDS, were able to hold off full-blown AIDS longer if they had high levels of B_{12}. "The question is, how fast can your system adapt to an adverse situation, such as infection, by making more DNA?" Dr. Pinto says. "When B_{12} is in short supply, your body slows down and can't defend itself as well."

Friend of Folic

Vitamin B_{12} works hand in hand with folic acid, which also helps to make DNA. One form of folic acid circulates throughout the body. When B_{12} removes a piece of the molecule from this circulating form, the folic acid becomes available for other reactions. As it goes about its business, B_{12} uses the stolen piece of molecule for some of its own important functions.

Since B_{12} and folic acid are so closely linked, a deficiency of one can leave the other in cold storage. You may be getting plenty of folate (the food form of folic acid) in your diet, for instance, but if you're coming up short on B_{12}, the folate stays inside cells, trapped in its inactive form.

The Amino Acid Shuffle

Vitamin B_{12} and folic acid are also necessary for amino acid synthesis, meaning that they need to be there when your body sends the wrecking ball up against the proteins in food so they can then reassemble those proteins to create new structures.

This demolition and reconstruction work is going on all the time. If your body wants to take those scrambled eggs you had this morning and turn them into useful energy and hearty body cells, B_{12} and folic acid have to be on hand to do their part. They help to ensure that the protein parts—amino acids—are present in the proper amounts to make new proteins.

Nerves of Steel

Vitamin B_{12} also maintains the fatty sheath, called myelin, that surrounds and protects nerve fibers and promotes their normal growth, Dr. Pinto says. Like insulation around copper wires, this sheath allows your radiating network of nerves to send their electrical messages without short-circuiting. When B_{12} is missing, the myelin sheath breaks down, which eventually leads to nerve damage. It may even lead to brain shrinkage, researchers have discovered. A study done at Britain's Oxford University found that people with the lowest blood levels of B_{12} and the highest levels of biochemicals associated with B_{12} deficiency had about six times more brain shrinkage, as measured by MRI over the course of 5 years, than people with the highest B_{12} levels.

One important finding: No one in this study was ever technically B_{12} deficient. In other words, even the people with the most brain shrinkage had blood levels that most doctors would consider within a "low-normal" range. Here again, it points out the importance of getting a dosage of B_{12} that keeps you in a strong middle range. Don't just let your doctor tell you it's "normal." Ask for a copy of your test results and look at them yourself to make sure your level is 400 or above.

Should You Have a B₁₂ Test?

Doctors are usually pretty good about checking blood levels of B_{12} when a patient shows signs of anemia or severe nerve damage, but sometimes the early signs of deficiency can escape a doctor's notice. Among the less noticeable symptoms of vitamin B_{12} deficiency are numbness and tingling in the feet or hands, loss of balance, and memory loss or disorientation.

"Doctors should be testing people when they have these symptoms," says Dr. Allen, "And if B_{12} is in the low-normal range, they should do a follow-up test that measures two additional things, methylmalonic acid and homocysteine. This test is very useful because it helps us accurately diagnose a deficiency and distinguish between a deficiency of B_{12} and one of folic acid.

"Too many doctors still follow the old textbook rule from 15 years ago," Dr. Allen says. "They don't give their patients B_{12} injections unless their blood levels are below 200 ng/ml, and that's clearly a mistake. It is now clear that many people who have levels in the 200 to 400 range require treatment or further evaluation."

As the redevelopment authority inside your body, B_{12} can make trouble for your heart if it goes on strike. Along with folic acid and B_6, it is needed to break down an amino acid by-product called homocysteine. When you don't have enough, blood levels of homocysteine rise, "and high levels of homocysteine seem to increase your risk for heart disease and stroke even more than high cholesterol does," Dr. Pinto says.

Homocysteine damages the cells lining the blood vessels, creating rough spots that attract cholesterol deposits and issue invitations for blood to start clotting. Exactly how much of the three B vitamins you need in order to prevent this problem isn't known. In one study where people received daily doses of 400 micrograms of B_{12}, 1 milligram of folic acid, and 10 milligrams of B_6, homocysteine levels dropped significantly.

So far, researchers have found that high levels of homocysteine are associated with heart disease and that B vitamins can help lower homocysteine levels. They are trying to complete the circle by showing that lowering homocysteine levels with B vitamins can also lower heart disease risk, says Dr. Allen.

bee propolis

Whenever we go to work, make a trip to the supermarket, or just step outside to smell the roses, we risk picking up germs and bringing them back to the nest. They're darn near impossible to avoid.

The same goes for bees. As tens of thousands of bees buzz in and out of the hive each day, they pick up germs along the way and take them back to the colony. Thanks to a sticky brown substance called propolis, however, bees keep the insides of their hives germ free.

Bee propolis is the resin that bees collect from the buds and wounds of trees and other plants and mix with beeswax. In warm weather, propolis is sticky and soft and can be used to fill holes or spread over surfaces like shellac. In cool weather, the propolis hardens and becomes brittle. The bees use it to caulk, seal, line, and strengthen the hive, but they also use it to ward off contamination and germs in the hive. That's because propolis, also known as Russian penicillin, has antibacterial properties.

It's this ability to fight bacteria that makes it an intriguing supplement for humans. The use of propolis as medicine dates back to the time of Aristotle, about 350 BC.

The Greeks used propolis for abscesses, while the Assyrians used it to heal wounds and tumors, according to Steve Nenninger, ND, a naturopathic doctor in New York City. The Egyptians used it for mummification—and so do bees, says Theodore Cherbuliez, MD, a physician in Scarsdale, New York, and president of the American Apitherapy Society, a nonprofit organization that advances the investigation of the healing uses of products from the beehive. If a mouse crawls into the hive for warmth in the winter, bees will sting it to death. Then, since they can't physically remove the mouse, they will mummify it with propolis to protect the health of the hive. "Imagine the inside of a beehive, says Dr. Cherbuliez. "It's hot, humid—an ideal milieu to grow bacteria on that dead mouse. Propolis prevents this from happening."

Proponents today use propolis to treat a variety of illnesses, including colds, flu, and sore throats; skin problems; cold sores; wounds and bruises; stomach ulcers; burns; hemorrhoids; gum disease; bad breath; and tonsillitis. They also promote it for boosting immunity.

Propolis extract does have antimicrobial activity against a variety of bacteria, and some viruses, such as herpes simplex 2, which causes genital herpes and some cases of oral herpes. It also fights organisms that cause dental cavities and periodontal disease. When applied topically, propolis reduces inflammation and accelerates epithelial repair. (Epithelial cells are "lining" cells such as skin and mucous membranes.) And yes, propolis has been used in a placebo-controlled study (a study comparing it to a medical "blank") and was found to reduce the duration of colds. So it's definitely not all folk medicine and snake oil.

Stoked-Up Sticky Stuff

There are more than 300 components in propolis, including bioflavonoids, says Dr. Cherbuliez. Because propolis comes from a variety of plants, the amount and types of these components can vary by season and region.

Collecting propolis for human use is an arduous task. To get the purest product, beekeepers place small inserts in the hives. To bees, the inserts look like cracks. Thinking that their hive needs repair, the bees fill the inserts with propolis. Propolis can also be scraped out of the hive, but this yields an inferior product that may contain unwanted by-products.

SUPPLEMENT SNAPSHOT

▶Bee Propolis

May help: Wounds, infections, colds, cold sores, sore throats, skin problems, stomach ulcers, burns, hemorrhoids, gum disease, bad breath, and tonsillitis.

Special instructions: Take with food.

Cautions and possible side effects: Do not take if you have asthma; it contains allergens that can worsen asthma. Do not take if you are allergic to bee stings. May also cause a rash when handled.

Bee propolis is available in tablets, throat lozenges, chewable tablets with vitamin C, cough syrup, toothpaste, mouthwash, skin lotions, lipstick, throat spray, salve, and tincture. It's best to buy propolis from a supplement manufacturer that specializes in bee products, such as Beehive Botanicals. Such products are less likely to be contaminated.

beta-carotene, vitamin A, and carotenoids

Carrots. Squash. Broccoli. Kale. Orange and yellow vegetables. Dark leafy greens. They all contain beta-carotene (and other carotenoids).

Liver. Milk. Eggs. They all contain vitamin A.

At first glance, these two sources of nutrients seem far, far apart. One source is the plant world, the other is all animal. Once the beta-carotene from plant sources gets inside the body, however, it undergoes a transformation. Through a number of chemical processes, it can be converted into vitamin A. Once the transformation is complete and the body has all the vitamin A it can use, any extra beta-carotene can be used elsewhere in the body.

As for the supplement forms of these nutrients, they're often separate, but not equal. The problem is that the pure form of vitamin A, called preformed vitamin A, can create a number of nasty toxic effects if you take too much of it. Although beta-carotene isn't without its problems, low doses may be taken in supplement form.

The best source of vitamin A is a beta-carotene supplement or a multivitamin that contains a nontoxic amount of vitamin A along with an ample amount of beta-carotene. Both are readily available in drugstores and health food stores. And here's why you might want to pick some up—along with carrots; squash; broccoli; and dark green, leafy vegetables.

All the Roles of A

Vitamin A plays vital roles throughout the body. In our eyes, it helps maintain a crystal-clear outer window, the cornea. Without enough vitamin A, the cornea clouds over. "At the back of the eye, in the retina, vitamin A is part of the pigment that reacts chemically when struck by light and helps create the nerve impulse that goes to the brain and creates a visual message," says James Allen Olson, PhD, professor of biochemistry and director of the vitamin A research group at Iowa State University in

▶Beta-Carotene, Vitamin A, and Carotenoids

Daily Value: Beta-carotene—no DV; vitamin A—5,000 international units (IU) or 1,500 retinol equivalents (RE).

May help: Cancer of the lungs, stomach, esophagus, mouth, cervix, and colon; angina; genital herpes; colds and flu; osteoarthritis; and low immunity in people with HIV.

Good food sources: Beta-carotene—dark green, leafy vegetables; orange and yellow vegetables; and yellow fruits. (One large carrot—one of the best food sources—has about 10,600 IU.) Vitamin A—fortified milk and milk products, such as cheese, cream, and butter.

Who's at risk for deficiency: Cigarette smokers, alcoholics, and people who eat fewer than three servings a day of fruits or vegetables.

Special instructions: For maximum absorption, take supplements with meals that contain some fat. Do not take with meals or supplements that contain large amounts of pectin, a type of soluble fiber found in citrus fruits.

Cautions and possible side effects: Avoid taking more than 25,000 IU of beta-carotene in supplement form. There is evidence that it causes lung cancer in smokers taking 50,000 IU in supplement form. Smokers and recent ex-smokers are safest getting beta-carotene solely from foods.

Do not take preformed vitamin A supplements unless you are under a doctor's supervision. Taking more than 50,000 IU (15,000 RE) of preformed, animal-source vitamin A every day over a long period of time can lead to headaches, blurred vision, hair loss, joint pain, dry skin, drowsiness, diarrhea, and enlargement of the liver and spleen. Symptoms slowly disappear once the dosage is reduced. Do not take more than 5,000 IU a day if you are pregnant or trying to conceive. High doses can cause birth defects, especially during the first trimester. Pregnant women should monitor their vitamin A intake from all sources, including vitamin A–fortified foods such as cereals, vitamin supplements, and high vitamin A foods such as liver.

Ames. For this reason, vitamin A can help with the condition known as night blindness.

Without adequate vitamin A, your eyes recover very slowly after flashes of bright light at night, or you're unable to see in dim light. In Indonesia, where vitamin A deficiency is common, this condition is called chicken eyes because chickens can't see at night and go to roost when the sun goes down.

Vitamin A also has another basic function. "It helps cells to mature and develop certain definite characteristics and properties, a process called cell differentiation," Dr. Olson says. It acts as a kind of traffic cop for cells in a developing embryo. As the cells start to divide and multiply, vitamin A helps guide them in the direction they need to go, putting this one on its way to becoming a muscle cell, steering another one toward becoming a liver cell, and so on.

Vitamin A helps maintain the surfaces of the skin, the mucous membranes lining the nose and throat, and the tissues lining the intestines, bladder, and other internal cavities. All of these benefits can help boost immunity, since mucous membranes help prevent invasion by bacteria and viruses.

The vitamin also plays a direct role in immunity by helping the immune cells change into the special forms necessary to fight off infection. "One special kind of cell, called a T-helper cell, which helps to direct other immune cells, is very sensitive to vitamin A status," Dr. Olson says. "There's no question that the immune system doesn't function very well with inadequate vitamin A, and you don't necessarily need to be clearly deficient for this to happen."

Vitamin A even helps bones. It's involved in the dismantling and reforming of bone, an important part of making new bone. However, excessive vitamin A intake can actually hurt your skeleton. It seems to suppress osteoblast activity (the process of building your bone), stimulate osteoclast formation (the process of losing bone), and reduce vitamin D's ability to maintain normal calcium levels in the blood.

The Many Beta Benefits

Given the many roles of vitamin A in the body, it's fortunate that we can get it from so many sources—plant as well as animal. While the transformation from beta-carotene into vitamin A is chemically complex, it doesn't take long to happen.

Beta-carotene is what's known as a precursor of vitamin A, which means that it's an essential part of the production process. As your body needs vitamin A, it can split beta-carotene in half, producing two molecules of vitamin A. Alternatively, the beta-carotene might split other ways, leaving one molecule of vitamin A.

In either case, the presence of beta-carotene leads to the production of vitamin A when it's needed. "When the body is lacking vitamin A, more beta-carotene is converted to vitamin A by an enzyme in the intestines as well as elsewhere, in other tissues in the body," says Susan Taylor Mayne, PhD, director of cancer prevention and control research at the cancer center at Yale University School of Medicine.

Apart from the role it plays in vitamin A production, beta-carotene gives you other benefits that have been studied by researchers. Studies often involve other forms of plant chemicals, including beta-carotene, that are known as carotenoids.

For years, researchers have seen a growing body of evidence that suggests that the more foods we eat that contain beta-carotene and other carotenoids, the less likely we are to develop certain types of cancer. It looks as if these nutrients may help prevent cancers of the lung, stomach, and esophagus. There's also been some evidence that beta-carotene might lower the risk of developing cancer of the cervix and colon, as well. Mouth and throat cancers may also be on the hit list.

"A reduction in the risk of lung cancer really stood out, followed by mouth and throat cancer," says Dr. Mayne. "Again, beta-carotene and other carotenoids showed very strong preventive activity. In fact, an international group of researchers reviewed this data, and the evidence of a protective effect remains very compelling."

Given these results, scientists have tried to find some evidence of how carotenoids can produce a protective effect in our bodies. What they've found is that carotenoids act as antioxidants. Like vitamins E and C, carotenoids can neutralize free radicals, the free-roaming, unstable molecules that can damage cells. Once these antioxidants are incorporated into the fatty membranes around and inside of cells, they help protect the whole cell, including its genetic material. By protecting your cells from damage, beta-carotene can help protect you from various diseases.

Making Good Neighbors

Beta-carotene and other carotenoids may also help to regulate the proteins that enable cell-to-cell communication. "Every cell in the body has the ability to communicate with its neighbors, as though it were calling out across the backyard fence," Dr. Mayne says. This ability to communicate is thought to play a role in inhibiting cancer.

When normal cells are grown in the laboratory, they won't pile up on top of one another, she says. "Once they have filled up the top of a layer in a cell culture system, they send messages to each other that say, in effect, 'We are done growing.' This makes all the cells stop."

To cancer researchers, that's a fascinating effect, because cancer cells don't stop growing, and that's the problem. "In cancer cells, that communication goes awry, and they just continue to grow and grow," says Dr. Mayne.

In their frenetic growing process, the cancer cells eventually pile up, forming tumors. As the pileup continues, the cells eventually invade the space of normal, healthy cells and generally take over the neighborhood. If beta-carotene and other carotenoids really are a key link in cell-to-cell communication, maybe they can help to keep cells from overgrowing. At least, that's what researchers think.

Starting with some studies in the 1980s and 1990s, however, doctors began to see that the scenario is even more complex. While some doses of beta-carotene in certain forms may have the cancer-preventive effect that we want, there are many variables. In fact, in certain high-risk groups, certain kinds of beta-carotene in high doses may tilt the balance the other way and actually increase the risk of one kind of cancer.

The Carotene Conundrum

A study conducted in Finland showed an unexpected outcome among heavy smokers, ages 50 to 69, who took 20 milligrams (33,200 international units, or IU) a day of beta-carotene for 5 to 8 years. Compared with other smokers who had similar lifestyles but took no beta-carotene, the people who took the supplements had an increased rate of cancer. In fact, they had an 18 percent higher incidence of lung cancer than the heavy smokers who did not take supplements. This study also found an 11 percent increase in deaths from heart disease or stroke among the smokers who were taking beta-carotene.

Another study, called the Carotene and Retinol Efficacy Trial, was conducted at a number of US medical centers that specialize in the prevention of lung cancer. Again, the study focused on very high-risk groups—in this case, heavy smokers and asbestos workers who were also smokers. But scientists had to end the study almost 2 years earlier than planned because the supplement seemed to increase health risks. The supplemented group, who were taking 30 milligrams (50,000 IU) a day of beta-carotene in combination with 25,000 IU of vitamin A (five times the Daily Value), were showing a 28 percent greater risk of developing lung cancer. They also had a 25 percent higher risk of death from heart disease. "It's hard to draw conclusions from this study, since it was stopped early and used a combination of nutrients," Dr. Mayne says. "But the data did indicate that there was the possibility of harm from beta-carotene, and little likelihood of benefit."

In a third study, the Physicians' Health Study, participants took 50 milligrams (83,000 IU) of beta-carotene every other day. Although the study went on for 12 years, the researchers found that beta-carotene had no effect—either beneficial or harmful—on the risk of cancer or cardiovascular disease. This study included relatively fewer smokers, however.

These results were not what scientists would have expected, given the positive results of earlier studies with people involving foods rich in beta-carotene and animal studies involving supplements. "There's no doubt that now there are more questions than answers about beta-carotene," says Dr. Mayne.

What's the Right Dose?

What does the uncertainty about beta-carotene mean to you if you are wondering whether to take a supplement?

Well, if you don't smoke, you probably shouldn't worry. Those who were adversely affected were heavy smokers, and they were taking large amounts of supplements. "The only evidence of possible harm we have is in people who smoke more than one pack a day of cigarettes," Dr. Mayne says.

Researchers still don't know why harm occurs in this select group, but the very large doses are certainly a factor. "Antioxidants can promote free radical formation rather than inhibit it under certain circumstances, which could occur in someone with lots of oxidative damage going on in their body," Dr. Mayne says. "In smokers, there's a lot of oxidative damage."

A heavy smoker's mouth, throat, lungs, and blood are constantly being exposed to chemical reactions that involve oxygen, Dr. Mayne points out. When oxygen is involved, trouble can follow. "These compounds can damage the cell membranes, which hinders the cell's ability to function properly. And they can go right through the cell membrane and chemically react with the cell's genetic material, setting the stage for cancer."

"It's possible that one dose of beta-carotene might offer protection from oxidative damage, while a higher dose could promote it, especially in already-damaged cells," Dr. Mayne says. Still, for smokers, the best advice is this: Quit smoking, and get your beta-carotene and other carotenoids from foods, not supplements.

Judicious Approaches

People at risk for vitamin A deficiency can benefit from beta-carotene supplements. In the United States, most people get enough vitamin A from food; worldwide, vitamin A deficiency is a common cause of blindness. Those most likely to have low supplies are children from poor families, who may not get enough vitamin A–fortified milk or beta-carotene–rich fruits and vegetables. In some areas of Africa and Asia, both children and adults die as a result of a lack of vitamin A, usually from infections.

Others who may suffer from vitamin A deficiency are alcoholics, people who can't absorb fat properly, and people with liver disease. (Vitamin A is stored in the liver.) If you don't get enough zinc, an essential trace mineral, you can also become deficient, because your body needs zinc to make a protein that carries vitamin A in your bloodstream from the liver to other organs. If zinc's not there, vitamin A is not used effectively.

bioflavonoids

Hidden inside vegetables, fruits, flowers, herbs, and grains are certain pigments that seem to do a lot more than add color to the scene. Once thought to be lacking in nutritional value, the compounds—called bioflavonoids—are known to perform lots of colorful activities. Among their powers: anti-inflammatory, antiallergenic, antiviral, and anticancer properties.

Bioflavonoids were discovered in the 1930s by Albert Szent-Gyorgyi, a Hungarian-born American chemist who won a Nobel Prize in medicine for his work with vitamin C. He found that when combined with vitamin C in his animal studies, a substance in the rinds of citrus fruits, which he named citrin, helped strengthen the small blood vessels called capillaries. When he traced the active ingredients in citrin, Szent-Gyorgyi discovered a group of compounds that he named vitamin P, which was later renamed bioflavonoids.

Subsequently, doctors began using these compounds to treat various bleeding problems, such as bruising. In 1950, though, a committee of experts decided that they were not actually vitamins, since no studies could prove that they are essential to our health. And in the late 1960s, the FDA also determined that bioflavonoids were not vitamins. While that is true, it doesn't mean that they have no value.

With the publication of new research, medical experts regard these substances as powerful antioxidants, providing protection against the free-roaming, unstable molecules called free radicals. That's a significant contribution because free radicals have been linked to cancer, heart disease, arthritis, and other ailments. Supplements are now being used to prevent and treat fragile capillaries, bleeding gums, varicose veins, hemorrhoids, bruises, diabetes, heavy menstrual bleeding, glaucoma and other vision problems, and many other conditions.

Between the date of Szent-Gyorgyi's original discovery and today, nearly 4,000 bioflavonoids have been identified. Selected from this vast array, a much smaller number are commonly found in supplements.

One that has been studied is quercetin, found in grapes, green tea, tomatoes, onions, kale, green beans, and strawberries. Other supplements contain rutin, which comes from buckwheat and a number of other plants. A third widely available bioflavonoid is hesperidin, which is derived from the rinds of oranges, lemons, and other citrus fruits.

You'll also see supplements called proanthocyanidins, or PCOs, which are primarily from red wines and grape seed extract. In the United States, Pycnogenol is a registered trademark name for a PCO from a different source—the bark of the French maritime pine tree.

Some bioflavonoid supplements contain both hesperidin and rutin. A combination of rutin and vitamin C is sold as vitamin C complex, says Michael Janson, MD, president of the American College for Advancement in Medicine, based in Laguna Hills, California, and author of *The Vitamin Revolution in Health Care*. The combination makes sense because bioflavonoids and vitamin C work together to provide protection from free radicals, says Dr. Janson. He adds, however, that it's usually less expensive to take vitamin C and bioflavonoid supplements separately.

SUPPLEMENT SNAPSHOT

▶ Bioflavonoids

Individual names: Quercetin, rutin, hesperidin, and proanthocyanidins, among others.

May help: Allergies, asthma, carpal tunnel syndrome, bruises, gout, high cholesterol, varicose veins, hemorrhoids, low immunity, arthritis, and sciatica. With vitamin C, used for gingivitis, colds and flu, canker sores, cold sores, menopausal discomforts, heavy menstrual bleeding, vaginitis, and genital herpes. May also strengthen capillaries, enhance connective tissue repair, decrease risk of heart disease and stroke, and help prevent cancer.

Good food sources: Rinds of oranges, lemons, and other citrus fruits; blueberries, blackberries, black cherries, onions, kale, green beans, broccoli, endive, celery, cranberries, tomatoes, red bell peppers, apples, green and black tea, grapes, and red wine.

Special instructions: Take with food.

Cautions and possible side effects: Generally regarded as safe.

A Case for Quercetin

Among the bioflavonoids, quercetin is perhaps the most highly regarded as a supplement to reduce inflammation and relieve asthma and allergies.

The main causes of run-of-the-mill allergy symptoms are histamine and leukotrienes, biochemicals that are released by your immune system to defend your body against invading allergens. For many allergies, antihistamine drugs do just what their name implies: They help prevent histamines from getting into your cells and causing symptoms such as congestion and sneezing, says Elliott Middleton Jr., MD, professor emeritus of medicine at the State University of New York at Buffalo.

In preventing allergy symptoms, quercetin and other bioflavonoids act somewhat differently. Instead of blocking the pathways into the cells, they inhibit the manufacture and release of histamine and leukotrienes in the first place, explains Dr. Middleton. Plus, it seems that they can inhibit the action of these allergy-causing chemicals even after they've been released.

Because of quercetin's antiallergy properties, some naturopathic doctors regularly prescribe supplements. During hay fever season, Jennifer Brett, ND, a naturopathic doctor at the Wilton Naturopathic Center in Stratford, Connecticut, recommends quercetin for many of her patients, particularly those who are allergic to ragweed and leaf mold. According to Dr. Brett, quercetin helps reduce her patients' allergy symptoms, including itchy eyes, runny noses, and scratchy throats. She's found that it's also effective for people who have asthma, which is sometimes touched off by allergic reactions. If they take the bioflavonoid, Dr. Brett says, they don't need to rely as much on inhalers for relief.

Something for the Heart . . . And More

Quercetin and other bioflavonoids have also been targeted for biodetective work because of their ability to prevent heart disease and strokes. When Dutch scientists studied the eating patterns of 805 men between the ages of 65 and 84, they discovered that those who consumed the most bioflavonoids—specifically from tea, onions, and apples—were less likely to die from a heart attack than those who ate less. The more bioflavonoids the men consumed, the lower their risk of heart attack. Those who got the most preventive payback were consuming the equivalent of 4 cups of tea, an apple, and ½ cup of onions a day.

In another study from the Netherlands, researchers gathered health and dietary information from 552 men between the ages of 50 and 69. Fifteen years later, during follow-up examinations, the researchers found that those who consumed a high amount of bioflavonoids—mostly from black tea—had a 73 percent lower risk of stroke than those with a low intake.

Bioflavonoids appear to reduce the risk of cardiovascular disease by making small blood cells called platelets less sticky, explains Joe Vinson, PhD, professor of chemistry at the University of Scranton in Pennsylvania. Sticky platelets can cause blood clots that ultimately result in heart attacks. Bioflavonoids also act as antioxidants and may prevent the oxidation of LDL cholesterol, which is believed to be a leading cause of atherosclerosis (hardening of the arteries).

Preventing Cancer and Cataracts

These multitalented pigments also show some promise in cancer prevention, according to Dr. Middleton. So far, the evidence comes from animal and laboratory studies in which bioflavonoids were used. That research shows that certain bioflavonoids, such as those in green tea, grapefruit, parsley, artichokes, broccoli, and other plants, can cause apoptosis (a fancy term for cell death) in cancer cells.

Cataract prevention is another area where bioflavonoids, particularly quercetin, may help. When cataracts develop, obscuring normal vision, substances called sugar-protein complexes are deposited on the lens of the eye. According to Dr. Janson, quercetin reduces the activity of an enzyme that leads to these deposits. When the deposits are reduced, there's less risk of developing cataracts.

Finally, bioflavonoids are believed by some to enhance vitamin C activity in situations where the vitamin alone is ineffective and to improve the strength of blood vessels and connective tissue. You can get the benefit of those actions in a number of ways. Stronger blood vessels mean less bruising, and they offer some protection against the development of varicose veins and hemorrhoids. There's also less chance of developing bleeding gums.

Bioflavonoids may strengthen and repair connective tissue by stimulating the synthesis of collagen, the fibrous protein that helps hold cells together. They also inhibit the breakdown of collagen, which means that connective tissue between your cells is more likely to stay strong and unbroken. This benefits the nervous system and may reduce allergy symptoms, such as inflammation.

The Pluses of Getting Enough

While the many benefits of bioflavonoids are being explored, experts are still trying to decide whether most of us can benefit from supplementation. Some say that we get all the bioflavonoids we need from our diets and that supplementing provides no additional benefits. Others argue that supplements provide extra protection and help fill the gaps when our diets are lacking.

"There are many good things in your food that you can't isolate in a supplement," says Dr. Vinson, who believes that bioflavonoid supplements aren't usually necessary.

Dr. Janson agrees that food is the preferred source of bioflavonoids, but he recommends supplementation as well. "Therapeutic doses for allergies, for example, are higher than you can get from diet. If people eat a wide variety of plant-based foods, they'll probably get a good supply of bioflavonoids. But I still believe there are benefits to supplementation." Based on this view, Dr. Janson regularly prescribes bioflavonoids to his patients.

If you're going to take a supplement, try a mixed berry supplement or mixed greens supplement as a powder that you mix into a liquid. This provides a nice, whole foods mix of bioflavonoids in a larger dose than you would get in capsules.

biotin

You may regard biotin merely as a cure for your brittle nails—it's been shown to thicken fingernails as well as the hooves of horses and pigs—but this B vitamin means more to our bodies than simple beauty care.

Biotin has a daily job that it does with great reliability in our bodies: It helps us use carbohydrate, fat, and protein to produce the energy that allows us to stay alive. It also helps to make the tissues that form our bodies. Biotin may be especially beneficial to newborns and people with diabetes.

One of the major roles of this vitamin is very simple. It helps to attach a carbon and two oxygen molecules, called a carboxyl group, to other molecules. "This is a basic step in a lot of the chemical reactions that go on in our bodies," says Donald McCormick, PhD, chairman of the department of biochemistry at Emory University in Atlanta. "It happens when we break down carbohydrates for energy, when we use amino acids that come from protein, and when we use fats for energy. So biotin is working all over our bodies, all the time. It is critical for good health."

Are You Absorbing This?

Luckily, most people never become deficient in biotin. Among adults, people who are most likely to be deficient are those with absorption problems. People who have Crohn's disease, an intestinal disorder, may be deficient because they don't absorb enough biotin from food. Anticonvulsant medications can also promote biotin deficiency.

Some infants have a genetic inability to use biotin. Lacking the support of this hardworking vitamin, they develop skin problems, such as an oily, flaky rash around their ears, noses, and mouths and on their buttocks. Eventually, they may also develop muscle weakness and potentially fatal nerve damage.

"Evidence of a biotin deficiency is most likely to be seen first where there are rapidly regenerating cells, such as those that lead to the formation of skin and hair," Dr. McCormick says. Even if you don't have a biotin deficiency that affects your health, the lack of this vitamin might be evident in some parts of your body. One study found that an additional 2,500 micrograms a day of biotin helped to strengthen and thicken brittle fingernails.

"Hair and nails contain a lot of a type of protein called keratin, which gives them their hard structure, and keratin production indirectly requires biotin," Dr. McCormick says. Certain fatty acids that our bodies use to make hair and nails can't be utilized unless biotin is on hand.

In fact, all animals need biotin. In furry animals such as mink and fox, a deficiency leads to a condition called spectacle eyes—baldness around the eyes. Horses and cattle that are short on biotin have hoof problems.

A Diabetes Connection?

In several studies, biotin supplementation has been shown to enhance the performance of insulin, the hormone that plays a critical role in helping your body incorporate blood sugar. The supplements can also increase the activity of an enzyme, glucokinase, which the liver uses early in the process of utilizing blood sugar, says Michael Murray, ND, a naturopathic doctor and coauthor of *Encyclopedia of Natural Medicine*.

SUPPLEMENTSNAPSHOT

▶Biotin

Daily Value: 30 micrograms.

May help: Thin, brittle nails and seborrheic dermatitis; may also help lower blood sugar in some people with diabetes.

Good food sources: Brewer's yeast, molasses, egg yolks, milk, liver, soybeans, walnuts, peanuts, wheat bran, and cauliflower.

Who's at risk for deficiency: People with intestinal absorption problems and babies with problems metabolizing biotin.

Special instructions: Take in divided doses throughout the day.

Cautions and possible side effects: Generally regarded as safe.

One study that looked at biotin supplementation in people with type 1 (insulin-dependent) diabetes found significant improvements in blood sugar control. Another study looked at the potential benefits of biotin supplements in people with type 2 (non-insulin-dependent) diabetes. Every day for a month, Japanese researchers gave 9 milligrams of biotin to 18 people with type 2 diabetes. After 30 days, the participants' blood sugar fell to nearly half its original levels. Researchers have also shown high-dose biotin to be very helpful in the treatment of severe diabetic nerve disease, Dr. Murray reports.

A Little Goes a Long Way

Two things make biotin deficiency rare. For starters, you need only a small amount—300 micrograms, or about one-third of a milligram. Second, many foods contain some biotin, although only a few—such as egg yolks, molasses, and soybeans—are rich sources. Ounce for ounce, the very top sources are two old-time "health foods"—royal jelly, a substance secreted by bees, and brewer's yeast.

Bacteria in our intestines also make biotin, although just how much they make—and how much of it we absorb—remains a mystery, according to Dr. McCormick. "Most of these bacteria are in the colon, and we just don't absorb much biotin in that part of our intestines."

black cohosh

In the late 1800s, when many women were embarrassed to consult male doctors about "female problems," they found comfort in Lydia Pinkham's Vegetable Compound, a patent medicine advertised to cure everything from nervous prostration to a prolapsed uterus.

Pinkham, a grandmotherly type from Lynn, Massachusetts, first shared her mixture of ground herbs and alcohol with neighbor women. Her son urged her to market the formula with her picture on the bottle, and within a few years, the compound was the best-selling medicine of the era. Pinkham was exalted as the "savior of her sex."

One of her principal herbs was black cohosh, a native plant with a long folk history of relieving menstrual cramps and easing childbirth. Whether women found relief from the herb or from the 18 percent alcohol content in the compound is a matter of debate.

Not for Women Only

Pinkham's wasn't all hooch and no medicine, however. Black cohosh is a powerful relaxant and antispasmodic for both nerves and muscles. It is especially good at relieving cramping in smooth muscles, which include the uterus.

All of these properties are helpful to women who have problems with their reproductive systems: excessive bleeding, irregular periods, delayed menstruation, severe menstrual cramps, and the hot flashes of menopause. Black cohosh works as a regulator or normalizer of the female reproductive system by helping to restore hormone balance, says Stanley W. Beyrle, ND, a naturopathic doctor at the Kansas Clinic of Traditional Medicine in Wichita.

"When it comes to gynecological complaints, there isn't a better herb than black cohosh," says Dr. Beyrle. "It's always one of my base herbs in any herbal formula for females."

Although it has a reputation as a woman's herb, black cohosh may have therapeutic benefits for both sexes. As an anti-inflammatory, it has been used to reduce pain and swelling in people who have rheumatoid arthritis, sciatica, osteoarthritis, neuralgia, or inflammation as a result of joint and muscle injuries.

"Anything that reduces inflammation, cramping, and swelling can reduce pain," says Dr. Beyrle. "That makes black cohosh useful for many conditions."

A Forest Herb

A member of the buttercup family, black cohosh is a native plant found in eastern deciduous forests from Ontario to Georgia. In North America, most black cohosh root is still harvested from the wild. In Europe, supplies come from herb farmers.

Native American women made a tea from the plant's resinous roots and rhizome to soothe menstrual cramps and promote menstruation. Black cohosh was also important in folk medicine as a childbirth aid that eased delivery by stimulating the uterus. Native Americans and American colonists also valued it as a treatment for rheumatism and sore throats.

SUPPLEMENT SNAPSHOT

▶Black Cohosh

Botanical name: *Cimicifuga racemosa.*

Origin: Found in eastern deciduous forests from Ontario to Georgia.

May help: Bronchial, stomach, and muscle spasms; rheumatoid arthritis; osteoarthritis; sciatica; neuralgia; muscle and joint injuries; breast cancer; premenstrual syndrome; leg cramps, endometriosis; menstrual cramps; heavy menstrual bleeding; irregular periods; and hot flashes and other menopausal discomforts.

Cautions and possible side effects: Do not take while pregnant. Do not take while breastfeeding or for longer than 6 consecutive months without a doctor's supervision. May cause occasional stomach upset, diarrhea, abdominal pain, headache, and lowered heart rate and blood pressure.

As early as 1787, the plant attracted the interest of Europeans. Eclectic physicians, a 19th-century branch of early American medicine, made black cohosh one of their central healing botanicals for women. From 1820 to 1926, the herb was listed as an official drug in the *United States Pharmacopoeia.*

Like many phytomedicines, however, it eventually fell out of favor with the American medical community. It continued to be used in Europe, and today, in Germany, it is a government-approved treatment for premenstrual syndrome, painful menstruation, and nervous conditions connected to menopause.

Hormone Harmony

The herb has many active ingredients, but an isoflavone called formononetin is the critical one for women. Formononetin and other compounds in the root and rhizome are able to bind to estrogen receptors in the uterus and other tissues, particularly the brain (pituitary).

If you have fluctuations in estrogen—as is the case during menopause—the herb acts like a hormone modulator. If you have too much estrogen, which is frequently the case when menstruation is painful and cramping is severe, the phytoestrogens block estrogen from binding at those receptor sites, says Kathleen Head, ND, a naturopathic doctor in Sandpoint, Idaho, and senior editor of *Alternative Medicine Review.*

Besides replacing estrogen, black cohosh also eases the symptoms of menopause by inhibiting the production of luteinizing hormone (LH). LH levels tend to increase in the body at the same time that estrogen levels plummet. Hot flashes may be linked to high levels of this hormone.

The results of one clinical study seem to reinforce black cohosh's effectiveness in menopause. Researchers studied 60 women under age 40, all of whom had had hysterectomies. Because their uteruses had been removed, these women experienced premature menopause-like symptoms. Some were given black cohosh extract, while others were treated with various estrogen replacements.

The study found no difference between the two treatments. The black cohosh appeared to be equally as effective as its pharmaceutical counterparts. As with most herbs, however, the beneficial effects took longer to appear—as much as 4 weeks to have an effect. The pharmaceutical drugs tended to work much faster. "It's really a useful treatment during menopause," says Dr. Head, "but it's mild, and it may take time before it starts to work."

Quash That Cramp

The antispasmodic effect of black cohosh is much more immediate. Dr. Beyrle recommends the herb for patients who've sprained their backs, strained muscles, or have cramping and pain from arthritis. Pain from an injury often comes from tightness and soreness in a muscle, he says.

"I routinely use black cohosh in an herbal pain formula," he says. "If you can get those muscles to loosen up and relax, you can give someone relief from pain."

The herb has also been used to relieve stomach cramps, as well as to quell coughing and relax constricted blood vessels in cases of whooping cough, bronchitis, and asthma. Sometimes, herbalists combine black cohosh with valerian or other sedative herbs to create a botanical tranquilizer for the central nervous system.

As a single supplement, black cohosh is available in tablets, capsules, and tinctures. Follow the dosage directions on the label.

brewer's yeast

Wouldn't it be wonderful news for beer-lovin' adults if a nice cold brew turned out to be the answer to all of their health problems? We can just hear the doctor now: "Got a cold? Have a Bud," or "Allergies acting up? Try a Heineken."

A beer drinker's dream—but not true of the brew. There's no beer that will fulfill our nutritional needs. But there is a related substance, brewer's yeast, that can help some of what "ales" us.

Available as a powder and in flakes or tablets, brewer's yeast is a slightly bitter-tasting ingredient that's used in brewing beer. It's also a by-product of beer making. The yeast itself—a tiny fungus—is grown on grain, usually barley.

Brewer's yeast is a rich source of many nutrients, including protein, some B vitamins, phosphorus, and chromium. The protein content of yeast accounts for slightly more than half of its weight.

It's this variety and abundance of nutrients that have made brewer's yeast such an enduring supplement, says Michael Janson, MD, president of the American College for Advancement in Medicine, based in Laguna Hills, California, and author of *The Vitamin Revolution in Health Care.*

A Big Sweet Tooth

Yeast is a living, single-cell organism. It's grown on anything sugary, including sugarcane sap, yeast extract, malt extract, or just a handful of salt and sugar, says Richard M. Walmsley, PhD, senior lecturer in the department of biomolecular sciences at the University of Manchester Institute of Science and Technology in England.

Like humans, a single yeast cell has a life span, but it will divide about 20 times before it dies. Within days, these 20 divisions and the divisions of all of the offspring give rise to millions of yeast cells.

There are many kinds of yeast. They all acquire their nutrients the hard way, says Michael J. Conboy, a researcher in the department of biological sciences at Stanford University. They require many of the same vitamins and amino acids that humans need, but because they often grow on foods that are lacking in certain nutrients, like grains and fruit, they are forced to manufacture their own amino acids and vitamins biochemically. In doing so, the yeast cells become a much more complete food for anyone who eats them, Conboy explains.

Among the many varieties of yeast are baker's, brewer's, and nutritional yeast. Baker's yeast, the secret ingredient that makes bread rise, contains living cells and is also a good source of vitamins and minerals. The live cells are killed during the baking process, but the B vitamins that are accumulated by them are still present in the baked bread. The live cells in brewer's yeast are also destroyed during the brewing process, but the dead cells still have nutritional value.

The terms *brewer's yeast* and *nutritional yeast* are sometimes used interchangeably, but they are not exactly the same. Basically, nutritional yeast is any yeast grown for the specific purpose of being a food supplement, Conboy explains. While it might be a brewer's yeast, it could also be yeast from another species.

Brewer's yeast is used as a nutritional yeast when it's grown in the presence of vitamin B_{12} and other nutrients. It can have a wide range of nutritional values, depending on the species of yeast and on what medium it was

SUPPLEMENTSNAPSHOT

▶Brewer's Yeast

May help: Diabetes, hypoglycemia, high cholesterol, eczema, nervousness, fatigue, and constipation.

Special instructions: Take on an empty stomach unless indigestion occurs, in which case you should take it with food.

Cautions and possible side effects: If you have diabetes or hypoglycemia, consult your doctor before taking. Do not take if you have candidiasis, gout, or high blood levels of uric acid. Use with caution if you have a known allergy to molds. Rarely, may cause occasional flatulence or digestive upset.

grown in, such as grain or sugarcane sap. Some yeasts are grown with a high chromium content, for example, while others have a high selenium content.

Brewing Up Healthy Benefits

If we get most of the vitamins and minerals we need from our diets, is there any reason to make brewer's yeast a regular supplement? Possibly not, says Dr. Janson. "But I like my nutrients to come from a variety of sources," he adds, noting that foods such as brewer's yeast may contain undiscovered nutrients that do have some benefits. "Think of brewer's yeast as an additional supplement, not as a replacement for whole foods and a comprehensive supplement program."

When it's grown with vitamin B_{12}, brewer's yeast is the supplement of choice for some vegetarians, especially vegans (strict vegetarians who eat no meat, fish, poultry, eggs, or dairy products). "There are very few natural vegan sources of B_{12} except certain forms of brewer's yeast," says Jennifer Brett, ND, a naturopathic doctor at the Wilton Naturopathic Center in Stratford, Connecticut.

Many vegetarians take vitamin and mineral supplements rather than brewer's yeast, Dr. Brett says. The doses contained in these supplements are known, while the amounts of specific nutrients found in yeast will vary. Each type of yeast has varying amounts, and the variations are also affected by how old the yeast is, she says.

Brewer's yeast also has been used to prevent and reduce the symptoms of diabetes. That's because it contains chromium, a mineral that has been shown to regulate blood sugar (glucose), says Richard Anderson, PhD, lead scientist in the nutrient requirements and functions laboratory at the USDA Beltsville Human Nutrition Research Center in Maryland. Chromium works together with insulin to help transport blood sugar across cell membranes and into cells, where it can be burned for energy.

The chromium in brewer's yeast may also help raise HDL cholesterol, the "good" kind, and reduce LDL cholesterol, the "bad" kind, says Dr. Anderson. Some of the chromium found in brewer's yeast is thought to be glucose tolerance factor, a combination of chromium, nicotinic acid (a form of niacin), and amino acids.

If you're supplementing with brewer's yeast simply because of its chromium content, though, you might want to take a chromium supplement instead, suggests Dr. Anderson. "With brewer's yeast, you don't know what you're getting, because the nutritional quality varies from batch to batch and supplier to supplier," he cautions.

Dr. Brett, however, has had success with prescribing brewer's yeast to her patients who have a personal or family history of diabetes or hypoglycemia (low blood sugar). She has found that her patients get much better long-term control of their symptoms when they take brewer's yeast than when they take a chromium supplement. Why? "It's possible that the nutrient is more bioavailable from the yeast, and therefore more effective," she says.

Since chromium may affect blood glucose and insulin levels, people with diabetes or hypoglycemia should consult their doctors before supplementing their diets with brewer's yeast.

Brewer's yeast has also been used to treat eczema, nervousness, fatigue, and constipation. Interestingly, some pet owners believe that brewer's yeast somehow helps their four-legged friends repel fleas and ticks, although there is no scientific evidence that it works.

In general, brewer's yeast has the strong taste of yeasty bread or sweet bread dough. Some people find that brewer's yeast grown on sugar beets is sweeter and more appealing, says Dr. Brett. As flakes or a powder, it can be stirred into juice, especially grape juice, and soups; sprinkled over salads, popcorn, cottage cheese, or yogurt; or added to casseroles and any dish made with tomato sauce. Heating makes the flavor of brewer's yeast stronger, so it's best to add it to foods as they are being served, advises Dr. Brett. If you find the taste unpleasant, try taking the tablets instead, says Dr. Anderson.

bromelain

Kitchen wizards know that you can't make a gelatin dessert with fresh pineapple. The natural enzymes in this prickly fruit prevent the gelatin from setting, leaving the amateur cook with a runny mess.

What's bad for Jell-O may be good for you, however. Bromelain, the enzyme found in pineapple, has been credited with a number of health benefits, including aiding digestion, speeding wound healing, and reducing inflammation.

Bromelain is found in both the fruit and stem of the pineapple, but the enzyme in supplements comes from the stem.

An Inflammation Tamer

More than 200 scientific papers have been written about bromelain since it was first introduced as a health-boosting substance in 1957. Much of the research has focused on its anti-inflammatory effects. Whether you have a sprained ankle, a nasty bruise, sinusitis, or any other type of inflammation, bromelain may help you heal faster, says Greg Kelly, ND, a naturopathic doctor in Stamford, Connecticut. In fact, he routinely recommends that his patients take bromelain before and after surgery to speed the healing process. "I would consider using bromelain for any type of inflammation for which you might use aspirin," he says.

Bromelain inhibits the release of certain inflammation-causing chemicals, explains Alan L. Miller, ND, technical advisor for Thorne Research in Sandpoint, Idaho, and senior editor of *Alternative Medicine Review*. It also activates a chemical in the blood and tissues that breaks down fibrin, a protein-sugar complex that is partly responsible for blood clotting.

By breaking down fibrin, bromelain produces another benefit: It reduces swelling. That's because fibrin prevents injured tissues from draining, and when they can't drain, they swell. "Bromelain is most beneficial when used after trauma such as surgery or injury," says Dr. Miller. "I also prescribe it for colds, flus, and ear infections to loosen thick mucus so it can drain or be coughed up."

Bromelain may also keep platelets from sticking to each other and to blood vessel walls, which is a major factor in atherosclerosis (hardening of the arteries). Bromelain helps prevent platelet clumping by decreasing the release of a chemical that causes them to stick together.

Treating Troubled Tummies

If you ate more steak and potatoes for dinner than your stomach was prepared to digest, you might want to try a bromelain supplement to quell the discomfort. It is a digestive enzyme that helps break down protein, thus aiding digestion, says Dr. Kelly.

Bromelain also appears to be helpful for people with food allergies, especially allergies to wheat and other grains, says Dr. Kelly. In one Japanese study, bromelain was added to wheat flour, which was then used to make bread. The enzyme changed the structure of a protein in the wheat and allowed people with wheat allergies to eat the bread without having an allergic response.

Some research has shown that bromelain also holds promise for increasing the potency of antibiotics, and it is used that way in several

SUPPLEMENTSNAPSHOT

▶Bromelain

May help: Digestive disorders, inflammation, wound healing, colds and
   flus, ear infections, atherosclerosis, food allergies, muscle soreness,
   phlebitis, lupus, gout, intermittent claudication, osteoarthritis, and
   rheumatoid arthritis; may also increase the effectiveness of antibiotics.

Good food source: Pineapple.

Special instructions: As a digestive aid, take with meals; for all other
   uses, take on an empty stomach.

Cautions and possible side effects: May cause nausea, vomiting,
   diarrhea, skin rash, and heavy menstrual bleeding; may increase the risk
   of bleeding in people taking aspirin or anticoagulants (blood thinners).
   Do not take if you are allergic to pineapple.

countries outside the United States. In one study, combined bromelain and antibiotic therapy was given to 53 hospitalized patients with a variety of infectious ailments. For every disease studied, there was a significant reduction in disease symptoms when the patients received the combined therapy as compared to antibiotics alone.

Dr. Kelly concedes that the studies are dated, but he reviewed the evidence and found it convincing. Since bacteria have become increasingly resistant to antibiotics, using bromelain to increase a drug's potency makes sense, he says.

Doing Your Homework

Manufacturers of bromelain supplements really make you do your math, because the supplements are measured in milk-clotting units (mcu) or gelatin-dissolving units (gdu); 1,200 gdu are equal to roughly 2,000 mcu per gram. Check the label carefully. Some brands list the mcu by the pill and others by the amount per gram. If the label lists only the weight in milligrams, it may be an inferior product.

Dosages for bromelain vary, depending on the reason that you're taking it. Look for standardized supplements so you know that you are getting the same potency from batch to batch. You can buy either capsules—which do not contain any binders or fillers—or tablets.

If you're lactose intolerant, read the labels or check with the manufacturer to find out whether a particular product is mixed with lactose. Manufacturers are not required to list lactose with other ingredients on the label, says Dr. Miller, but some products offer the information or specify that the product is lactose free.

vitamin C

During the days of Columbus, sailors who joined the crew of a seagoing ship knew that they had only a 50 percent chance of coming home alive. The danger wasn't that they might fall off the edge of the Earth or be eaten by sea monsters. Instead, it was that they might contract a dreadful disease, unnamed at the time, that would make their gums bleed, loosen their teeth, cause bruises and bleeding under their skin, and ultimately, kill them. Only men on short voyages, especially around the Mediterranean Sea, seemed able to avoid these symptoms.

At that time, no one knew that the disease was scurvy, caused by a deficiency of vitamin C. On long ocean voyages, the cook used up the fresh fruits and vegetables first, then served only cereals and meats, which contained no vitamin C, until the ship returned to port. That sometimes meant that the crew went for months without this essential vitamin.

Even though James Lind, a British physician, showed in 1747 that oranges and lemons could prevent scurvy, it was another 50 years before the British navy mandated a daily ration of lime juice on all vessels (thus giving British sailors the traditional nickname "limeys"). And it took another 200 years before the component of citrus that protected against scurvy, vitamin C, was isolated. Its scientific name, ascorbic acid, reflects its antiscurvy past.

Our C Rations

These days, we get so much vitamin C from foods that we never have to worry about scurvy or lime juice rations. A lot of us even keep bottles of vitamin C on hand so we can down a couple of hundred extra milligrams if we feel a cold coming on. In fact, vitamin C is the most popular vitamin supplement in the United States. And while it may be best known for its cold-fighting powers, that's just one of its vital roles in the body.

Body Building

Vitamin C helps to form the fibrous structural protein known as collagen, the single most important protein of connective tissue and, literally, the stuff that holds us together.

SUPPLEMENTSNAPSHOT

▶Vitamin C

Also known as: Ascorbic acid.

Daily Value: 60 milligrams or, for smokers, 100 milligrams.

May help: Bacterial and viral infections, including colds and flu, HIV, and urinary tract infections; cancer; gingivitis; genital herpes; asthma; emphysema; angina; cataracts; sunburn; bedsores; diabetes-related organ damage; depression; impotence; intermittent claudication; phlebitis; infertility; high cholesterol; heavy menstrual bleeding; muscle soreness; osteoarthritis; menopausal discomforts; chronic inflammatory diseases such as lupus and rheumatoid arthritis; recovery from surgery or injury; and exposure to toxins.

Good food sources: Broccoli, Brussels sprouts, cabbage, citrus fruits, collard and turnip greens, guavas, kale, parsley, all bell and hot peppers, and strawberries.

Who's at risk for deficiency: Smokers and people exposed to cigarette smoke; people with viral or bacterial infections, diabetes, high cholesterol, cardiovascular disease, cancer, or chronic inflammation; and people who take aspirin or barbiturates regularly.

Special instructions: Take larger amounts in several spaced doses throughout the day. Take with adequate amounts of water.

Cautions and possible side effects: Safe at a wide range of doses, although more than 3,000 milligrams a day can cause diarrhea; if this occurs, cut back until the diarrhea stops. If you're taking high doses, cut back to 100 milligrams at least 3 days before a physical exam or tests, as high amounts can interfere with some tests, including those for blood in the stool and sugar in urine. Large doses may interfere with anticoagulants (blood thinners). Supplements made from a corn base may cause a reaction in people allergic to corn.

The Rationale behind Megadosing

Some doctors recommend so-called megadoses of vitamin C—amounts far higher than the Daily Value—to literally flood the body with the vitamin during certain illnesses.

The thinking is this: Many illnesses involve damage from free radicals, which are unstable molecules that affect healthy cells. Once it gets started, the damage can cause a chain reaction that quickly depletes areas of inflamed tissue of vitamin C and allows the damage to spread even more.

"I am trying to literally pickle the tissues involved in the disease in order to neutralize all the free radicals," says Robert Cathcart, MD, a physician in Los Altos, California, who is a longtime practitioner of megadosing. "I want to push the vitamin into cells and flood the tissue to stop the chain reaction of free radical damage. This is not a nutritional effect. Rather, it is a pharmacological effect."

Dr. Cathcart recommends and has successfully used large doses of vitamin C in the form of ascorbic acid. In this form, the vitamin isn't buffered—that is, no chemicals have been added to help the body absorb it. The ascorbic acid, he says, can help with many kinds of health conditions, from the common cold to life-threatening viral hepatitis.

Normally, he recommends that his patients take the vitamin to bowel tolerance (meaning until it begins to produce loose stools), and then back off a bit until the loose stools stop. His reasoning: When people are sick, they tend to tolerate a lot more ascorbic acid than they do when they are healthy. The one exception is people with bowel problems, who may not be able to take much ascorbic acid orally. In these cases, Dr. Cathcart administers a form of the vitamin intravenously.

"Vitamin C lets these fibers cross-link, or weave together, to make them strong," explains Robert Jacob, PhD, a research chemist in micronutrients at the USDA Western Human Nutrition Research Center in San Francisco.

When these fibers don't cross-link, we get the symptoms typical of scurvy: We start to fall apart. Our teeth loosen because our gums can't hold them in anymore; our gums bleed, and we develop little pinpoints of blood under our skin as blood vessels break down and release blood. If we

For a bad cold or the flu, for instance, Dr. Cathcart might recommend that patients take 2 to 12 grams of ascorbic acid every 15 minutes until they reach bowel tolerance. The time frame varies from person to person, but tolerance could occur within 4 to 8 hours, Dr. Cathcart says. For a condition like severe mononucleosis, he says, one woman was able to tolerate 200 grams of ascorbic acid before she reached bowel tolerance.

"When you reach that point," Dr. Cathcart says, "generally, your symptoms quickly vanish." How long you need to take high amounts to keep your symptoms at bay depends on many variables and could range from a few days to months. Some people take several grams a day indefinitely.

While there is some research to indicate that taking additional vitamin C can help shorten the duration of a cold, there is little evidence to support the use of large amounts for illnesses such as mononucleosis, hepatitis, cancer, or AIDS, says Balz Frei, PhD, professor of biochemistry and biophysics and director of the Linus Pauling Institute at Oregon State University in Corvallis. "I'm not saying that it doesn't work or that the theory behind this isn't sound. I'm saying that there is currently not enough scientific evidence to conclude that megadoses of vitamin C provide health benefits beyond those of more moderate doses of the vitamin," he says.

As for everyday or antiaging use of vitamin C, Dr. Cathcart believes that the amount individuals need is based on their own "free radical load." "If you have a chronic illness or inflammation, if you've abused your body with alcohol or smoking, or if you look old for your age, you probably can use more than someone who's healthier," he says. For a vitamin regimen tailored to your needs, see your doctor.

get hurt, we don't heal, because the body relies on collagen to fill the gaps in wounds. If we break a bone, it doesn't heal, either, because bones regenerate by depositing minerals such as calcium on a matrix of collagen.

Some doctors believe that a low intake of vitamin C does more than aggravate the symptoms of scurvy, says Balz Frei, PhD, professor of biochemistry and biophysics and director of the Linus Pauling Institute at Oregon State University in Corvallis. A shortage may also worsen symptoms of osteoporosis, cancer, and heart disease.

Fat for Fuel

One of the first symptoms of vitamin C deficiency is fatigue, and one reason for that may be an often-overlooked function of this vitamin, says Dr. Frei. "Vitamin C is required for the synthesis of a compound called carnitine, which transports fatty acids into the mitochondria, the tiny powerhouses that generate energy inside cells," he explains. "If you don't have enough vitamin C, you can't synthesize enough carnitine, so you can't convert all the fatty acids into usable energy."

While it's true that carbohydrates are the main source of energy for most of our body parts, fatty acids are the major sources for the production of energy in the heart and skeletal muscles. These areas are particularly vulnerable to a carnitine shortage, Dr. Frei says.

Vitamin C also helps your body convert the amino acid tyrosine into two important hormones, epinephrine and norepinephrine. Both are released by the body in response to stress. "These hormones are responsible for mobilizing energy and activating a lot of metabolic pathways so that you can respond to stressful situations in a physical way," Dr. Frei explains. "They produce the fight-or-flight response."

In fact, our adrenal glands, which produce these two hormones, have a higher concentration of vitamin C than any other organ in the body. "It's well established that if you're under physical stress, such as during an infection or after surgery, you need more vitamin C," Dr. Jacob says. "There's less evidence to indicate that psychological stress also raises vitamin C needs, but since psychological stress also makes the adrenal glands crank up production, it makes sense that you would need more vitamin C."

Stopping the Thieves

In the annals of research, vitamin C has won considerable renown as an antioxidant. That means that it helps keep a lid on chemical reactions that involve oxygen, explains Dr. Frei—reactions that go on all the time, all over our bodies. We have oxygen in our lungs, but blood carries it to every cell, where it is used as part of the process of energy metabolism. These chemical reactions have the potential to create molecular particles called free radicals. A free radical lacks an electron, which makes it unstable, so it tries to "steal" an electron from some other molecule. Then that molecule is minus an electron and becomes a free radical, causing a kind of free radical domino effect.

Vitamin C breaks up this cycle of larceny. "It can give up one of its electrons without becoming a dangerous free radical, so every time a molecule of vitamin C does that, it helps to stop a whole string of electron pilfering," Dr. Frei explains. That's important because free radical damage is thought to be involved in many diseases and conditions, including inflammation, viral infections, cancer, heart disease, and even aging.

Vitamin C can also regenerate vitamin E, another important free radical scavenger, by giving it an electron.

As an antioxidant, vitamin C helps many parts of the body function better. When immune cells are called into action, for instance, they use a lot of oxygen and produce free radicals and oxidants that can damage cells and surrounding tissue. Vitamin C helps protect these cells.

In your lungs, this versatile vitamin helps you breathe more easily by fighting off the onslaught of oxidants you inhale, says Dr. Frei, especially if you are a smoker. In your liver, it helps to protect the cells as they break down toxins. And in your stomach, vitamin C is secreted in gastric juices and helps to neutralize potential cancer-causing substances called nitrosamines, which are found in some lunch meats and smoked foods. However, vitamin C combined with iron should be avoided in people with stomach inflammation.

How Much Is Enough?

Only about one out of every four Americans gets less than the Daily Value for vitamin C, which is 60 milligrams. They are people who simply don't eat fruits and vegetables, Dr. Frei says.

The bigger question today is how much vitamin C is optimum for good health. Dr. Frei believes that everyone should get a minimum of 200 milligrams, and in fact, studies show that in healthy people, 200 milligrams daily produces tissue saturation. It's about as much as most parts of your body can hold.

There are some decent arguments that can be made for some people's need for higher amounts, however. Smokers and people exposed to cigarette smoke; people with viral or bacterial infections, diabetes, high cholesterol, cardiovascular disease, cancer, or chronic inflammation; and people who take certain drugs such as aspirin or barbiturates on a regular basis may need more vitamin C, Dr. Frei says.

calcium

Chalk, eggshells, milk, and bones have something in common: All get their dense white color from calcium. They're loaded with it.

Sharing this natural resource sometimes leads to some strange lend-lease arrangements. Bones and eggshells are often ground up for calcium supplements that go into livestock feed; then, from milk and other dairy products, we pick up some of the calcium that we need for better bones and other body-building biology projects. If we don't get quite enough, we can turn to supplements that are often made from the basic geological substrata—the same mineral deposits that are sometimes used to make chalk.

We have more calcium in our bodies than we do any other mineral, and we're right to associate it with bones because that's where 99 percent of it is found. It's vital throughout our lifetimes for building strong bones and teeth.

Calcium is used for much more, however. It's also dissolved in the fluids in the body, those inside cells and those that bathe cells. There, it helps muscles spring into action and aids proper blood clotting. It assists nerves in transmitting impulses and helps launch hormones and enzymes on their journeys to inner organs.

Usually, the dissolved calcium in our bodies never gets so low that these important functions are impaired, but our bodies sometimes behave like poachers during lean times. Robbing Peter to pay Paul, they take calcium from bones as needed to make sure that the vital functions go on.

Like a Rock . . . Not

Bones aren't the inert, rocklike objects that we might imagine them to be. They are in a constant state of flux, dissolving and forming new bone all the time.

As bones begin to form, calcium salts form crystals on a grid of strands of a protein called collagen. These crystals invade the collagen and gradually lend more and more strength and rigidity to the developing bone. Bones reach their peak mass—when they're strongest and most dense—in your late twenties. That's why it's so important to get enough calcium early on: The denser your bones are at their peak, the longer they'll stay strong.

SUPPLEMENTSNAPSHOT

▶Calcium

Supplement forms: Calcium carbonate, citrate, citrate malate, lactate, gluconate, and aspartate; dicalcium phosphate; bone meal; oyster shell; and dolomite.

Daily Value: 1,000 to 1,300 milligrams.

May help: Osteoporosis, high blood pressure, insomnia, menstrual cramps, muscle cramps, pregnancy-related high blood pressure, and restless legs syndrome.

Good food sources: Milk and milk products, sardines (with bones), kale, calcium-fortified orange juice, sea vegetables, and sesame seeds.

Who's at risk for deficiency: People who don't eat many dairy products, those who don't get adequate vitamin D, women who are pregnant or breastfeeding, and people over age 50.

Special instructions: Divide your daily dose into two smaller doses, no more than 500 milligrams each. If you use calcium citrate, lactate, or gluconate, you can take it between meals without absorption problems, and it also won't interfere with absorption of iron and other trace minerals. All other forms of supplemental calcium are best absorbed when taken with food. Avoid taking supplements at the same time as large amounts of wheat bran. To further aid absorption, get 800 international units of vitamin D daily from fortified foods or supplements; it's not necessary to take the supplements together.

Cautions and possible side effects: If you have had calcium oxalate kidney stones, check with your doctor before taking calcium. The supplements may slightly increase your risk of getting stones again. Supplements from natural sources—oyster shells, dolomite, or bonemeal—may be contaminated with lead or other toxic metals; check labels for refined or purified sources. High doses may cause constipation.

What's in the Bottles?

Calcium comes in so many forms, even as a supplement, that choosing among the varieties may be confusing. Here's a clue: When you're reading labels, look for the "elemental calcium" listing to tell you how much you're really getting, says Robert E. C. Wildman, PhD, professor of nutrition at the University of Delaware in Newark. Most labels include this listing, he adds.

If the label does not indicate how much elemental calcium is in each tablet, you can use the table below. If you're taking a 500-milligram tablet of calcium carbonate, for example, you can see that it contains 40 percent elemental calcium—which translates into 200 milligrams of calcium from each tablet. Here are the typical percentages of actual calcium in supplement products.

Supplement	Elemental Calcium (%)
Calcium carbonate	40
Dicalcium phosphate	38
Bonemeal	31
Oyster shell	28
Dolomite	22
Calcium citrate	21
Calcium lactate	13
Calcium gluconate	9

You don't absorb all of the elemental calcium that's in a tablet, Dr. Wildman points out—only about 30 to 40 percent. (In fact, calcium citrate malate, which is available mostly in fortified orange juice, is perhaps the best-absorbed form.) If you take a supplement with food, a tablet of calcium carbonate is the most efficient way to get what you need. With supplements like calcium citrate, lactate, or gluconate, you'll need to take more tablets to equal the amount of calcium in a single dose of calcium carbonate.

The shipments of calcium need to continue well beyond that peak, however. "After that time, continuing to get enough calcium will help to reduce the rate of bone loss that occurs with aging," says Richard Wood, PhD, chief of the mineral bioavailability laboratory at the Jean Mayer USDA Human Nutrition Research Center on Aging at Tufts University in Boston.

Calculate Your Calcium Needs

Although calcium calculations may seem like higher math, there's a simple way to figure out what you need. As a starting point, let's say you get about 500 milligrams, which is the equivalent of about 2 cups of milk, and you're aiming for the 1,200 milligrams that are recommended for many people. You'll need to make up the shortfall with 700 milligrams of supplemental calcium each day, says Robert E. C. Wildman, PhD, professor of nutrition at the University of Delaware in Newark.

If you know that your intake isn't average—or you just like to play with figures—take the custom-tailored route.

1. Add up your daily servings of calcium champs—foods that you eat every day that supply substantial calcium. The champs most likely to be consumed daily (in single-serving amounts) are 8 ounces (1 cup) of 1 percent or fat-free milk, 8 ounces of low-fat or nonfat yogurt, 8 ounces of calcium-fortified orange juice, 8 ounces of low-fat or nonfat calcium-fortified soy or rice milk, and two 1-ounce slices of reduced-fat or fat-free cheese.

After you've determined which of these you eat regularly, count 300 milligrams of calcium for each serving (or check labels, since calcium content can vary by brand).

2. To this number, add 200 milligrams for women and 300 milligrams for men. (This is an estimated calcium total for all the other foods you eat throughout the day.)

3. If you take a multivitamin/mineral supplement, add the amount of calcium that you get from that. (Don't assume that a multi will cover your needs; most have too little calcium to make up average shortfalls.)

4. Subtract the total of steps 1, 2, and 3 from your daily requirement, 1,200 milligrams. Anything over zero is your daily shortfall and is the amount you should take in a supplement, says Dr. Wildman.

For Muscles and Nerves

Calcium is also vitally important when it comes to properly functioning muscles, explains Lisa Ruml, MD, a physician in Wharton, New Jersey. To contract and then relax, a muscle depends on the presence of calcium.

Can Calcium Supplements Cause Heart Problems?

A study from New Zealand in 2010 found that people who took 1,000 milligrams of calcium in addition to whatever calcium they got from foods had a 30 percent increased risk of having a heart attack or of dying suddenly, compared to people who took a placebo.

Nobody knows for sure why this happened (there were no autopsies or invasive diagnostic procedures done), but one plausible connection is that the higher blood levels of calcium in supplement-takers caused calcium to build up in artery-clogging plaque, the researchers say.

So should you give up your calcium supplements? Not exactly—although you may have to alter your dose and the amounts of other nutrients you take in.

The supplement-takers in this study got an average of 1,800 milligrams of calcium a day from both foods and supplements, points out Andrew Weil, MD, director of the Center for Integrative Medicine at the University of Arizona, in Tucson, and author of *Eight Weeks to Optimum Health*.

"Calcium ions in the cell move from one spot to another very quickly, and that changes the electrical charge of certain proteins in the muscle cell so that the proteins change shape," she explains. These proteins tighten up and, in effect, pass along the tightening action to increase the tension.

As proteins shorten the muscle cells, the muscle contracts. When the calcium ions move back to their former positions, the proteins ratchet down from their state of peak tension, and the muscle relaxes. If you have too little calcium in your cells, however, the muscle cells tend to stay in the tightened position. You'll become more prone to muscle cramps.

Along with other electrically aggressive minerals like potassium, calcium also allows our nerves to transmit messages. Because the electrically charged calcium ions in cells rapidly shift position, an electrical charge is handed along the chain of nerve cells. The result is that a small electrical current travels along the nerve. Once the current reaches the end of the nerve, it triggers the release of a neurotransmitter, a chemical that allows the message to be relayed to another cell.

In the heart, calcium's role in both muscle contraction and nerve transmission comes into play. Calcium interacts with potassium and sodium

That's more than the recommendation of about 1,000 milligrams of calcium a day. Dr. Weil recommends that people figure out how much calcium they are getting from their daily diet (a glass of milk is usually about 300 milligrams) and then supplement to get up to about 1,000 milligrams a day. So if you eat about 500 milligrams a day, then only take a 500-milligram supplement. He recommends taking calcium citrate, a form that is easily absorbed.

Other nutrition experts point out that the New Zealand study also had patients take only calcium, but for your body to use the mineral properly you also need vitamins D and K. Low blood levels of both vitamins increase your risk for arterial calcification. And magnesium is needed for calcium-regulating hormones such as parathyroid hormone, so your body can balance out its calcium levels. Experts are recommending that you get the recommended amounts of vitamins D and K and at least 500 milligrams of magnesium for every 1,000 milligrams of calcium you get.

over and over again in a carefully orchestrated sequence to produce a heartbeat. You would have to be seriously ill to be so low on calcium that it affects your heart, but it does happen. Doctors sometimes use drugs called calcium channel blockers to slow down and regulate heartbeat in people with high blood pressure, Dr. Ruml says. "These drugs temper the shift of calcium in and out of cells," she explains. Normally, however, getting more calcium isn't going to help—or hurt—your heart.

Bowel Binder

In the intestines, calcium can combine with other nutrients and foods—such as saturated fat—to create compounds that cannot be absorbed by the body. In one study, a group of people getting 1,000 milligrams or so of calcium a day from fortified foods and 1,000 milligrams from supplements excreted twice as much saturated fat as people getting normal amounts of calcium. They also had an 11 percent drop in harmful LDL cholesterol.

Calcium may also play a role in preventing colon cancer by binding with cancer-promoting fats and bile acids, the digestive fluids secreted by the liver, says Dr. Wood. This neutralizes the toxic effects of the fats and acids, and if all goes well, they are excreted more rapidly, along with intestinal cells that might be cancer generators. But don't count on miracles, he says. "The effects are fairly modest and occur only at amounts well above normal intake."

Calcium also helps to prevent the absorption of toxic minerals such as lead by interfering with cellular transport, says Dr. Wood. Unfortunately, it can also interfere with minerals that we may need more of, such as iron, zinc, copper, and manganese. That's why some doctors recommend that you not take calcium supplements with meals.

Coming Up Short

Women in the United States average between 700 and 800 milligrams a day of calcium. Men get nearly 1,000 milligrams, which is the DV. Some experts recommend higher amounts to protect against a deficiency, which results in more calcium being withdrawn from bones than is deposited.

Usually, you don't know how frail your bones have become until you develop a condition called osteoporosis (the term means "porous bones"). At worst, your bones can become as riddled with holes as a termite-infested log and so fragile that simply bearing your own weight causes them to break.

Even if it's not that bad, invisible damage can take its toll, eventually producing evidence that your skeleton has been starved of calcium. If you develop tiny fractures in your spine, you also end up with the bent-over stance called dowager's hump, which many women accept as a sign of old age. Moreover, with osteoporosis, one fall can produce complicated and serious fractures. These are all good reasons to take calcium seriously and make sure that you're getting enough.

cat's claw

When you hear about all of the potential medicinal plants in a tropical rain forest, you probably picture an inconspicuous fern beneath the damp forest canopy or a dainty water lily floating in a steamy swamp. How about a tree-climbing, 100-foot vine that's 12 inches around, with thorns as sharp and tenacious as a jaguar's claws?

Cat's claw is one of the newly discovered herbs of the Amazon. It's actually new, however, only to Western civilization, since the Peruvian Indians of the region have used the vine medicinally for centuries.

If you follow the news on cat's claw, you might think it's the cat's meow. It's been called a superb immune system booster, a vigorous antioxidant, a plant able to flush chemical toxins from the body, and a kind of scrubber that removes plaque buildup in clogged arteries.

Health food stores in North America brim with products that contain cat's claw, but there really isn't much known about this herb. The labels make many claims that may be exaggerated, warns Eran Ben-Arye, MD, a researcher at the natural medicine research unit at Hadassah University Hospital in Jerusalem.

"Right now, all we have are anecdotal reports and very preliminary findings regarding the herb's immunological and antifungal properties," Dr. Ben-Arye says. "Cat's claw may have very good potential as a medicine, or it may not. We just don't know yet."

Putting Teeth into Immunity

In the burgeoning marketplace of herbal products and nutritional supplements, cat's claw has gained a reputation as a cure-all for conditions such as lupus, arthritis, bursitis, fibromyalgia, chronic fatigue syndrome, and chemical and environmental allergies.

Although there are many theories about how it fights these conditions, the one most often cited is stimulation of the immune system, says Tirun

Gopal, MD, an obstetrician and gynecologist who practices holistic and Ayurvedic medicine in Allentown, Pennsylvania.

"It's used mostly for degenerative diseases where there is a significant loss of immunity," says Dr. Gopal. When people have diseases like cancer, lupus, or rheumatoid arthritis, their immune systems take a hard knock, leaving them open to secondary infections from colds and flus. Such infections—manageable for healthy people—can be life-threatening for people battling a chronic illness, he says.

"I've found that cat's claw can make the body more tolerant and better able to fight an infection, especially at its initial onset," he says. "You can use cat's claw by itself or with echinacea and astragalus—two other immune system stimulators—to boost its effectiveness."

The Jaguar's Claw

Historically, the Peruvian Indians made a tea from the root and inner bark of the plant to treat arthritis, tumors, ulcers, and inflammation. But since the Indians have an oral rather than a written tradition, the methodologies and uses of the plant remain obscure.

The first references in literature to this woody vine date back to the late 1700s, but it wasn't until the 1970s that an Austrian doctor drew attention to the herb in the West. The name cat's claw, or *uña de gato* in Spanish, comes from the vine's sharp, curved thorns that resemble the claws of a jaguar or cat.

SUPPLEMENTSNAPSHOT

▶Cat's Claw

Botanical names: *Uncaria tomentosa, U. guianensis;* also known as *uña de gato.*

Origin: Found in the Peruvian rain forest.

May help: Heart disease, low immunity, bursitis, rheumatoid arthritis, chemical poisoning, fibromyalgia, chronic fatigue syndrome, and lupus.

Cautions and possible side effects: Don't use if you have hemophilia or are pregnant. May cause headache, stomachache, or difficulty breathing; also has contraceptive properties.

Chemical analysis has revealed that the plant contains several important medicinal ingredients. Some of its alkaloids are known to be immune stimulants, and the plant appears to stimulate the activity of T cells, a type of white blood cells, says Dr. Gopal. These blood cells hunt down and act against virus-infected cells and tumor cells.

One alkaloid in particular seems to reduce blood pressure and may reduce the risk of stroke and heart attack.

The herb also contains compounds called glycosides that exhibit antiviral and anti-inflammatory activity. Some researchers suggest that cat's claw is effective at relieving swelling. "Because of this anti-inflammatory effect, some people have advocated its use with rheumatoid arthritis," comments Dr. Gopal.

Three of the glycosides in the herb have antioxidant activity, meaning that they have the ability to scavenge free radicals, the free-roaming, unstable molecules that cause aging and cell damage. An Italian study in 1992 suggested that cat's claw can also stop cells from mutating, which may mean that it could have value as a cancer treatment.

As good as all of this sounds, it's important to remember that these analyses and studies have been done using laboratory tests. No published study has looked at how the herb works in the human body, says Dr. Ben-Arye. "Even though there have been some important ingredients found, we have no idea if the herb and those ingredients are actually beneficial to people," he says.

In other words, looking at the individual active ingredients can only partially explain why cat's claw works as well as it does. The healing power may actually come from a combination of these chemicals working together, says Dr. Ben-Arye.

Soap for Your Innards

Although the science may still be inconclusive on cat's claw, many herbalists and health professionals believe that this Amazonian plant has healing properties. Julie Clemens, ND, a naturopathic doctor in Sagle, Idaho, says cat's claw is one of her workhorse herbs. She prescribes it frequently, usually as part of a detoxifying therapy.

Dr. Clemens believes that many lifestyle diseases—arthritis, diabetes, headaches, and chronic constipation—are a result of chemical toxicity. The chemicals come from the environment, diet, or a person's lifestyle choices, such as smoking and drinking, she says.

"What eventually happens is that your body is unable to process and eliminate the toxins at the same rate that they are coming in," she explains. "That can cause all types of problems."

Cat's claw has been used to cleanse and detoxify the intestinal tract, says Dr. Clemens. Typically, she prescribes cat's claw to an overweight person who has high blood pressure, problems with digestion and stomach acidity, and an unhealthy lifestyle. Her aim is to lower the toxic load, start cleaning plaque out of the arteries, and convince the person to make healthier lifestyle choices, she says.

"Cat's claw works on the entire body. I like to call it an internal scrubber. Think of it as soap for your insides," she says.

Get the Real Cat

The popularity of cat's claw has grown so quickly that supplies of the herb are not consistent. Only the inner bark and root have medicinal value, but analyses of some cat's claw products have found outer bark, stems, and twigs mixed in.

The popularity of the herb has caused the Peruvian government to declare it a threatened species and to ban the harvesting of the root. Today, people are leaving the root, taking only the inner bark, and allowing the plant to recover.

In North America, cat's claw is available as a tincture, in capsules, and in raw bark form for brewing tea. Cat's claw tea tends to be very bitter, so most people prefer capsules. "I'd look for a product that contains at least a 0.3 percent alkaloid content," says Dr. Clemens.

Although you may hear cat's claw referred to as *uña de gato,* that can be a generic name for more than 20 herbs from Peru, some of which are toxic. Cat's claw belongs to the genus *Uncaria,* of which there are some 60 species in the world. Only two, however—*U. tomentosa* and *U. guianensis*—from Peru are known to have the medicinal value discussed here.

cayenne

*Capsicum is a pure, energetic, permanent stimulant,
producing in large doses vomiting, purging, pains in the
stomach and bowels, heat and inflammation of the
stomach, giddiness, a species of intoxication, and an
enfeebled condition of the nervous power.*

—King's American Dispensatory, *a 19-century herbal
medical text*

When a medicinal herb makes your gut growl like that, it brings new clarity to the old adage "The cure is worse than the disease." Of course, dosage matters. Who knows how much capsicum, better known as cayenne pepper, brought on such a purging?

In the case of cayenne, a little is good, but more usually isn't better, says Priscilla Evans, ND, a naturopathic doctor at the Community Wholistic Health Center in Chapel Hill, North Carolina. "In small amounts, it is often beneficial, but by its very nature, cayenne is an irritating herb," she says.

Whether eaten as a food or taken as medicine, cayenne pepper has been used for centuries to treat asthma, fevers, sore throats, respiratory infections, and digestive problems. It can relieve flatulence and stimulate the stomach and gastrointestinal tract, and it may also reduce blood cholesterol and decrease a tendency to form blood clots.

Many of these actions stem from the ability of cayenne to stimulate the circulation and generate heat, says Dr. Evans. "Cayenne is found in many herbal formulas to get the blood moving."

Stops a Charging Bear

Cayenne is native to tropical America. Also called chile pepper or red pepper, it comes from the dried fruit of several species and hybrids of plants in the Solanaceae family.

The main active ingredient in cayenne is capsaicin, the stuff that makes hot peppers hot. In concentrated form, cayenne is so irritating that it's bottled in self-defense sprays that are advertised as being strong enough to stop a charging grizzly bear. Other constituents in cayenne include carotenoids, vitamins A and C, and volatile oils. The carotene molecules are potent antioxidants.

In 1552, an Aztec herbal text recommended cayenne as a treatment for toothaches and scabies, a skin disease caused by parasites. Subsequently, it was introduced to Europe, where it was used to reduce swollen lymph glands caused by tuberculosis, which was then known as the king's evil.

By the 19th century, doctors and herbalists prescribed cayenne as a general stimulant, believing that it "made the blood go round" and restored "internal heat." In the early 20th century, it was used as part of the cure for alcohol and opium withdrawal. Doctors reasoned that the quickened action of the circulation increased the rate of blood cleansing and purification.

Mucus Mover

Because cayenne acts as a diaphoretic (which means that it makes you sweat), it was an herbal mainstay for general cleansing of the body, breaking fevers, and fighting infection.

"When you eat something hot like cayenne, your nose runs, you sweat, and all your fluids get moving," says Dr. Evans. That's a good thing when you have a cold or flu and your mucous membranes are swollen and inflamed. Breaking up stagnant and congested mucus brings some relief

SUPPLEMENT SNAPSHOT

▶Cayenne

Botanical names: *Capsicum frutescens, C. annuum,* and other species.

Origin: Native to tropical America.

May help: Blood clots, asthma, fever, sore throat, respiratory infections, flatulence, and high cholesterol and triglycerides.

Special instructions: Take with food.

Cautions and possible side effects: May cause a burning sensation in the gastrointestinal tract in high doses or for some sensitive people.

from cold symptoms, says Dr. Evans, but even better, it brings fresh blood to the site of the infection. Fresh blood contains infection fighters from the immune system—white blood cells and leukocytes—that fight viruses and other foreign invaders.

Cayenne is frequently found in herbal cold and flu combinations, especially those with immune stimulants like echinacea and goldenseal, says Dr. Evans. "Cayenne helps the action of these other herbs by stimulating circulation and therefore the delivery of the herbs," she adds.

Its stimulating effects may also be good for your heart, says Pamela Herring, ND, a naturopathic doctor at the Naturopathic Clinic of Concord in New Hampshire.

People in cultures that consume large amounts of cayenne appear to have lower rates of cardiovascular disease. There's evidence that frequent consumption of cayenne reduces levels of cholesterol and triglycerides (another type of blood fat) in the bloodstream. High levels of either can lead to atherosclerosis (hardening of the arteries) and blockages in the blood vessels.

Cayenne also appears to decrease the tendency to form blood clots and reduce the bunching up of blood platelets around plaque buildup in the vessels.

Dr. Herring believes that the herb's antioxidant properties and circulation-enhancing effects benefit the heart muscle. "Cayenne really stimulates the whole cardiovascular system," she says.

Fire Down Below

Cayenne is available in pills, capsules, and tinctures. You can take it by itself or in combination with other herbs. You can also add it to foods as a spice.

When you take a capsule, you're likely to feel a bit of heat in your belly. For that reason, it's best to take it with food and start out with just one or two capsules a day, advises Dr. Herring. Sensitivity to cayenne varies from one person to the next.

chromium

This essential trace mineral is vital to health. In fact, the evidence is stronger than ever that chromium deficiency plays a fundamental role in the development of type 2 (non-insulin-dependent) diabetes. Supplementation, experts say, may partly reverse some of type 2's effects.

Getting to Insulin and Arteries

In our bodies, chromium improves insulin effectiveness, says Richard Anderson, PhD, lead scientist in the nutrient requirements and functions laboratory at the USDA Beltsville Human Nutrition Research Center in Maryland. Insulin is a hormone secreted by the pancreas; it helps our bodies use blood sugar (glucose) by binding to receptor sites on the membranes of cells. This primes the cell in a way that allows it to take in blood sugar.

Chromium improves insulin function in two ways: It increases the sensitivity of receptor sites so that when insulin binds with the site, the cell is strongly activated and takes in lots of blood sugar. Plus, it increases the available number of insulin receptor sites on cells.

Keeping insulin and blood sugar levels normal is important because high levels of either—or both—can cause circulation problems that may lead to clogged arteries.

In studies, supplemental chromium has helped people with glucose intolerance, or insulin resistance—an early sign of diabetes for many people. A study conducted by Dr. Anderson in China showed that chromium supplements can reduce blood sugar and insulin levels in people with full-blown type 2 diabetes.

People with diabetes have a high risk of developing heart disease, but chromium may help reduce that risk, as well, says Dr. Anderson. "High insulin levels have a direct damaging effect on the cells lining the arteries, so anything that keeps the level of insulin normal is helpful," he says. Also, since chromium is needed for your body to use fats just as it's needed to help your cells incorporate blood sugar, it helps clear fats out of your bloodstream. In several studies, people who were given supplemental chromium had drops in total cholesterol and "bad" LDL cholesterol and increases in "good" HDL cholesterol.

Chrome-Plated Muscles?

Promotions for chromium supplements often imply that chromium can help you lose fat and gain muscle. The reasoning behind this claim is based on chromium's insulin-enhancing effect. Insulin builds up muscles and other tissues, promotes utilization of amino acids and the production of protein, and retards protein breakdown. In theory, at least, this would

SUPPLEMENTSNAPSHOT

▶Chromium

Supplement forms: Chromium picolinate, nicotinate, aspartate, and chloride.

Daily Value: 120 micrograms.

May help: Glucose intolerance, type 2 diabetes, and high cholesterol.

Good food sources: Broccoli, turkey, ham, and grape juice.

Who's at risk for deficiency: People who eat large amounts of refined sugar and carbohydrates and those who have diabetes, are insulin resistant, or are fighting infection or recovering from injuries.

Special instructions: Take chromium picolinate, nicotinate, or aspartate; chromium chloride is the least absorbable form. Avoid the form called glucose tolerance factor (GTF), a combination of chromium, nicotinic acid, and amino acids, which may vary so much in composition that it is not a reliable source.

Cautions and possible side effects: Don't take more than 200 micrograms a day without medical supervision, although doses up to 1,000 micrograms daily seem to be safe. If you have diabetes or hypoglycemia, consult your doctor before taking. If you have diabetes, the upper limits are 400 to 600 micrograms a day, but have your doctor carefully monitor your blood sugar levels.

mean that people getting optimal amounts of chromium would be able to build more muscle than people whose chromium intake was low.

In reality, though, the truth is a little harder to pin down. In some studies—mostly of young, hard-training athletes—those taking chromium supplements sometimes saw some favorable changes in body composition. They had less fat and more muscle than comparable athletes not taking supplements. In a number of other studies, however, supplementation appeared to offer no advantage.

"Now that several of these studies have been done, it seems that the real gains in body composition don't start to appear until the fourth month," Dr. Anderson says. And even the "real gains" aren't what the ads might have you expect. You might see 1 to 2 percent more muscle and 1 to 2 percent less fat, with no change in body weight. "For highly trained athletes, that edge may make the difference," Dr. Anderson says.

If you don't exercise hard, Dr. Anderson adds, chances are that you'll see less of an effect. "Don't expect chromium supplements to do as much for your body as exercise does," he says. "Don't think that chromium alone is going to take you from a size 16 to a size 8 dress."

The Short Story

It's clear that few people are getting the Daily Value of 120 micrograms of chromium. In fact, studies show that the average diet contains about 25 micrograms of this important mineral, and even balanced diets designed by dietitians contain less than 50 micrograms.

Some nutritionists argue that people simply don't need more chromium than they get from foods—that 25 micrograms a day may be sufficient. Others, including Dr. Anderson, believe that people are less likely to develop diabetes and heart disease if they get 200 micrograms or more— the amounts that were found helpful in his studies. Moreover, he recommends as much as 400 to 600 micrograms for people who have diabetes.

If you are taking insulin for diabetes and you want to start taking high doses of chromium, check with your doctor and make sure that he keeps close tabs on your blood sugar levels, because your insulin needs will probably drop, Dr. Anderson says.

What about trying to help prevent diabetes by monitoring your chromium levels?

Unfortunately, says Dr. Anderson, there's no good way to test for chromium deficiency. "The only way to find out if supplemental chromium is going to be helpful to you is to try it under a doctor's supervision and see if it improves your blood sugar, insulin, and cholesterol levels," he says.

Your doctor can get a reading of these levels before you start taking supplements. After you've been taking the supplement for a while, the doctor can take a second reading for comparison.

coenzyme Q_{10}

When a 19-year-old college student from Houston experienced short-ness of breath and a racing heartbeat, his doctors diagnosed dilated cardio-myopathy, a condition characterized by an enlarged and weakened heart. They also told him that he would someday need a heart transplant.

Then he went to see Peter Langsjoen, MD, a cardiologist in Tyler, Texas, who recommended a little-known substance called coenzyme Q_{10} (CoQ_{10}). Within a few weeks of starting to take CoQ_{10}, the student required fewer prescription heart medications. Eventually, his heart size and function returned to normal.

"This is someone who, before CoQ_{10} came along, would most certainly have gone downhill," says Dr. Langsjoen. "It's clearly lifesaving."

Similar stories, coming directly from medical practitioners, have drawn public attention to this naturally occurring compound that our cells need to produce energy. Proponents credit CoQ_{10} with protecting the heart, strengthening the immune system, boosting energy and endurance, nor-malizing blood pressure, and healing periodontal disease.

Getting to the Heart of the Matter

CoQ_{10} is made by the body and stored in the liver, kidneys, pancreas, and heart. We also get it from a variety of foods, especially liver and other organ meats. It is found in all cells, but it's most highly concentrated in heart muscle cells because they use the greatest amount of energy.

Most of us have plenty of CoQ_{10} in our bodies until around the age of 30. About then, our bodies lose the ability to manufacture it at the same levels, so the natural supply begins to diminish.

Apart from the decline in production that accompanies aging, there are other reasons for a shortage of CoQ_{10}. Certain conditions, such as viral illnesses and shock, can rob us of this compound, says Dr. Langsjoen.

CoQ$_{10}$ deficiency is especially common in people with various types of heart disease. In fact, the more severe the heart disease, the lower the levels of CoQ$_{10}$ found in heart muscle cells. Doctors don't know, though, whether the deficiency is one of the contributing causes or whether the reduced level of CoQ$_{10}$ is the result of heart disease, says Dr. Langsjoen.

"CoQ$_{10}$ is definitely a factor in heart health because we know without a doubt that when you replenish it and restore levels to where they should be, heart function improves. If you let levels slide down again, heart function worsens," he explains.

This substance may improve the function of the heart by enhancing energy production, improving the ability of the heart to contract, and providing powerful antioxidant protection. The activity of CoQ$_{10}$ helps prevent the buildup of oxidized LDL cholesterol, the "bad" kind of cholesterol that starts to block arteries when it's exposed to certain kinds of oxygen molecules. Because CoQ$_{10}$ provides antioxidant protection, it helps prevent this oxidizing process, and in so doing, it helps keep LDL cholesterol from blocking your blood vessels.

SUPPLEMENT SNAPSHOT

▶Coenzyme Q$_{10}$

Also known as: CoQ$_{10}$.

May help: Gingivitis, chronic fatigue syndrome, Parkinson's disease, heart disease, high blood pressure, high cholesterol, congestive heart failure, mitral valve prolapse, angina, and arrhythmia; may provide some protection during heart surgery; may boost immunity and improve physical performance.

Good food sources: Liver and organ meats are possible sources but are not recommended because of their high fat and cholesterol content.

Special instructions: Take supplements, preferably gelcaps, with food. Take tablets or capsules with a little peanut butter or other food that contains fat to aid absorption.

Cautions and possible side effects: Rarely, a slight decrease in the effectiveness of the blood thinner warfarin (Coumadin) has been observed. No other known side effects.

It may also speed recovery after heart surgery. When patients take CoQ_{10} for several days prior to surgery, they recover faster and better, with fewer complications, according to Dr. Langsjoen.

Unfortunately, some of the medications that are beneficial for heart disease patients actually deplete the body's supply of CoQ_{10}. Among the thieves are cholesterol-lowering statin drugs and beta-blockers such as propranolol (Inderal) and metoprolol (Toprol XL).

For prevention and recovery—and to counteract its depletion due to heart drugs—a number of doctors are now touting the many benefits of CoQ_{10} supplements. It can help almost any disease related to the heart muscle, they say, including such problems as recurrent chest pain (angina) or irregular heart rate (arrhythmia). Some studies also suggest that it may enhance the benefits of cholesterol-lowering drugs, help lower blood pressure, and improve heart health for those with congestive heart failure, a condition in which the heart is unable to maintain normal blood circulation.

The CoQ_{10} Controversy

Critics and skeptics argue that many studies of CoQ_{10} have been flawed or poorly controlled. Many of them have not been double-blind, for example. Considered the definitive form of medical research, a double-blind study is one in which neither the researchers nor the subjects know who is receiving the actual treatment. That's ideal because neither of them can influence the outcome by wishing for a positive result.

In experiments that don't use the double-blind method—like the CoQ_{10} studies—there's a lot of room for bias. Another criticism of the research is that some study periods have been too short to be conclusive.

One popular use for the supplement is as a booster for aerobic endurance, especially among younger adults. It actually provides little in the way of benefit to athletes. If you're young and healthy, chances are that your body already has all the CoQ_{10} it needs, says Dr. Langsjoen.

On the other hand, there's no question that your body's supply of CoQ_{10} is depleted with aging. It seems to make sense that—all other things being equal—you would continue to have a "younger" heart if you used a supplement that provides some of the missing ingredient.

How to Get Your CoQ₁₀

If you decide to give CoQ₁₀ a try, stick with the gelcaps that come mixed with oil for better absorption. If you do buy tablets or capsules, take them with a small amount of peanut butter or other food that contains fat to help absorption, suggests Dr. Langsjoen.

As for the recommended dosage, Dr. Langsjoen says that most people have a good response with 60 to 120 milligrams twice a day. The appropriate individual dosage can best be determined by measuring blood levels of CoQ₁₀, although there are currently few commercial laboratories that offer this test. To determine your dosage, ask your physician, who should also test your heart function at least twice a year if you're taking CoQ₁₀.

copper

Shiny new pennies remind us of copper's value as currency, but it would take many bagfuls to buy a week's worth of groceries. In our bodies, however, a little copper goes a long way. It's an essential part of many enzymes, which spark the chemical reactions that sustain life.

Copper-containing enzymes have diverse roles. They help us form strong, flexible connective tissue; produce energy; use iron; and manufacture cholesterol. "Copper has a direct effect on our bones, skin, heart, liver, blood, kidneys, thyroid, immune system, and just about every part in between," says Judith Turnlund, PhD, RD, a trace mineral specialist at the USDA Western Human Nutrition Research Center in San Francisco.

Like a Chain-Link Fence

If you examine a chain-link fence, you'll see that each strand of wire knits with the adjacent one, forming a strong mesh. In our bodies, copper helps link the long strands of proteins that make up the connective tissues throughout our bodies. It literally helps to hold us together.

"A copper-containing enzyme cross-links collagen, the body's most important connective tissue, which is used to make skin, bones, lungs, and many other tissues," says Leslie Klevay, MD, a doctor of hygiene and research medical officer at the USDA Human Nutrition Research Center in Grand Forks, North Dakota. Copper also cross-links elastin, a fiber that can stretch and rebound. It is found mostly in the skin and blood vessels.

Copper-deficient animals have weakened hearts and blood vessels and may die of heart failure. Lacking copper, the heart or the aorta, the main artery from the heart, may burst, Dr. Klevay says. Also, copper-deficient animals have bone defects that are very similar to osteoporosis. These dangers may lie in wait for humans, too. That's one reason why nutritionists keep an eye on this significant trace mineral.

Enzymes That Lean on Copper

Two copper-containing enzymes are essential for our bodies to be able to use another important mineral—iron. These enzymes help move iron out of storage in cells lining the intestines or liver and transport it to the bone marrow, where it becomes part of the red blood cells produced there.

"If you don't have enough copper, your body simply can't use iron," Dr. Klevay says. Babies born with the inability to use copper and people who are copper-deficient develop anemia (insufficient red blood cells) because the copper shortage creates an iron shortage. When iron is in short

SUPPLEMENTSNAPSHOT

▶Copper

Daily Value: 2 milligrams.

May help: Bacterial, viral, and fungal infections and high cholesterol.

Good food sources: Chocolate, legumes, mushrooms, nuts, peanut butter, seeds, shellfish (especially cooked oysters), and whole grains.

Who's at risk for deficiency: People who take more than 30 milligrams a day of zinc, because zinc may be absorbed instead of copper; people who take more than 100 milligrams of vitamin C at the same time as copper supplements; people who don't eat copper-rich foods or who take nonsteroidal anti-inflammatory drugs; and people who consume large amounts of fructose, a component of both fruit and table sugar that can interfere with copper absorption.

Special instructions: Take as part of a multivitamin/mineral supplement that contains up to 2 milligrams of copper and less than 100 milligrams of vitamin C. If you want to take more vitamin C, take it separately; vitamin C interferes with copper absorption and utilization. Iron and zinc can interfere with absorption if taken in amounts greater than the Daily Value.

Cautions and possible side effects: Excess copper from supplements or from water (from copper pipes) can cause health problems. Signs include vomiting and diarrhea. Taking less than 10 milligrams occasionally is considered safe, but do not take more than 2 milligrams on a regular basis. Consult your doctor before taking higher amounts.

What Are Trace Minerals?

If you check the label on your multivitamin/mineral bottle, you may find some unfamiliar ingredients that seem somewhat suspicious, including such items as nickel, molybdenum, manganese, and vanadium. Some high-priced "designer" multis even contain silver or gold.

These are all trace minerals. Like iron and copper, some of them, such as molybdenum and manganese, are essential to human health in tiny amounts. "Both are enzyme activators," says Forrest Nielsen, PhD, director of the USDA Human Nutrition Research Center in Grand Forks, North Dakota. These minerals are necessary for certain vital chemical reactions that take place in your body.

Molybdenum is important because it activates the enzyme that produces uric acid—the substance that helps carry excess nitrogen out of your body when you urinate. Manganese is a component of an enzyme that plays a role in preventing degenerative disease.

Lots of other trace minerals, even those found in multivitamins or sold singly, haven't been proven to be essential. There's some evidence that nickel, silicon, boron, and vanadium might be, but scientists still don't know for sure. And the jury's still out on minerals like germanium.

We get more than enough of certain trace minerals, such as molybdenum and silicon, in our diets, Dr. Nielsen says. Others, such as manganese

supply, the body doesn't produce enough hemoglobin, the protein in red blood cells that carries oxygen.

Along with iron, copper is also needed for many reactions that transform the food we eat into energy that our bodies can use. In a series of chemical reactions, the food is broken down and transported to cells. Inside the cells, tiny powerhouses called mitochondria change the food into energy-containing molecules that can either be stored or hacked apart to release energy. This process involves a kind of assembly line of proteins, Dr. Klevay explains, and "the final protein in this line must contain two or three molecules of copper or the job of energy production stops before it is completed."

The activity of the copper-containing enzyme lysyl oxidase and prolyl oxidase, which cross-links collagen, is highest in cells that use the most energy—those in the heart, brain, liver, and kidneys.

and boron, may be in short supply. Either way, it's okay to take the 10 to 25 micrograms of any of these that you might find in a multivitamin/mineral tablet, he says. They won't hurt you, and they may even be helpful. Some trace minerals come from unprocessed foods like whole grains and certain vegetables and fruits, but if you're not likely to eat these foods, the supplements can easily make up any deficit.

What's not safe is using large amounts of trace mineral supplements in an attempt to achieve druglike effects. Vanadium, which supposedly builds muscle or prevents diabetes, and germanium, which has been said to prevent cancer and build the immune system, are sold singly. These supplements have shown little evidence of benefit, Dr. Nielsen says, and no studies have assessed the long-term effects of high amounts.

"I am concerned because vanadium is toxic if you build up a high enough quantity in your body," says Dr. Nielsen. Furthermore, germanium might be contaminated with germanium dioxide, an inorganic form that can cause kidney damage. Worldwide, some 20 to 30 people have died from kidney damage caused by inorganic germanium. While it's true that you can order it from Internet sources, that doesn't mean that you should. "This is not something to take lightly," Dr. Nielsen says.

Another copper-dependent enzyme, superoxide dismutase, plays a role as an antioxidant. Like vitamin E, it can neutralize the free-roaming, unstable molecules called free radicals. It circulates inside cells, soaking up free radicals that are produced as the cells break down waste products. Or it rushes to help immune cells called phagocytes, which "digest" bacteria that they swallow whole. With copper as an essential part of its wiring, superoxide dismutase helps cells stay young and protect themselves from bacterial, viral, fungal, and free radical onslaughts.

The Cholesterol Connection

Copper research has led to some close scrutiny of cholesterol metabolism. "Over 20 independent laboratories around the world now show that copper deficiency raises cholesterol levels in animals," says Dr. Klevay.

When people are deprived of copper, their cholesterol levels shoot upward, similar to what happens in animals that are deprived of the mineral.

At least three enzymes seem to be involved, but the most important is HMG-coA reductase, found in the liver. Studies have found that this enzyme is overactive in copper-deficient animals. "What's so interesting about this is that the newest cholesterol-lowering drugs, called statins, also act on HMG-coA reductase," Dr. Klevay explains. "They are specifically designed to inhibit its activity, which lowers cholesterol very efficiently."

Does that mean that people with high cholesterol aren't getting enough copper in their diets? "I think it's certainly a possibility for some people, but it has yet to be studied," Dr. Klevay says.

A Penny Short?

Severe copper deficiency is extremely rare, and it takes more than a poor diet to cause it. Still, some researchers believe that marginal copper deficiency is more common than we know and that people may develop chronic illnesses such as heart disease and osteoporosis as a result. Supporting the connection to osteoporosis are two studies that were done with women who took copper supplements. Both showed that the women's bone density improved when they had supplementation.

Most people get less than 1.5 milligrams a day of copper from foods, which is less than the Daily Value of 2 milligrams. You can increase your copper intake to recommended amounts by making appropriate food choices, Dr. Klevay says. Copper from foods is tolerated better than supplemental copper, so "you don't want to go overboard with supplements," he cautions.

creatine

Cruise the ingredients lists in the "sports performance" section of any health food store or study the drink selection at a gym's beverage bar and you'll find creatine—an energy-enhancing amino acid that many athletes think is the best thing to come along since dumbbells.

Supplementing with creatine helps people perform at their maximum energy level for their level of fitness. It won't turn you into the Incredible Hulk, but it can help you to make the most use of the muscle you do have, especially during repeated short bursts of exercise (such as during interval training) or sports where you have quick start-and-stop motions.

Your own body makes some creatine, about 1 to 2 grams a day, primarily in your liver, kidneys, and pancreas. Dietary sources, such as fish and meats (especially red meat), supply an additional 1 to 2 grams. For example, 1 pound of fresh uncooked steak contains about 2 grams of creatine. Vegetarians get much less dietary creatine than carnivores do, so vegetarian athletes are one group that often benefits by getting more creatine. But can creatine help the everyday person just trying to stay healthy and fit? Read on.

Creatine is critical to a type of energy stored in our muscles, called phosphocreatine. Phosphocreatine is a precursor to the energy molecule adenosine triphosphate, or ATP. Higher levels of creatine are thought to enhance the ability of muscles to renew ATP for short 10- to 20-second energy bursts and to improve recovery time from intense exercise.

ATP fuels all cells, including muscles, and is used up quickly when muscles are operating at maximum intensity. That's because only a small amount of ATP is stored in muscle cells. In fact, the total amount of ATP in the body provides just enough energy to perform at maximum exertion for a few seconds. You know what this is like if you've ever tried to race up a flight of stairs, overtake a competitor in a bike race, or lift a car off a screaming baby! You simply cannot sustain it, and you have to back off. What's happening is that ATP can't be regenerated fast enough to meet your body's demands.

That's where supplemental creatine enters the picture. It allows your muscles to make more phosphocreatine, so you have more energy for longer periods of time and may attain an edge if you're performing any kind of activity that requires quick bursts of speed or power.

A Boon for Athletes

Because supplemental creatine helps regenerate ATP more quickly, numerous studies show that it can help athletes recover faster during repeated, short, maximal energy bursts. It also seems to be beneficial for exercise of longer duration with alternating intensity, such as you would experience during interval training.

Creatine may also help delay the buildup of lactic acid that occurs in muscles during intense exercise. It's lactic acid that makes your muscles burn during or after a workout. Lactic acid can limit the amount of intense exercise you can do because it makes you want to stop. Creatine helps minimize lactic acid, allowing you to go longer and harder.

Weighty Evidence

A number of studies back up proponents' claims that creatine improves short-burst performance and strength. In one study by Richard Kreider,

SUPPLEMENTSNAPSHOT

▶Creatine

May help: Enhance athletic performance and allow athletes to recover faster and increase muscle mass; muscular dystrophies and Parkinson's disease; exercise tolerance in people with congestive heart failure.

Good food sources: Red meat and fish.

Cautions and possible side effects: Can cause dehydration, muscle cramps, weight gain, and stress on kidneys. Take with plenty of water. Do not use supplemental creatine if you have kidney disease or a disease that increases your risk for kidney disease, such as diabetes or high blood pressure.

PhD, of the University of Memphis, 25 NCAA Division 1A football players were divided into two groups. One group took creatine and the other took a placebo. During a 4-week supplementation period, the athletes participated in a standardized training program that included weight lifting, high-intensity sprinting, and football agility drills. At the end of the study, the creatine group had greater gains in weight-lifting volume, sprint performance, and weight gain.

In another study, researchers at Pennsylvania State University investigated the influence of creatine supplementation on muscle performance during repeated sets of high-intensity resistance exercise. Groups performed bench presses and jump squats before and after taking either 25 grams of creatine or a placebo.

At the end of the test period, researchers found that performance was unchanged for the men in the placebo group. The creatine group, however, had significant improvement in peak power output during jump squats and bench presses after only 1 week on the supplement.

Benefits for Muscle Disorders

Because of its ability to improve muscle performance, researchers have tried supplemental creatine in cases of congestive heart disease, muscular dystrophies, and other diseases that affect muscle strength.

Your heart is, basically, a big hollow muscle. In congestive heart failure, that muscle gets weaker and weaker. In patients with congestive heart failure, both phosphocreatine and ATP levels in the heart muscle are lower than in people with normal cardiac function. Higher phosphocreatine levels appear to improve congestive heart failure by stabilizing the sarcolemma, the cell membrane that allows muscle cells to receive and transmit nerve messages that tell it to contract and relax. Creatine also helps to prevent oxidative damage and improves microcirculation in muscles, allowing tiny capillaries to deliver blood to muscle cells.

In adults and children with various types of muscular dystrophy, taking creatine short-term seems to improve muscle strength and daily life activities.

In people with early Parkinson's disease who do not need medications for symptom control, some evidence shows that taking 10 grams a day of creatine can slow the rate of disease progression compared to a placebo. In people with more advanced Parkinson's, taking a dose of 20 grams a day for 6 days followed by 4 grams a day for 18 months may allow them to take a smaller dose of symptom-controlling drugs such as dopamine.

Creatine can also help some rare genetic metabolic disorders that interfere with energy metabolism, such as gyrate atrophy of the choroid and retina, which causes blindness, and McArdle's disease. People with McArdle's can't convert the storage form of glucose (glycogen) into APT, so they don't have a steady supply of cellular energy.

Is It Safe?

Creatine has been around for more than 100 years, and while not all experts agree that it's very useful for the nonathlete, most do agree that creatine is relatively safe. Creatine has been safely used daily for up to 5 years in dosages of about 0.03 grams per kilogram of body weight—a typical maintenance dose for an athlete. Creatine is allowed by the International Olympic Committee, the National Collegiate Athletic Association, and professional sports. Annual consumption of creatine in the United States is estimated to exceed 4 million kilograms.

Some Downsides

The biggest downside to creatine for most people is that it can lead to muscle strains, cramping, dehydration, nausea, diarrhea, and weight gain that's mostly the result of water retention. You need to be careful while using it if you are sweating a lot and losing a lot of water.

And the most serious risk is kidney damage in people with compromised kidney function. Creatine does put some stress on kidneys. It's not recommended for people younger than age 18, during pregnancy, or for people at high risk for kidney damage due to diabetes or high blood pressure. If you take any medication, check with your doctor first, as creatine may affect how your kidneys process certain drugs.

Loading Up

Athletes and people using creatine for health problems typically take it in two phases, beginning with a "loading" phase. A typical loading program is about 20 grams per day (0.3 grams per kilogram of body weight) for 5 days. An alternative loading program uses 3 grams per day for 28 days.

The loading phase is followed by a maintenance dose of 0.03 grams per kilogram of body weight daily. Any time you are using creatine, you should be drinking at least 64 ounces of water each day.

Some research suggests that using it off and on may be more effective than continuous low-dose use. You "load" with it, just as you would carbo-load before a competition. Also, there is a "ceiling" for creatine, where getting more doesn't help at all, it just dehydrates you. Don't take more than the recommended dosages.

Pay attention if you are using sports drinks. Many of them contain both carbohydrates and creatine. In fact, combining the two boosts muscle levels of creatine by about 60 percent, so it's a good way to help you absorb creatine but it's not such a good way to maintain adequate hydration. Drink plenty of plain water, too.

curcumin (turmeric)

Curcumin has only recently come into the spotlight—and under scientists' microscopes—but this compound found in the yellow spice turmeric has already generated a good bit of excitement. Researchers at MD Anderson Cancer Center in Houston, Texas, are looking at it for an intravenous cancer treatment. The National Cancer Institute is funding 40 human trials using curcumin to possibly help prevent and treat colon, pancreatic, rectal, and other cancers. Other research is testing the compound on asthma, psoriasis, and depression. And scientists at UCLA have been testing curcumin on Alzheimer's patients.

All this fuss is about a spice that's used the world over, especially in African and Indian cuisine. Turmeric is related to ginger, and like ginger, it's the root that's ground up to make the spice. If you've ever had yellow rice, often served with red beans, then you've eaten turmeric.

Turmeric's major active constituents are curcuminoids, including curcumin (diferuloylmethane) and others. Traditionally, turmeric has been used to treat upset stomach, gallstones, flatulence, respiratory infections, fever, cancer, diabetes, and depression. It's been mixed into a paste and used to treat skin conditions from leprosy to ringworm to infected wounds.

Several studies have demonstrated that curcumin is a powerful anti-inflammatory, says Bharat Aggarwal, MD, chief of the cytokine research laboratory in the department of experimental therapeutics at MD Anderson Cancer Center. "It has the ability to turn off something called nuclear factor-kappa B," he says. This is a "master switch" in the nucleus, or control center, of a cell, which seems to be a primary mediator for inflammation. "It is present in every cell in the body, without exception, and it controls more than 500 different genes, and all of those genes are linked with chronic inflammation and chronic disease," Dr. Aggarwal says.

A Cancer Cure?

Cancer needs nuclear factor-kappa B to grow, Dr. Aggarwal says. "When you turn it off, cancer cells die," he says. "We have yet to find a cancer that is not killed by curcumin, because virtually all types of cancer have an active need for nuclear factor-kappa B." Of course, these are laboratory experiments, done with cancer cells in culture. Killing cancer cells once they've developed in your body is more complicated, and what works in a cell culture doesn't always work in the body. Dr. Aggarwal acknowledges that large, blinded trials that compare curcumin to other treatments and placebos are needed to truly establish its effectiveness.

Still, based on preliminary research, curcumin appears to interfere with the cancer process at an early point, impeding multiple routes of development: It reduces the inflammatory response and inhibits the proliferation of tumor cells, which induces their self-destruction and discourages the growth of blood vessels feeding tumors. These effects can shrink tumors and slow the growth of cancer, Dr. Aggarwal says. At the same time, curcumin does not harm nonmalignant cells. "What has been mind-boggling to me is that curcumin kills only tumor cells, not normal cells," he says. "There are not too many drugs that can do that. And we would like to know the mechanism of how it selects a tumor cell over a noncancerous cell."

SUPPLEMENT SNAPSHOT

▶Curcumin (Turmeric)

Scientific Name: *Curcuma longa.*

May help: Alzheimer's disease, certain types of cancer, diabetes and diabetes-related kidney and retinal damage, other inflammatory conditions such as inflammatory bowel disease and rheumatoid arthritis, postexercise muscle soreness, and osteoarthritis.

Good food sources: Turmeric powder.

Cautions and possible side effects: Use with caution in patients with gallstones, as turmeric can cause gallbladder contractions. Large doses can interact with blood-thinning medications, so talk with your doctor before taking turmeric if you're on one of these drugs. Discontinue taking turmeric at least 2 weeks before surgical procedures.

Turmeric may also help prevent cancer by aiding the liver in the process of breaking down or inhibiting activation of some cancer-causing chemicals, such as carbon tetrachloride and benzenes. It seems to increase levels of natural detoxifying enzymes in the liver, such as glutathione.

A Spicy Help for Diabetes

If you have diabetes, you might want to consider sprinkling turmeric into your everyday meals or taking a curcumin supplement. Research indicates that curcumin may prevent kidney damage, a common complication of diabetes, says Subrata Chakrabarti, MD, a professor of pathology in the School of Medicine at the University of Western Ontario. Animals with diabetes that were fed curcumin for 8 weeks had less "leaky" kidneys. In other words, the membranes in their kidneys that filter blood to produce urine were more likely to remain intact. Their urine also contained less protein and lower levels of several key enzymes that signal kidney tissue breakdown. And under a microscope, the kidneys also showed less tissue damage, Dr. Chakrabarti says. Curcumin has also shown some success in animal models in preventing diabetic retinopathy, the main cause of blindness in adults.

Can Curcumin Help Alzheimer's Disease?

In India, where people use turmeric like we use salt, Alzheimer's disease rates are among the world's lowest, Dr. Aggarwal says. In a study of mice genetically altered to develop Alzheimer's, curcumin inhibited the accumulation of destructive beta-amyloid protein in the brain—the "tangles" that are the hallmark of the disease. What's more, the spice also broke up existing plaques. These findings suggest that curcumin is more effective in inhibiting plaque formation than many other drugs being tested as Alzheimer's treatments, the researchers concluded. Unfortunately, the few human trials that have been done have been disappointing, but research is continuing.

Is Turmeric for You?

If you like Indian food, the answer is easy: yes! Any excuse to eat it is good enough. In a traditional Indian diet, people get 100 to 200 milligrams a day of curcumin, Dr. Chakrabarti says. That's enough to be preventive, but it's not enough to be curative if you have an inflammatory condition such as diabetes, ulcerative colitis, or nephritis. If you have any of these diseases, you'll need to get extra curcumin. Most people do this simply by taking turmeric capsules. You can also take curcumin extract, and the best are standardized to contain about 95 percent curcuminoids.

Turmeric is not very absorbable, and only a small percentage of turmeric is curcumin, so researchers have developed a form of turmeric that is more absorbable. It's called liposomal (or, sometimes, phytosome) curcumin, and it's composed of tiny, fat-enclosed spheres of curcumin that are more easily absorbed than the usual stuff. In one study, liposomal curcumin was 20 times more absorbable than the regular curcumin found in turmeric. However, it is quite expensive compared to regular turmeric.

Dr. Aggarwal recommends taking about 500 milligrams a day of turmeric as a preventive measure against cancer and other chronic diseases, and he says people with cancer can safely work their way from 500 milligrams up to about 8 grams (8,000 milligrams) a day, with medical supervision. "I have seen some people do this and they are doing quite well," he says. (See the Web site www.curcuminresearch.org for more on their stories.)

vitamin D

For a long time, vitamin D's function seemed pretty straightforward: It was calcium's wingman, the nutrient that the bone-builder needed in order to do its job. It regulated calcium levels throughout the body, making sure there was enough of this critical element in the blood.

Now we know that vitamin D has many more jobs than just that. In fact, it affects everything from mood regulation to cancer prevention. "Osteoporosis, heart disease, hypertension, autoimmune diseases, certain cancers, depression, chronic fatigue, and chronic pain have all been associated with vitamin D deficiency," says John Cannell, MD, director of the Vitamin D Council, a nonprofit organization. Because of this, the "sunshine" vitamin has rocketed to superstar status in the last few years.

And like any good superstar, vitamin D is generating a good deal of controversy, especially about how much we really need. A committee from the Institutes of Medicine's Food and Nutrition Board issued a report in 2010 that recommended that people up to age 70 get 600 international units (IU) a day of vitamin D, and that people over age 70 get 800 IU a day. (It said there was not enough evidence to recommend higher doses and that there were also concerns about the safety of higher doses.)

But some world-renowned vitamin D experts, including Michael Holick, MD, PhD, professor of medicine, physiology and biophysics at Boston University School of Medicine, argue that there is more than enough evidence to support taking more. Dr. Holick, for example, personally takes 3,000 IU a day and advises his patients to do the same. Andrew Weil, MD, director of the Center for Integrative Medicine at the University of Arizona, in Tucson, and author of *Eight Weeks to Optimum Health,* recommends 2,000 IU a day of vitamin D_3 (the most easily absorbed kind). And Dr. Holick notes that the committee also increased the safe upper limit to 4,000 IU for adults. That's the amount another vitamin D expert, Bruce Hollis, PhD, director of pediatric nutrition at the Medical University of South Carolina, recommends to every adult. As you can see, that's a wide variation among experts.

But let's back up here and review both the historical use of vitamin D and the newer research findings.

How It Works

Vitamin D is called "the sunshine vitamin" because we can make it when sunlight hits our skin. Ultraviolet B rays from the sun convert one

---

SUPPLEMENT SNAPSHOT

▶Vitamin D

Daily Value: 600 international units (IU) for people ages 1 to 70; 800 IU for people 71 and older. (Some experts believe these amounts should be higher.)

May help: Osteomalacia, osteoporosis, chronic back pain, fibromyalgia, heart disease, high blood pressure, autoimmune diseases, psoriasis, seasonal affective disorder (SAD), depression, and cancer.

Good food sources: Fatty fish, such as mackerel and salmon, and fortified milk and milk products. (Food sources are not adequate to supply all the vitamin D you need.)

Who's at risk for deficiency: People who don't eat much dairy and who aren't exposed to sunlight; those who use sunscreen at all times; breastfed babies of vitamin D–deficient mothers; people who have chronic intestinal absorption problems, such as celiac disease; people taking anticonvulsants; and people with chronic liver or kidney disease.

Cautions and possible side effects: People with hyperparathyroidism should only take vitamin D under the care of a knowledgeable endocrinologist. (Secondary hyperparathyroidism can be caused by vitamin D deficiency.) Granulomatous diseases such as sarcoidosis, granulomatous TB, and some cancers can also cause vitamin D hypersensitivity. These people should not take vitamin D except when under the care of a knowledgeable physician.

type of chemical compound in our skin, called previtamin D_3, to a substance called cholecalciferol. This in turn is converted twice more, in the liver and kidneys, into activated vitamin D, calcitriol.

Though it's called a vitamin, in the body, vitamin D is a hormone. It has a direct effect on organs such as the intestines, kidneys, brain, and bones. The cells of these organs have receptor sites just for vitamin D. And all of these organs respond to the vitamin in various ways.

The Bone Vitamin

Vitamin D's main claim to fame used to be that it allowed calcium, and the lesser-known but important phosphorus, get access to the bones. As these essential minerals are deposited into protein "scaffolding," the bones mineralize, or harden.

Vitamin D makes calcium and phosphorus available in three ways. In the intestines, it sends cells the message, "Absorb more calcium and phosphorus." In the kidneys, the instruction is, "Don't pee out that calcium and phosphorus—recirculate it." And when blood levels of calcium begin to drop, vitamin D sends bone cells the message, "Start breaking down bone and get that calcium into the bloodstream."

That final message is important because calcium is needed throughout our bodies to maintain normal muscle and nerve function. And if you have plenty of calcium but not enough D, you can still end up with a calcium deficiency.

Even in adults, whose bones are formed but constantly remodeling, vitamin D deficiency causes a condition called osteomalacia, which is characterized by pain, weakness, and fragile bones due to poor bone mineralization. One study found that up to 30 percent of people with hip fractures had osteomalacia, which can be present along with osteoporosis. People with chronic back pain, especially if they also have muscle weakness, may also have osteomalacia.

The traditional line has been that doses of more than 2,000 IU a day for several months can cause high blood levels of calcium, kidney stones, and calcium deposits in heart and kidney tissues. But recently the safe upper limit was raised to 4,000 IU a day, and some experts believe that this amount may be necessary simply for most people to maintain their current blood levels of vitamin D.

An Autoimmune Helper

Bones aren't the only parts of our bodies that vitamin D befriends. Researchers are finding more and more links between a growing list of health problems and vitamin D deficiency.

For instance, vitamin D deficiency has been associated with an increased risk for autoimmune diseases such as scleroderma, rheumatoid arthritis, and type 1 (insulin-dependent) diabetes, Dr. Hollis says. When you are deficient in vitamin D, you generate an immune cell (T helper type 1) that attacks your own body.

Other research has found that high daily doses of vitamin D dramatically cut the relapse rate in people with multiple sclerosis (MS). A study at the University of Toronto found that for every 10-nanogram-per-milliliter increase in blood vitamin D level in a patient, there was an associated 34 percent decrease in the rate of MS relapses. "Research seems to show that vitamin D deficiency is associated with a higher risk for autoimmune disease and greater severity if you already have such a disease," Dr. Cannell says.

Cancer and Vitamin D

Vitamin D deficiency is also implicated in the development of cancer, Dr. Cannell says. One of the vitamin's roles in the body is to help cells to properly differentiate (or mature into) their final, healthy forms. Vitamin D increases the self-destruction of mutated cells that, if allowed to replicate, could lead to cancer. It helps to reduce the spread and reproduction of cancer cells. And it reduces the growth of new blood vessels from preexisting ones, which is a step in the transition of dormant tumors turning into cancerous ones.

In fact, two meta-analyses (in which data from multiple studies is combined) conducted by the Moores Cancer Center at the University of California at San Diego suggested that raising blood levels of vitamin D could prevent half of the cases of breast cancer and two-thirds of the cases of colorectal cancer in the United States, according to study author Cedric Garland, DrPH. For breast cancer alone, Dr. Garland says, "the serum level associated with a 50 percent reduction in risk could be maintained by taking 2,000 international units of vitamin D_3 daily plus, when the weather permits, spending 10 to 15 minutes a day in the sun."

Keep in mind, Dr. Cannell says, "that although current research indicates vitamin D to be an effective tool in the fight against cancer, it should be used in addition to regular chemotherapy or surgery." And it's still too early to say for certain what dosages or blood levels really are best.

A Brighter Outlook

Research has also shown that vitamin D deficiency is associated with poor mood and depression. Getting supplemental vitamin D, or even getting more sun, seems to help seasonal affective disorder (SAD), a kind of low-grade inertia that some people develop during wintertime.

As for depression, it is too early to say for sure if vitamin D might help, Dr. Cannell says. Still, there are plenty of vitamin D receptors in the brain, and there are a number of ways it could work, he says. For instance, vitamin D provides an amino acid called tyrosine, needed for the production of several neurotransmitters that help regulate mood. If you suffer from depression, Dr. Cannell suggests getting your vitamin D levels checked and working with your doctor if you come up low.

Do You Need More Vitamin D?

Maybe. Many more people than previously thought are deficient or low in vitamin D, even by conservative standards. But the only way to know for sure is to get your blood level checked, and that's a pretty easy thing to do, Dr. Cannell says. For starters, make sure your doctor orders the right test. "A 25-hydroxy-vitamin D—or 25(OH)D—test is the only blood test that can diagnose vitamin D deficiency accurately," Dr. Cannell says. (A 1,25-dihydroxy-vitamin D test, which some doctors mistakenly order, cannot.) Ask for a copy of the test results—don't just let the doctor tell you it is "normal." Find out what the level is.

Then what? Experts disagree on what is an optimal blood level. Some health authorities consider a level of 20 to 30 ng/ml good. Others, including many experts, think that is too low and like to see 30 to 50 ng/ml, or even 50 to 80 ng/ml. The best level for you should be for you and your doctor to decide together.

DHEA

Back in the 1990s, when it first became popular, DHEA was touted as an anti-aging miracle. It's still used mostly for age-related concerns, more by women than men. And it does seem to have some mood-elevating, libido-enhancing, and even wrinkle-reducing effects. "It was called the fountain of youth because it can cause gray hair to regain its natural color," says Jacob Teitelbaum, MD, author of *From Fatigued to Fantastic* and director of the Fibromyalgia and Fatigue Centers, a national group of clinics. But it can also cause baldness if you take too much! There's no doubt that DHEA is a double-edged sword, with both benefits and side effects to be weighed.

Let's start with what it is: DHEA (short for dehydroepiandrosterone) is a hormone that's made naturally in the body, in the adrenal glands and in the testes, in men. (Very small amounts are also made in the liver and brain.) It's a precursor for a number of other hormones, mostly androgens and testosterone. "Supplemental DHEA is a major precursor for androgens in women and a minor precursor in men, who have much more to begin with," Dr. Teitelbaum says.

In fact, research does suggest that DHEA supplementation seems to change hormone balance differently in men and women. In men who take DHEA, there is an increase in the levels of estrogen in the blood and not much of an increase in androgens. In women, the opposite is true. When they take DHEA, there is an increase in blood levels of testosterone, but less of an increase in estrogen.

Antiaging Abilities

DHEA is promoted mostly as an antiaging supplement, and there is some evidence that it can help some aspects of aging. For instance, taking DHEA orally seems to increase skin thickness, oil production, and skin hydration, and to decrease age spots in older men and women. It seems to improve erectile dysfunction and overall sexual satisfaction in men whose erectile dysfunction is related to high blood pressure. DHEA also seems to improve sexual arousal in postmenopausal women, but not premeno-pausal women.

In women, DHEA has more estrogenic effects, but unlike traditional hormone replacement therapy, it stimulates both female and male hor-mones. Taking what is considered to be a large dose of DHEA for a woman (50 to 100 milligrams a day) seems to improve bone mineral density in older women and men with osteoporosis or low bone density in young women with anorexia, who tend to have low DHEA.

Help for Chronic Fatigue Syndrome and Fibromyalgia

Doctors who use DHEA for chronic fatigue syndrome and fibromyalgia (also called CFS and FM, these are conditions where people feel constantly tired and in pain) suspect that there is an imbalance in a hormone-regulating

SUPPLEMENTSNAPSHOT

▶ DHEA

Also known as: Dehydroepiandrosterone. Also sold as DHEA-S, a precursor to DHEA, and as Prestara, a prescription synthetic DHEA.

May help: Some aspects of aging, such as reduced bone mineralization, energy and depressed mood, vaginal atrophy, hot flashes, and reduced sex drive; lupus; some causes of erectile dysfunction; chronic fatigue syndrome; and fibromyalgia.

Cautions and possible side effects: High doses can cause masculin-ization in women, including acne, darkening of facial hair, and hair loss. There is concern that high doses can promote growth of hormone-sensitive cancers such as breast, ovarian, or prostate cancer. Can worsen polycystic ovary syndrome and cause insulin resistance at high doses. Large doses, such as those taken with SLE, have been reported to cause mania and hypersexuality. May worsen bipolar disorder. Men and women under 35 should avoid DHEA supplements because they could suppress the body's natural production of DHEA; deficiencies in this group are rare.

feedback loop called the hypothalamic-pituitary-adrenal (or HPA) axis in the body, Dr. Teitelbaum says. The HPA axis controls levels of many hormones, including cortisol (the main stress hormone), and there's some research to suggest that this system can get out of whack in people with CFS or FM. "I find that it helps people to feel better and I will suggest it if I find that someone's blood level is lower than I like it to be," Dr. Teitelbaum says. The DHEA brings that loop back into balance. If you have CFS or FM, talk to your doctor about testing your hormone levels, and ask if DHEA is something you should look into.

Autoimmune Additive

DHEA may also help some symptoms of systemic lupus erythematosus (SLE), an autoimmune disease better known as lupus. In one study, taking DHEA along with conventional treatments reduced the frequency of flare-ups and allowed a reduction in the dosage of steroids normally used to treat this disease. It also helped decrease the symptoms of muscle aches and oral ulcers and improved bone mineral density in people with SLE being treated with high-dose steroids. "DHEA seems to reduce or balance out the toxicity of prednisone, the drug normally used to treat lupus," Dr. Teitelbaum says. It also sometimes allows a lower dose of prednisone to be used. But the high doses of DHEA that are effective—200 milligrams a day—should not be used without medical supervision, Dr. Teitelbaum says. "And, unfortunately, not many mainstream doctors know much about using DHEA," he says. "You may need to find a holistic practitioner."

Respect, and Help, for Mother Nature

Even if you think you could be helped by getting supplemental DHEA, it's not something you should just go out, buy, and start taking, Dr. Teitelbaum says. "It's not like a lot of supplements that have a wide safety range and that, if you body doesn't need it, you'll just excrete it. This is one where, if you take it and you don't need it, you can get toxic. You can get too high a level fairly easily, especially in women."

He recommends that you get your blood levels checked first, to find out if they are low. The blood test is for DHEA sulfate, or DHEA-S, the storage form of DHEA. If your DHEA-S level is low (under 120 mcg/dL for females or 325 mcg/dL for males), he recommends beginning treatment with 5 to 25 milligrams of DHEA a day and slowly working up to what feels like an optimal level to you. (At that level, your mood may improve and you may feel more energy, but you won't be hyper or impulsive.) For women, he suggests keeping the DHEA-S level around 150 to 180 mcg/dL, which is the normal range for a 29-year-old female. For men, he keeps the DHEA-S level between 350 and 500 mcg/dL, which is the normal range for a 29-year-old male. "The low ends of the normal range are normal only for people over 80," he says. If you have side effects, such as facial hair or acne, which are uncommon, check your blood levels of DHEA-S and decrease your dose.

Some doctors, such as Ray Sahelian, MD, a physician in southern California and author of *DHEA: A Practical Guide,* suggest keeping the dose lower and taking breaks from DHEA. "At this point, I am only comfortable with the temporary use of this hormone," Dr. Sahelian says. "I would say 5 to 10 mg for 1 or 2 weeks at a time is okay. And then I would suggest a break from it for at least 3 or 4 weeks," he says. "My main concern is cancer. We just don't know whether this could be promoting cancer somewhere down the line." He's most likely to recommend DHEA to older female patients who complain of loss of sex drive. "It can provide certain benefits," he says. "It can increase a sense of well-being and increase libido."

But isn't it torture to feel better and then have to stop taking the very thing that makes you feel better? "Not really," Dr. Sahelian says. "It is kind of like a car that is stalled. It can give you the motivation to go out and exercise, eat well, do the healthy things that need to be done for long-term improvements. DHEA can be in tissues for a long time, even when blood levels are low, and it can stimulate protein synthesis and other actions that go on for a while and continue to help people feel better."

Getting the Good Stuff

Like many dietary products, DHEA is plagued by quality control issues. In one test of over-the-counter products, DHEA content ranged from 0 to 150 percent of the labeled amount. There are more than 300 DHEA-containing products listed in one natural medicines database, so you can imagine how difficult it is to try to figure out which one to buy. That's another good reason to see a holistic health care practitioner before taking DHEA. Most know which brands are consistently reliable and can select among top quality brands that are available only through a health care practitioner. They can also advise you on dosage. You can also get DHEA at some compounding pharmacies.

vitamin E

Vitamin E got itself a reputation as a "sex vitamin" early on. When it was being tested on laboratory animals, it gave every sign of deserving that reputation.

When male animals were deprived of vitamin E, their testicles shrank. In pregnant female animals with vitamin E deficiency, the fetuses were reabsorbed into the uterus, preventing the animals from bearing young. Giving the animals even a single drop of vitamin E–rich wheat germ oil restored their fertility. In fact, vitamin E got its scientific name, tocopherol, from this particular ability. It means, "to bring forth offspring."

Today, most vitamin E research focuses on much broader roles, such as preventing heart disease and cancer. And since most people don't get enough vitamin E from foods to protect themselves from these diseases, it wasn't long before favorable reports on vitamin E began to affect sales of the supplements. Soon, sales of vitamin E were catching up with those of vitamin C, the biggest-selling single-supplement nutrient in the United States.

A Heart Helper

In the case of heart disease, two studies from Harvard University involving a total of about 135,000 health professionals found that those who took daily supplements of vitamin E were one-fourth to one-third less likely to develop heart disease than those who didn't take supplements. They took at least 100 international units (IU) daily over a period of at least 2 years.

A study done in England, called the Cambridge Heart Antioxidant Study, showed that people with heart disease who took at least 400 IU of vitamin E daily had about one-quarter the risk of having nonfatal heart attacks as people who took look-alike pills (placebos) that didn't contain any vitamin E.

Researchers in another study found that among male smokers who took 50 to 75 IU a day of vitamin E, the incidence of prostate cancer was reduced by about one-third. There were 41 percent fewer deaths from prostate cancer among the men who took vitamin E when compared with those who didn't.

Many other studies point to areas in which vitamin E looks promising. In Boston, for instance, Tufts University researchers discovered that 200 IU a day of supplemental vitamin E could reverse age-related declines in immune function. Researchers at Columbia University in New York City

SUPPLEMENT SNAPSHOT

▶Vitamin E

Supplement forms: D-alpha-tocopherol, d-alpha tocopheryl acetate, and d-alpha tocopheryl succinate.

Daily Value: 30 international units.

May help: Heart disease, angina, cancer, multiple sclerosis, diabetes, Alzheimer's disease, cataracts, emphysema, high cholesterol, intermittent claudication, infertility, impotence, genital herpes, bedsores, leg cramps, muscle soreness, phlebitis, menopausal discomforts, HIV, osteoarthritis, and chronic inflammatory diseases such as lupus and rheumatoid arthritis.

Good food sources: Walnuts; almonds; spinach; turnip greens; mustard greens; kohlrabi; kale; dandelion greens; and unrefined, cold-pressed olive, nut, wheat germ, or vegetable oils.

Who's at risk for deficiency: People who can't absorb fat properly and those with Crohn's disease or cystic fibrosis.

Special instructions: For doses higher than the Daily Value, take in divided doses with meals that contain some fat. Take a natural form (d-alpha-tocopherol or d-alpha tocopheryl acetate or succinate).

Cautions and possible side effects: Use only with medical supervision if you are taking anticoagulants (blood thinners), ginkgo, or fish-oil supplements; if you take aspirin regularly to help prevent heart disease; if you have high blood pressure, heart disease, or cancer; if you smoke; if you have had a stroke; or if you are at high risk for stroke. Although vitamin E is commonly sold in doses of 400 IU, one small study showed a possible risk of stroke in doses over 200 IU.

found that people with Alzheimer's disease who took 2,000 IU a day were able to delay certain problems associated with the disease. Those who took the supplement were able to go 7 months longer before they lost their ability to groom or feed themselves or had to make a switch from their own homes to nursing homes.

Vitamin E has also shown promise for the treatment of rheumatoid arthritis. European researchers have found that people with rheumatoid arthritis who take 800 IU a day of vitamin E report less pain than those who go without it.

Playground Supervisor

Vitamin E apparently has only one major role in the body, but that one is a whopper. "It functions as your body's major fat-soluble antioxidant," says Maret Traber, PhD, principal investigator at the Linus Pauling Institute and associate professor of nutrition at Oregon State University in Corvallis. Vitamin E is found throughout our bodies in the tissues that contain fat, including the protective membranes surrounding cells and their nuclei, which contain the cells' genetic material.

This all-important vitamin is also found in the fatty sheaths that wrap around and insulate nerves and in molecules called lipoproteins, which circulate in our blood. "In these places, vitamin E helps to neutralize molecular particles called free radicals that are produced as a normal part of reactions that involve oxygen," Dr. Traber says.

These reactions, called oxidation-reduction reactions, go on all the time. Problems occur, though, when a chemical reaction generates a free radical. "A free radical is a molecule that has an unpaired electron, making it unstable," Dr. Traber says. Because the imbalance makes it hungry for an electron, it steals one from some other molecule.

Stopping a Chain Reaction

Unfortunately, that means that another molecule is short an electron, so it becomes a free radical that in turn strives to pluck an electron from some other unlucky molecule nearby. The effect is a chain reaction of free radical damage, kind of like a game of tag that's gotten out of control.

This innocent game leads to trouble. Cell membranes are damaged, sometimes beyond repair. Cell contents leak out, and the cell dies. Or, if the damage occurs in the membranes inside a cell, the cell's genetic material is harmed.

If the damage occurs in the membrane of the cell's power plant, the mitochondria, trouble multiplies like a fight at a hockey game. Free radicals normally generated inside the mitochondria leak out into the cell. Cellular unrest spreads like wildfire.

Vitamin E can stop all of this by donating one of its own electrons to a free radical. When that happens, there's no chain reaction. Vitamin E stops the outbreak of electron grabbing dead in its tracks. You could think of it as a playground supervisor for that rowdy game of tag.

High-Speed Chase

Vitamin E moves with uncanny speed throughout the fluid cell membrane. Because it moves so quickly, it can help protect about 1,000 of the molecules that make up the membrane, Dr. Traber says. Once it neutralizes a free radical, the vitamin E twists within the membrane so that its free radical part is exposed to the watery solution surrounding the cell. There, it meets up with any vitamin C that's available, and vitamin C is an award-winning ally in this process. It regenerates vitamin E by giving up one of its own electrons, allowing vitamin E to go right back to work.

Many diseases, and even aging, seem to be associated with free radical oxidative damage, Dr. Traber says. Cancer, for instance, may be started by free radical damage to a cell's genetic material. Heart disease may begin when free radicals oxidize LDL cholesterol, the artery-clogging kind of free-floating fat that doctors monitor most closely. In effect, the free radicals turn this fat rancid. In so doing, they initiate what is thought to be an early step toward heart disease.

Also, it seems that inflammation anywhere in the body—joints, nerves, or connective tissues—may well involve out-of-control free radical damage, Dr. Traber says. That's why vitamin E and other antioxidants, such as vitamin C, are being studied for their effects on such a variety of conditions.

Supplements Are Essential

The amounts of vitamin E that studies suggest provide protection from heart disease or enhance immunity can't be gotten from even an exemplary diet. The Daily Value for vitamin E is 30 IU, but estimates of an optimal dose really start at around 100 IU. You'd have to eat 58 cups of boiled spinach, 6 cups of peanuts, 1½ cups of corn oil, or 3 tablespoons of wheat germ oil to get close to that amount.

If you are watching your weight and reducing the amount of fat in your diet, you are even less likely to get close to the DV for vitamin E. In one study of people who had cut their fat intake below 30 percent of calories, daily vitamin E intake dropped from 14.5 to 9.5 IU.

Even the DV, however, is only a measure of what it takes to prevent a deficiency, while most of us—and most doctors—are interested in how much vitamin E we might need to significantly improve health. There's a huge gap between the DV and what researchers call the optimal value. And when it comes to discussing optimal value, there's even more divergence of opinions and recommended amounts.

While some researchers recommend from 100 to 400 IU a day, a number of clinicians recommend even higher amounts for people age 45 and older or for those with chronic diseases. One study, from researchers at the University of Texas Southwestern Medical Center in Dallas, found that the minimum dose of vitamin E required to significantly reduce LDL oxidation was 400 IU a day. Doses up to 1,200 IU—which is 40 times the DV—provided additional benefits. Taking 200 IU a day did not significantly reduce LDL oxidation, they found. Given this wide range of results, Dr. Traber and other experts are involved in ongoing discussions about new guidelines for recommending vitamin E.

Is E for You?

Certainly, it's worth discussing with your doctor whether you should take vitamin E supplements, and of course, you'll want to ask about risks. One concern is that large doses of vitamin E might elevate the risk of bleeding problems and lead to hemorrhagic stroke, a fairly uncommon type. Unlike other strokes, it's caused not by a blood clot but by a bleeding or broken blood vessel in the brain.

The same study that saw a reduction in the risk of prostate cancer in men taking 50 to 75 IU of vitamin E also saw an increase in the number of hemorrhagic strokes in the men who took vitamin E. The percentage of men in the study who actually had strokes, though, remained fairly small.

"This is a finding that poses additional questions and requires further study," says Demetrius Albanes, MD, a senior investigator in the cancer prevention studies branch of the National Cancer Institute.

The link with hemorrhagic stroke is directly related to the way vitamin E works. One reason that vitamin E helps to reduce heart attack risk is that it interferes with little particles in the blood called platelets, which play a role in blood clotting. Platelets can clump together or stick to artery walls when they shouldn't, which can cause a clot that closes off an artery. Vitamin E helps to prevent that, but it could also prevent the platelets from sticking and clumping when they need to.

Until there are answers about vitamin E's real effects on the risk of bleeding problems, and until additional research supports vitamin E's beneficial effects on cancer and cardiovascular disease, Dr. Albanes suggests caution when you consider taking more than the Daily Value. Before giving you the go-ahead for large doses of vitamin E, your doctor can do a test that checks your bleeding time. With that test in hand, you're better able to discuss the benefits versus possible risks.

Choosing the Right Form

As for what form of vitamin E to take, research supports getting vitamin E in as close a form as possible to that found in nature. One of the best dietary sources of these natural forms of vitamin E is raw almonds, sunflower seeds, or walnuts.

In supplements, the closest to "natural" is a blend of all eight of the forms of vitamin E: alpha, beta, gamma, and delta tocopherols. (They may be listed on labels as "mixed tocopherols" of "mixed tocotrienols.") Most multivitamins contain only d-alphatocopherol, so you'll need to take a separate vitamin E supplement to obtain enough vitamin E in its different forms. Look for one that contains a good mix of vitamin E in its natural forms.

echinacea

When you catch a cold or the flu, it means that your body has been invaded by opportunistic microorganisms in the same way that an unsavory gang would take over a neighborhood. You need the cops to run them off and restore order to the land—and in your body, that's what white blood cells do.

They start in the passages of your nose and throat—that's where they launch their first attack against invaders. If they're successful, it stops right there and then. If not, prepare for a few days of misery.

And while they do a pretty good job most of the time, those white blood cells could use some backup. That's where certain herbs, like echinacea, can help. The beautiful North American Purple Coneflower acts as an immunostimulant, meaning it can kick your immune system into high gear.

Power Up with Early Intervention

The active components of echinacea fire up your body's early response system, which is the first line of defense against any organism trying to make a home in your body. Echinacea stimulates early responders called macrophages, which engulf invading cold and flu germs. In addition to gobbling up whatever they can, the macrophages produce biochemicals, called cytokines, that call in the rest of the immune system defense squad. When these other white blood cells arrive, macrophages show the posse the invaders they've captured, and white blood cells then crank out the antibodies that target the specific infection you have. It's like the macrophages tell the rest of your immune system: "These are the bad guys we want to get. Take it from here."

Because it revs up the first stages of the immune response, you need to take the herb at the very first inkling that you have a cold or flu. So take your first dose at the first sneeze or the initial tickle in your throat—and then keep taking it for the next 7 to 10 days. If you do so, you may be able to shorten the duration and lessen the symptoms of your illness, says Alison Lee, MD, a pain-management specialist and medical director of Barefoot Doctors, an alternative medicine practice in Ann Arbor, Michigan. During cold and flu season, it's probably smart to keep a bottle of it with you at all times, Dr. Lee says.

While it's famous as a cold stopper, it also has antiviral and antibacterial properties, so it speeds healing for skin ailments. It has been used to treat candida, a maddening yeast infection, and in some cases it's even used as a mouthwash to treat gingivitis.

Call It a Comeback

Echinacea has long been popular in Germany, but interest in it waned in the United States once antibiotics became widely available and it was no longer needed for saddle sores and snakebites. Now, though, with antibiotic resistance on the rise, echinacea has made a bit of a comeback, along with other herbal contenders, says David Winston, AHG, an herbalist and ethnobotanist with a practice in central New Jersey and coauthor

SUPPLEMENTSNAPSHOT

▶Echinacea

Botanical names: *Echinacea purpurea, E. angustifolia, and E. pallida.*

Origin: Native to the Great Plains and southern United States; currently scarce in the wild but cultivated in the United States and Europe.

May help: Colds, flus, upper respiratory infections, middle ear infections, chronic vaginal yeast infections (if used orally in conjunction with a topical anti-fungal), and psoriasis (used topically).

Special instructions: Use at the first sign of a cold or other infection, not as a long-term preventive.

Cautions and possible side effects: Not recommended for people with autoimmune diseases such as lupus, rheumatoid arthritis, or multiple sclerosis. Do not use if you are allergic to plants in the daisy family, such as chamomile and marigold. Consult your doctor before using for longer than 8 weeks.

of *Winston & Kuhn's Herbal Therapies and Supplements: A Scientific and Traditional Approach.* "It's an herb people are familiar with and use to treat colds and flu," he says.

Dozens of studies prove echinacea's effectiveness as an immune stimulator, and science seems to point to a group of polysaccharides, a combination of different kinds of sugar molecules, as an important active ingredient in echinacea. In addition, echinacea contains many other compounds that seem to have antiviral properties and a gearing-up effect on the immune system. "With herbs, it's not always possible to isolate all of the active ingredients, especially [an herb] that seems to have as many as echinacea," Winston explains. But the research on echinacea is leading to a better understanding of how it works, he points out.

Pick Your Fighters

In health food stores, you'll probably find dozens of echinacea products. The herb comes as a tincture, a freeze-dried extract in capsules or tablets, and a simple herb powder packaged in capsules. Some echinacea extract products are standardized for the active ingredient, echinacoside.

Despite the availability of methods to identify echinacea species, echinacea products are frequently mislabeled or may contain no echinacea at all. The claim "standardization" does not indicate accurate labeling. "I like tinctures best, and I would look for a product that says explicitly that the product contains the leaves and flowers of *E. purpurea* or the roots of *E. angustifolia,*" Winston says. A tincture that contains a good amount of active ingredients will produce a distinct tingling in your mouth and on your tongue. "That means it's stimulating your immune system," Winston says.

Be Generous with Your Dose

Research shows that people make a couple of mistakes when they take echinacea, Winston says. They don't take enough of it early on, and they stop taking it too soon. "You can start taking it if you are around a lot of sick people and don't want to get sick, like a schoolteacher in a classroom of coughing kids," he says, or, "you can take it when you first feel that tickle in the back of your throat that means you've got something." Start with 2 or 3 ml (40 to 60 drops, if you're using the tincture), every 2 to 3 hours. Don't skimp on it or it won't work, Winston says. Continue to take it until you feel pretty much recovered, or even a few days beyond that at a lower dosage. "It does not hurt to continue taking it for a while, and it does not stop working," he says.

If you have an autoimmune disease such as lupus or rheumatoid arthritis, you should be cautious, says Dr. Lee. "These diseases are partly due to an already overactive immune system. Anything that stimulates the immune system may, in theory, be harmful," she says. "You may be able to use echinacea really short-term, but I'd consider other choices, such as zinc."

enzymes

Driving from New York to Los Angeles takes several long days, even if you keep driving at a steady rate of speed. Hop on a jet, however, and you'll make the transcontinental trip in less than 6 hours.

Enzymes are the jet engines in our bodies. They take some plodding chemical processes and add considerable zip so our bodies get the job done, and fast. Enzymes accelerate nearly every chemical reaction.

In fact, high-speed action is written into the definition of an enzyme. It's any protein that increases the rate at which a chemical reaction occurs. Many of these chemical reactions happen in the mouth, stomach, and intestine, where enzymes immediately go to work on your morning toast and cereal and continue to assail every food that you put in your mouth all day long. Other enzymes speed up nerve impulses that make your heart pump, your head turn, and your hand pull away from a hot stove.

At a less obvious level, enzymes help form cell structures such as the genetic code (DNA) that determines everything from your eye color and height to the number of gray hairs you're getting—or losing. In fact, without enzymes to speed along the process, very few chemical reactions would proceed at a meaningful rate.

A lot of enzymes are needed to crack these many whips, and our bodies are home to an estimated 10,000 different ones. Each has a specific, nontransferable role. The enzyme that speeds digestion won't do a thing to help your nerves, and one that's dedicated to forming new cell structures is useless when it comes to driving nerve impulses.

Given their many intricate roles, however, there are good reasons to respect the enzymes that we have—and also to give them a helping hand from time to time. If any are missing or not doing their jobs, an appropriate enzyme supplement may be useful, says David B. Roll, PhD, professor of medicinal chemistry at the University of Utah College of Pharmacy in Salt Lake City.

Gut-Level Aid

The enzymes that seem to need the most assistance are those in our intestines. These digestive enzymes break down the food we eat so it can be stored in the liver and muscles, where other enzymes act upon it to produce energy. Digestive enzymes also make sure that the nutrients in our food are absorbed.

In the stomach and intestines, a variety of these digestive enzymes work on carbohydrates, fats, and proteins, breaking them into pieces that can be absorbed through the lining of the small intestine. The more food that's digested, the better, since your body relies on that energy supply.

If food is allowed to pass undigested through the small intestine and into the large intestine, bacteria will prey upon it, causing bloating and other intestinal problems, says Dr. Roll.

One food that many people have trouble digesting is milk. That might seem odd, since most of us grew up thinking that we had to drink three glasses a day. But a surprising number of adults have a condition called lactose intolerance, which means that they have trouble digesting a natural sugar that's in all milk, as well as other dairy products such as ice cream.

SUPPLEMENT SNAPSHOT

▶Enzymes

Individual names: Lactase, lipase, amylase, protease, alpha-galactosidase, bromelain, papain, pancreatin, and other digestive enzymes.

May help: Digestive problems such as irritable bowel syndrome and indigestion; lupus; and chronic fatigue syndrome.

Who's at risk for deficiency: The elderly, people with digestive disorders such as chronic pancreatitis, and those with cystic fibrosis.

Cautions and possible side effects: Alpha-galactosidase supplements alter the way you process sugar; if you have diabetes, check with your doctor before using. Do not use if you have galactosemia, a rare condition that causes an adverse reaction to all foods containing the sugar galactose. Do not take if you are sensitive to mold or penicillin; these supplements are often made from a type of mold.

Help for Intolerance

If you're lactose intolerant, you're actually short on an enzyme called lactase. Without that worker-bee enzyme in your intestines, you can't handle the lactose that accompanies the milk on your morning cereal. You need that enzyme to break down lactose into smaller sugars that are easier to digest.

Without lactase, lactose sits around too long in your small intestine. Left undigested, it is fermented by bacteria, causing gas, cramping, and bloating.

When people discover that they're lactose intolerant, it's usually because they have these symptoms. Once you know what the problem is, you can usually deal with it by avoiding dairy products or taking an enzyme supplement that can ease the symptoms. Available in tablets, drops, or treated milk and sold under brand names such as Lactaid and Dairy Ease, lactase enzymes take over the exact function of the missing natural lactase. The supplemental enzyme cracks the lactose sugars into smaller, more easily digestible components.

Bean Busters

As soon as intestinal gas is mentioned, you can be sure that the conversation will quickly turn to the lowly bean. Surely, this is a food—if ever there was one—that needs some firm coaching in the digestive process.

The fact is that, yes, most of us do have a hard time digesting beans. Here again, an enzyme supplement can come to our aid. It's an easy-to-take supplement that can also help with other gas producers such as broccoli, cabbage, and onions. These foods contain certain complex sugars that we cannot digest. The sugars ferment in the large intestine, causing gas and abdominal distress.

Alpha-galactosidase to the rescue. This supplement is highly effective and has been known to save many from social embarrassment. Products containing alpha-galactosidase include Beano, The Ultimate Florazyme, and Prevail Bean/Vegi Enzyme Formula.

In the small intestine, alpha-galactosidase supplements help break down the indigestible sugars found in certain foods. This benign action helps to stop gas before it starts.

The supplements come as drops or tablets, and dosage instructions are right on the bottle. If you get the drops, however, don't add them to foods during cooking, since high temperatures kill the active enzymes. Instead, add drops to your first bite of food.

Other Enzymes to Watch

While many of us don't need enzyme supplements to aid normal digestion, that may change as we age. "As we get older, we don't produce adequate amounts of some enzymes," says Dr. Roll. "In that case, supplements may be helpful for digestion."

Enzymes that deal with the gut-wrenching effects of lactose and beans are just two of many that can help with digestion and are available in supplement form.

Many supplements contain pancreatin, a combination of enzymes derived from the pancreas of a hog or an ox; some are made up entirely of pancreatin.

You can also find supplements made from natural enzymes that are extracted from tropical fruits—bromelain from pineapple and papain from papaya. Both help your body digest protein if you are lacking digestive enzymes. Some people who get bloating and cramps after eating high-protein foods like steak may benefit from these supplements.

Enzyme supplements designed to aid protein digestion must be enteric-coated so they can pass safely through the stomach and into the intestinal tract, where they perform their function, says Dr. Roll. Without the coating, the supplements would be digested in your stomach and therefore be useless.

feverfew

Feverfew, a common perennial known to gardeners for its feathery foliage and aromatic blossoms, has been used as a botanical medicine since AD 78. The herb earned its name because it was commonly used to lower fever, but today, it's more likely to be used by herbalists as a headache cure.

Some good evidence of feverfew's headache-healing powers emerged in the mid-1980s during a study at the City of London Migraine Clinic. All of the people included in the study were accustomed to taking crushed feverfew leaves for their headaches, but researchers wanted to find out scientifically whether the cure worked as well as people claimed.

To test its effectiveness, one group was given capsules of pulverized feverfew leaves and another was given capsules that looked exactly the same but contained no feverfew. (These were placebos.) Neither group knew what they were taking. The people in the placebo group experienced a return of their headaches, while those taking the real thing did not. The feverfew was apparently doing its job.

After the study was published in 1985, feverfew emerged from the obscurity of the garden and stepped into the limelight of botanical healing.

"I use it 100 percent of the time with my patients for migraines because it usually works," says Jennifer Brett, ND, a naturopathic doctor in Stratford, Connecticut. "It's a good alternative for people who have tried everything else."

An Herb for the Head

The modern view of this herb is fairly close to that of 16-century herbalist John Gerard. In 1597, Gerard recommended this member of the chrysanthemum family to "them that are giddie in the head" and suggested placing a poultice of the leaves on an aching noggin.

Ingesting rather than wearing the herb is the recommended course of treatment today, but it's clear that the early healers were on to something, says Steven Dentali, PhD, a natural products chemist with Dentali Associates in Troutdale, Oregon, and a member of the advisory board of the American Botanical Council. "This is really a case where the folk use coincided with the science," he says. "Feverfew appears to be a good alternative to the drugs now being used for migraines."

In previous centuries, feverfew wasn't just for headaches. Herbalists recommended it to relieve menstrual pain, expel the placenta after birth, treat arthritis, and break fevers. The common name is derived from *febrifugia,* which is Latin for "fever reducer."

"It does work for reducing fevers, but probably no one really uses it for that anymore," says Dr. Brett.

A Spasm Stopper

Just how feverfew works, scientists aren't certain. The leaves—the medicinal parts of the plant—are rich in parthenolide, a compound that makes the walls of the blood vessels in the brain less reactive to substances that cause them to contract and dilate. That's how migraines begin. The opening and closing of blood vessels may set off pain nerves and inflame the smooth muscles that line the blood vessels, says Alison Lee, MD, a pain-management specialist and medical director of Barefoot Doctors, an alternative medicine practice in Ann Arbor, Michigan.

SUPPLEMENTSNAPSHOT

▶Feverfew

Botanical name: *Tanacetum parthenium.*

Origin: Native to central and southern Europe.

May help: Migraines, menstrual pain, osteoarthritis, and rheumatoid arthritis.

Special instructions: For migraine prevention, take regularly; you may not see benefits for several months.

Cautions and possible side effects: Do not take if pregnant or breast-feeding. Chewing fresh leaves may cause mouth sores; take capsules containing powdered leaves, instead.

"Feverfew has a pronounced regulatory effect on these vascular muscles," she explains. "It seems to calm them down."

The herb may also inhibit the release of two inflammatory substances that cause the vessels to go into spasm in the first place—serotonin from blood platelets and prostaglandin from white blood cells. Because prostaglandin and other related substances are also culprits in the inflammation that occurs during painful bouts of rheumatoid arthritis, feverfew has been used in its treatment as well, says Dr. Lee. "If I have a patient who isn't a candidate for other anti-inflammatory treatments, I might recommend feverfew."

Since the herb can lessen or regulate the spasms of smooth muscles, it's not surprising that it also has a reputation for easing menstrual cramps. It also seems to prevent migraines that coincide with menstruation, adds Dr. Brett.

Give It a Chance

As a migraine preventive, feverfew is effective for 70 to 80 percent of the people who use it, says Dr. Brett. It takes time to work, however, and you may need to take it daily for two to five months before it has any effect.

"You can't just take a feverfew pill when you feel a migraine coming on. It won't do any good," she explains. "You have to take it over a long period."

You'll find capsules of powdered leaves in health food stores and drugstores. Look for a product with a parthenolide concentration of 0.2 percent or higher, says Dr. Dentali. Make sure there's an expiration date on the bottle, and always store the herb in the refrigerator, says Dr. Dentali, since some of the plant's chemical constituents are sensitive to warm temperatures.

fiber

Think about what you ate yesterday. How many high-fiber foods did you have? If you're like most Americans, probably not enough. The typical American diet includes only 10 to 15 grams of dietary fiber a day, but the Daily Value is 25 grams. For many of us, that means doubling our current intakes.

For more than two decades, scientists have been taking a close look at fiber and its potential health benefits. What they've found is that high-fiber diets may decrease the risk of colon and breast cancer; ease constipation and irritable bowel syndrome; and help prevent diverticulosis, hemorrhoids, high cholesterol, and diabetes.

Nature's Glue, Nature's Sponge

Fiber is the indigestible part of all plant foods, including fruits, vegetables, grains, and beans. It is not found in meat or any other animal foods. Most fiber-rich foods contain both soluble and insoluble fiber. Soluble fiber dissolves in water in your intestinal tract, forming a gluelike gel. It softens stools and slows down stomach emptying, allowing for better digestion and helping you feel fuller longer, an effect that may promote weight loss.

Soluble fiber has been credited with lowering blood cholesterol. It may also help people with diabetes by lowering the amount of insulin necessary to process blood sugar after a meal. When taken with plenty of water before meals, a soluble fiber supplement binds with water in the stomach and forms a gummy mass—and that's what makes us feel full.

Insoluble fiber is the champion of the gastrointestinal tract. It's a good natural laxative because it holds onto water and moves waste quickly through the intestines, says David Beck, MD, chairman of colon and rectal surgery at the Ochsner Clinic in New Orleans. It also adds bulk and softens stools.

In general, soluble fibers are found in higher concentrations in fruits, oats, barley, and beans. When shopping for soluble fiber supplements, you can choose from psyllium, gums, mucilages, glucomannan, or pectins, says Dr. Beck. Insoluble fibers are more abundant in vegetables, wheat, and cereals; supplements include wheat bran and flaxseed.

Although it's helpful to classify fiber as either soluble or insoluble, we need both kinds in our diets. And some fibers don't fit neatly into categories. Psyllium, for example, is a soluble fiber that promotes bowel movements—a benefit usually associated with insoluble fiber. And rice bran, an insoluble fiber, lowers blood cholesterol, which is a trait of some soluble fibers.

SUPPLEMENT SNAPSHOT

▶Fiber

Supplement forms: Psyllium, gums, mucilages, glucomannan, pectins, methylcellulose, calcium polycarbophil, flaxseed, and brans.

Daily Value: 25 grams.

May help: Colon cancer, breast cancer, heart disease, diverticulosis, hemorrhoids, constipation, diabetes, overweight, Parkinson's disease, irritable bowel syndrome, indigestion, high blood pressure, and high cholesterol.

Good food sources: All plant foods. The best sources include high-fiber wheat-bran cereals, beans, dried figs, peas, raspberries, bulgur, oatmeal, pears, sweet potatoes, oranges, apples, and barley.

Who's at risk for deficiency: Many Americans; average consumption is only 10 to 15 grams a day.

Special instructions: Do not take with food; always drink at least 8 ounces of water for each tablespoon of fiber that you take.

Cautions and possible side effects: Do not take if you have trouble swallowing. Talk to your doctor before taking any fiber supplement, especially if you have diverticulitis, ulcerative colitis, Crohn's disease, bowel obstruction, or any other serious gastrointestinal disorder, or if you are taking any medications. (Fiber blocks absorption of medications.) May cause bloating or constipation.

Moving Things Along

Some studies have shown a link between high-fiber diets and a decreased risk of colon cancer, says Dr. Beck. Since fiber increases the bulk of the stool, it may dilute cancer-causing substances there. It also moves waste faster through the digestive tract, leaving less time for potentially harmful or even cancerous substances in your stool to have contact with the lining of the bowel, he says.

Fiber, particularly insoluble fiber, is also thought to help prevent hemorrhoids and diverticulosis, a condition in which small sacs develop in weak areas of the intestinal wall. (Because fiber softens stools and speeds up the movement of waste through the intestinal tract, waste doesn't linger in the intestines and sacs don't have a chance to form.)

Fiber may also help ease the symptoms of irritable bowel syndrome, a condition characterized by alternating constipation and diarrhea, gas, and cramps. Sometimes fiber can make this condition worse, though, so talk with your doctor to see if fiber supplements are right for you.

While much research has focused on the link between fiber and gastrointestinal health, studies also show that dietary fiber may protect against breast cancer, according to David P. Rose, MD, PhD, DSc, chief of the division of nutrition and endocrinology for the American Health Foundation in Valhalla, New York. High fiber intake has been shown to reduce estrogen levels in the blood, he says. That's important because high levels of estrogen are associated with increased breast cancer risk.

Fiber may reduce estrogen by binding with it in the intestine before carrying it out of the body in the stool. Fiber may also help prevent the reabsorption of estrogen in the blood.

Be Heart Smart

Studies have shown that people who get the most fiber in their diets are less likely to have heart disease.

In a Finnish study of nearly 22,000 male smokers ages 50 to 69, men who ate the most fiber, averaging 35 grams daily, suffered one-third fewer heart attacks than those who ate the least fiber. To look at it another way, each 10 grams of fiber added to the diet decreased the risk of death from heart disease by 17 percent.

In a study of 44,000 male health professionals, those who ate more than 25 grams of fiber a day had a 36 percent lower risk of developing heart disease than those who ate less than 15 grams daily.

Soluble fiber gets a big chunk of credit for helping the heart because it has repeatedly been shown to lower blood cholesterol levels. It does so in several ways, says Tom Wolever, MD, PhD, professor of nutritional sciences and medicine at the University of Toronto. When we fill up on fiber, there is less room for high-fat, high-cholesterol foods. In fact, a growing number of studies show that a diet rich in soluble fiber will lower blood cholesterol levels by 6 to 8 percent, he says.

Soluble fiber has another cholesterol-lowering effect, Dr. Wolever says. It binds with bile acids, which affects the way the liver handles blood cholesterol. As a net result of this process, cholesterol levels go down.

This cholesterol-lowering effect of fiber seems to be limited to specific foods and supplements that contain a generous amount of soluble fiber, including pectin, guar gum, psyllium, oat bran, oatmeal, and legumes.

Do You Need a Fiber Supplement?

Health experts generally recommend that you get your fiber from food, not supplements, because food contains nutrients that supplements don't.

"I don't often prescribe fiber supplements, because I want people to change to a whole-foods diet," says William D. Nelson, ND, a naturopathic doctor at the Docere Naturopathic Centre in Colorado Springs. Patients who switch from processed and fast foods to whole foods, including whole grains, fresh vegetables, fruits, and beans, usually don't need supplemental fiber, he says.

Sometimes, though, we can't or won't get all the fiber we need. That's when supplements can help, says Dr. Beck. "Most of us are very busy. Fiber supplements allow us to worry less about what we're eating."

Whether you're adding more fiber-rich foods to your diet or taking fiber supplements, you need to increase your intake gradually. Since fiber isn't absorbed, it can ferment in the intestine, causing gas, bloating, cramps, and diarrhea.

Always drink at least 8 ounces of water with a fiber supplement, advises Dr. Beck. Fiber acts like a sponge, and if you don't drink plenty of fluids, it can swell and block part of the gastrointestinal tract. It can also block the esophagus, so experts recommend avoiding fiber supplements if you have trouble swallowing.

Too much fiber can block the absorption of minerals such as iron, calcium, and zinc. It could also cause calcium losses.

If you supplement, try to get your fiber from a variety of sources in addition to a high-fiber diet. Look for products like psyllium, apple and grapefruit pectin, guar gum, methylcellulose, and calcium polycarbophil. At your local health food store, you may also find wheat and oat bran tablets and multifiber tablets with ingredients like beet and carrot fibers.

Psyllium is a popular and inexpensive fiber supplement with a laxative as well as a cholesterol-lowering effect, says Dr. Nelson. This supplement is available in pill, capsule, or powder form. All forms are equally effective, but fiber capsules and tablets are more expensive than powders.

You'll have to take as many as 10 tablets or capsules to get the same amount of fiber you'd find in a tablespoon of psyllium seed powder, says Jennifer Brett, ND, a naturopathic doctor at the Wilton Naturopathic Center in Stratford, Connecticut. With so many pills to take, people tend to abandon them more quickly than they do powder supplements.

Psyllium causes gas and bloating in some people. If that happens to you, try flaxseed, which is easiest to take by grinding fresh flaxseed in a coffee bean grinder. Use it on cereals or in smoothies or baked goods. In addition to fiber, flaxseed contains lignans, compounds that may have anticancer, antibacterial, antifungal, and antiviral effects, says Dr. Nelson.

Be leery of marketing claims that fiber supplements containing chitosan (a form of chitin, which is a component of the shells of shellfish) promote weight loss, says Dr. Brett. "I've never seen any evidence that it works for weight loss," she says. Even if chitosan did remove fat from the body as its proponents claim, it would also bind with and remove fat-soluble vitamins that your body needs, she says.

Animal studies have shown that chitosan can absorb LDL cholesterol (the bad type) and reduce lipid concentrations, but further studies are needed to confirm any cholesterol-lowering action. As for a weight-loss effect, some animals in the studies actually gained weight when they were fed chitosan, while others lost.

fish oil

Imagine going to your favorite fast-food restaurant and ordering a blubber-packed whaleburger on a sesame seed bun instead of a flame-broiled burger. Sound unhealthy?

Maybe not.

Like some types of fish, whales and other marine mammals are high in a type of fat called omega-3 polyunsaturated fatty acids. Physicians working in the Arctic first began to uncover the heart-healthy benefits of omega-3s when they puzzled over why the Inuit Eskimos—who regularly dined on a high-fat, high-cholesterol diet of whale, seal, and fish—rarely developed heart disease.

Later, studies in Greenland confirmed that the rate of heart disease among the Inuits was much lower than that of Westerners, even though both diets provided similar amounts of fat.

The difference, scientists concluded, was due to the source of fat in the two diets. Whereas Westerners get their fat from land animals and plants, the Inuits get most of theirs from marine mammals and fish. Since this discovery, much research has focused on the role of the omega-3s and their impact on heart disease and other ailments.

Not All Fats Are Created Equal

Our bodies make most of the fat they need from the carbon, hydrogen, and oxygen atoms that are found in food. But they don't have any way to create omega-3s and another type of fatty acids, omega-6s. Both of these belong to a category called essential fats, and they come only from certain foods.

There are two forms of omega-3s. The first is made up of eicosapentaenoic acid (EPA) and docosahexaenoic acid (DHA). To get your fill of these, feast on fatty fish such as salmon and mackerel.

The second type of omega-3s is alpha-linolenic acid (ALA), which is provided by plant foods. Once it's inside your body, some ALA can be converted into EPA and DHA. Sources high in ALA include flaxseed oil, black currant oil, walnut oil, hemp seed oil, and canola oil.

The other essential fat that the body can't manufacture is known as omega-6, or linoleic acid. While omega-6 oils are vital to our health, we may be getting too much in our diets. Most vegetable oils today have very high amounts of omega-6s but not enough omega-3s, and that kind of imbalance could turn into risky business for our bodies.

Scientists think that in the diets of our ancestors, the ratio of the two types was nearly 1 to 1. While a ratio of 2:1 is considered healthy by experts, the omega-6/omega-3 ratio of most Americans is about 15 to 1. (In other words, *way* too high!) When linoleic acid dominates too heavily over omega-3s, it may jeopardize our health.

SUPPLEMENTSNAPSHOT

▶Fish Oil

Supplement forms: Omega-3 fatty acids, eicosapentaenoic acid (EPA), and docosahexaenoic acid (DHA).

May help: Heart disease, angina, high blood pressure, high cholesterol, asthma, breast cancer, colon cancer, lupus, multiple sclerosis, arthritis, gout, migraines, prostate problems, eczema, ADHD, and any sort of condition involving inflammation.

Good food sources: Mackerel, salmon, herring, sardines, arctic char, bluefish, chunk light tuna, and rainbow trout. Shellfish such as shrimp and crab also have some omega-3s.

Cautions and possible side effects: Increases bleeding time, possibly resulting in nosebleeds and easy bruising, and may cause upset stomach. Do not take if you have a bleeding disorder or uncontrolled high blood pressure, take anticoagulants (blood thinners) or use aspirin regularly, or are allergic to any kind of fish. Take fish oil, not fish-liver oil, which is high in vitamins A and D—vitamins that may be toxic in high amounts.

Fish Oils to the Rescue

The body uses both types of omegas to create a variety of short-lived, hormonelike substances called eicosanoids. These substances perform many functions, such as regulating blood pressure, controlling important aspects of the reproductive cycle, and inducing blood clotting, among other things.

Prostaglandins, one of the better-known types of eicosanoids, have an effect on the brain, blood vessel walls, certain blood cells, and blood platelets. They are involved in regulating almost every body function, including those of the digestive, nervous, and reproductive systems. Prostaglandins also influence the ways in which blood vessels expand and contract, and they help manage blood clotting.

When an overabundance of prostaglandins and other eicosanoids is set loose in the body, the result may be excessive blood clotting and narrowing of the arteries. That's where fish oils may act. EPA and DHA decrease the stickiness of the blood platelets involved in clotting, thus reducing the risk of a clot that could lead to a heart attack.

If omega-6s dominate and omega-3s are in short supply, eicosanoids can provoke inflammation, blood clots, and other problems. If omega-3s are plentiful, more anti-inflammatory messengers are made.

Prime Your Pump

Let's return to the Inuits. Studies have revealed that their omega-3-rich diet results in lower blood cholesterol, lower triglycerides (another type of blood fat), lower LDL cholesterol (the "bad" type), increased HDL cholesterol (the "good" type), and lower rates of heart disease. These Eskimos also have prolonged bleeding times. Ominous though that sounds, it is actually something that heart disease researchers like to see, because it means that blood is thinner and therefore flows more smoothly.

There's also evidence that fish consumption may make heart attacks less dangerous if they do happen. In one study, a number of men who had survived heart attacks went on a diet that was high in fish. Compared to male heart attack patients who just had normal diets, those in the fish-eating group were more likely to live longer.

How does fish oil help the heart? The omega-3s in fish oil may reduce the risk or even the severity of heart disease by influencing several factors, including blood clotting and blood pressure. Omega-3s may also reduce the risk that a person will have cardiac arrhythmia (irregular heartbeat), although in some people they can make the condition worse, so check with your doctor before taking fish oil for an irregular heartbeat.

When you eat foods that are high in omega-3s, that valuable fish oil becomes incorporated into the cell membranes of platelets, making them less likely to clump together. In a way, fish oil acts like a very weak form of aspirin, which also has a good reputation as a heart disease preventive and, like fish oil, is believed to decrease the clumping of platelets.

Aid for Arthritis

Various studies have tested fish-oil treatments for the symptoms of rheumatoid arthritis, the kind of joint-attacking arthritis that can begin as early as childhood. After analyzing data from the 10 best-conducted trials to date, researchers concluded that taking fish-oil supplements for at least 3 months resulted in modest but positive improvements—mainly a decrease in morning stiffness and tender joints.

The amounts of fish-oil supplements used in most clinical studies are high—about 3,000 to 5,000 milligrams, and sometimes more, of omega-3s daily. To get this much from your diet, you would have to eat at least 10 ounces of cooked rainbow trout. Most fish-oil supplements contain about 500 milligrams of omega-3 fatty acids in each 1,000-milligram capsule.

You may be able to benefit from smaller amounts of fish oil, as well. In one study, women who ate two or more servings of broiled or baked fish a week had about half the risk of developing rheumatoid arthritis as women who ate only one serving.

Fish oil appears to ease rheumatoid arthritis and a variety of other inflammatory diseases by suppressing inflammation. While no one seems ready to proclaim fish oil a cure, at least one study has shown that it helps reduce or even eliminate the need for the nonsteroidal anti-inflammatory drugs that are most commonly prescribed for the disease.

An Ocean of Uses

Fish oil may even prove beneficial in preventing and treating certain cancers. When it comes to reducing the risk of colon cancer, there's evidence

What's in a Name?

Fish-oil supplements are sold under many names, from the obvious, such as fish oil or omega-3, to the not-so-obvious, including supplements that feature docosahexaenoic acid (DHA) or eicosapentaenoic acid (EPA) prominently in the name. Chances are, most fish-oil supplements include a mixture of EPA and DHA, no matter what they're called. Usually, a closer look at the label will tell you.

Although they are often packaged together, they do possess different health benefits. EPA is more beneficial for promoting heart health. DHA, which is highly concentrated in brain tissues, promotes the proper functioning of brain and nerve tissues. DHA is used to help prevent age-related macular degeneration; to enhance brain development during pregnancy and infancy, and in preterm infants; and for treating depression, bipolar disorder, and attention deficit and hyperactivity disorder (ADHD).

As a preventive, most experts recommend getting 500 to 1,000 milligrams daily of omega-3 fatty acids, including both EPA and DHA. However, if you are treating a condition, you may need 1,000 to 3,000 milligrams a day, or more. Check with your doctor for the ideal dose for you.

that doses of about 2,500 milligrams a day might help with prevention. In one study, researchers found that this amount helped to reduce the abnormal cell proliferation associated with an increased risk for colon polyps and cancer.

Researchers are also looking into links between fish oil and reducing childhood asthma; helping women have healthier pregnancies and healthier babies; improving bone growth; and lengthening remission for patients with Crohn's disease (a chronic inflammatory gastrointestinal disorder) who are already in prolonged remission.

Fish oil might even influence the nervous system. For years, researchers have linked depression with low intake of fish oils. New research shows that supplementing with omega-3 fatty acids may lessen the symptoms of disorders such as depression and bipolar disorder.

Easy Does It

If you decide to supplement with fish-oil capsules, stick with a reasonable dose, says William S. Harris, PhD, professor of medicine at the University of Missouri in Kansas City. "You'll probably get good health benefits from taking one or two fish-oil capsules a day if you don't want to eat fish," he says. The American Heart Association currently recommends 1 gram daily for people with existing heart disease and notes that people with elevated triglycerides may need 2 to 4 grams per day.

If you eat fatty fish, you need to be aware that many fatty fish contain toxins such as mercury, dioxins, and other fat-soluble chemicals, which they ingest from smaller fish or from contaminated water. To check the mercury levels of various fish, see the Environmental Defense Fund's Seafood Selector (and Sushi Selector) at www.edf.org.

To prevent the same kind of contaminants in fish oil, make sure that you buy a brand that has been molecularly distilled. These days, most brands are and will say so on the bottle. And check the expiration date—pills can go rancid. (They'll smell fishy when they go bad.) Store fish-oil capsules in the freezer—this not only keeps them fresh, but it also reduces the not-so-fun side effect of fishy burps!

flaxseed

You've probably worn and touched more flax than you've eaten. Linen, that cool staple of summer wardrobes, is made from flax, as is linseed oil, which is used in paint and varnish. But the blue-flowered flax plant is cultivated for more than cloth and paint. Researchers have turned up some pretty convincing evidence that flaxseed and flaxseed oil may improve heart health, fight breast and colon cancers, boost the immune system, ease rheumatoid arthritis, cool down hot flashes, and provide other healthy benefits.

Flaxseed is one of the richest sources of alpha-linolenic acid (ALA), a plant source of omega-3 fatty acids. As mentioned in the fish-oils chapter, the omega-3s are one of two families of essential fatty acids that are necessary for growth and development and cannot be made by the body. Omega-3s are the building blocks of eicosanoids, hormonelike compounds that regulate blood pressure, clotting, and other bodily functions.

Other fatty acids, omega-6s, are abundant in vegetable oils such as corn, soybean, safflower, and sunflower oils, as well as in the many processed foods made from these oils. They're also available in meat from grain-fed livestock.

The discoveries about omega-3s and omega-6s are relevant to flaxseed as well as to fish oil. Our bodies function best when our diets contain a well-balanced ratio of these fatty acids, meaning no more than four times as much omega-6 as omega-3. But we typically eat 10 to 30 times more omega-6s than omega-3s, which is a prescription for trouble, says Artemis Simopoulos, MD, president of the Center for Genetics, Nutrition, and Health in Washington, DC, and author of *The Omega Plan*. This imbalance puts us at greater risk for a number of serious illnesses, including heart disease, cancer, stroke, and arthritis, he says.

As we've noted, an excess of omega-6 fatty acids, when not checked by a complementary amount of omega-3s, can lead to the overproduction of potentially inflammatory biochemicals called prostaglandins and leukotrienes.

A deficiency of omega-3s is linked to various skin disorders, arthritis and joint stiffness, irritable bowel syndrome, premenstrual syndrome, immune dysfunction, and depression, says Michael Janson, MD, president of the American College for Advancement in Medicine, based in Laguna Hills, California, and author of *The Vitamin Revolution in Health Care.* As the most abundant plant source of omega-3 fatty acids, flaxseed helps restore balance and lets omega-3s do what they're best at—balancing the immune system, decreasing inflammation, and lowering some of the risk factors for heart disease.

Seeds of Hope

These small brown seeds hold some big promise for combating breast and colon cancer. In animal studies, flaxseed has significantly reduced existing breast and colon tumors while stopping new ones from getting started. In one study, researchers at the University of Toronto were able to reduce tumor size by more than half in animals that were fed flaxseed over a 7-week period. Flaxseed and flaxseed oil reduced the growth of existing tumors, but another component of flaxseed, called lignans, appeared to help prevent the development of new ones.

SUPPLEMENT SNAPSHOT

▶Flaxseed

Botanical name: *Linum usitatissimum.*

Origin: Consumed in Europe and Asia since around 8,000 BC; introduced to North America during Colonial days but not widely used as food until the 1960s.

May help: Heart disease, heart arrhythmia, high cholesterol, angina, breast cancer, colon cancer, diabetes, stroke, lupus-related kidney damage, low immunity, irritable bowel syndrome, high blood pressure, fingernail problems, constipation, diarrhea, hot flashes, gout, migraines, asthma, osteoarthritis, rheumatoid arthritis, and dermatitis.

Special instructions: Take with food.

Cautions and possible side effects: Generally regarded as safe.

Lignans are plant-based compounds that can block excessive estrogen activity in cells, reducing the risk of certain cancers. Many plants have some lignans, but flaxseed has at least 75 times more than almost any other plant.

Lignans are phytoestrogens, meaning that they are similar to but weaker than the estrogen that a woman's body produces naturally. Therefore, they may also help alleviate menopausal discomforts such as hot flashes and vaginal dryness.

Flaxseed also appears to reduce the risk of heart disease and stroke. One way that ALA helps the heart is by decreasing the ability of platelets to clump together, a reaction involved in the development of atherosclerosis (hardening of the arteries), says Dr. Janson. ALA also lowers levels of dangerous LDL cholesterol and helps the body rid itself of blood fats called triglycerides, which, at high levels, can also be harmful to heart health.

Need more convincing? The ALA found in flaxseed oil has an anti-inflammatory effect that can help treat a number of illnesses, says Emily Kane, ND, a naturopathic doctor in Juneau, Alaska. In her practice, she recommends flaxseed oil for inflammatory diseases such as arthritis, irritable bowel syndrome, and asthma.

Flaxseed oil and lignans have also been credited with reducing inflammation of the kidneys experienced by some people with a condition known as lupus nephritis. Lupus is an autoimmune disease that affects the skin and other organs.

Flax Facts

Flaxseed oil comes in liquid and gelatin capsules, but you may want to skip the oil and just add ground flaxseed to your diet. Flaxseed is also an excellent source of fiber, whereas the oil has virtually none. Two tablespoons of ground flaxseed, the usual recommended daily dose, contain 3 grams of fiber—as much as you'll find in a slice of high-fiber bread. The fiber is beneficial for treating constipation and diarrhea, says Dr. Janson.

If you do go with oil, make sure it says that it contains lignans on the bottle.

Whether you decide to go with the seeds or the oil, keep the following tips in mind.

• Skip the gelatin capsules. Oil is less processed, more practical, and less expensive than capsules. With 1,000-milligram capsules, for example, you'd have to swallow about 10 capsules a day to equal 1 tablespoon of the oil. A typical daily dose for overall health is 1 tablespoon; therapeutic doses range from 1 to 3 tablespoons, depending on the severity of your condition and your weight, says Dr. Kane.

• Stick with flaxseed oil from the refrigerated section of your health food store. Buy only oil that comes in an opaque bottle, and store it in the refrigerator as soon as you get home. Or, if you don't plan to use it right away, keep it in the freezer. Flaxseed oil degrades quickly when exposed to heat and light.

• Look for oils certified as organic by a third party. Also, quality oils have a "pressing date" listed on the bottles. If the oil was pressed more than 6 months ago, don't buy it, says Dr. Kane.

• Use flaxseed oil for salad dressings instead of vegetable, olive, or other oils. The oil has a nice nutty taste, says Dr. Kane. She recommends the following salad dressing recipe: Combine ½ cup olive oil, ½ cup flaxseed oil, ⅓ cup freshly squeezed lemon juice, and 1 heaping tablespoon of prepared mustard. Shake well for a few minutes before serving. Refrigerate between uses.

• Never cook with flaxseed oil, since it's sensitive to heat.

• To avoid weight gain, be sure to take the high calorie content of oil into account when figuring your daily calorie intake.

• Grind whole seeds in your electric coffee grinder and sprinkle them on cereal, add them to smoothies, or mix them with yogurt or oatmeal.

• You can store whole seeds in a cool, dry pantry for up to one year. Use any ground flaxseed immediately or keep it in the freezer.

folic acid

Here's an easy way to remember the best sources of this essential B vitamin: think "foliage." Folic acid and its food form, folate, were discovered by researchers who waded through 4 tons of spinach to isolate enough of it to study.

You don't need to eat 4 tons of spinach to get all the folate you need in a day. If you have a yen for spinach, about 4 cups of the raw greens will provide the Daily Value of 400 micrograms. (Like your spinach cooked? You'll have to eat twice that amount, since up to half of the folate in foods is lost during cooking.) Or you can get a spinach-bowl's-worth of this nutrient in capsule form.

Genetic Engineering

Folic acid is essential for DNA and RNA synthesis. That means it has to be on hand for your body to make the genetic material—the blueprint—that allows a cell to grow and divide to make more cells. "Folic acid actually helps to make the building blocks, called bases, that are strung together like pearls to form the DNA," says Barry Shane, PhD, professor of nutrition and chair of the department of nutritional sciences at the University of California at Berkeley.

RNA is kind of a "working copy" of DNA. Parts of DNA can be copied to RNA when a cell has to make a certain kind of protein, for instance. The RNA then travels to the part of the cell where the protein can be made and hands over the instructions.

"More folic acid is needed for this process when cells are rapidly dividing, as they do during growth and development, and in areas where cells normally have a relatively short life, such as the intestines and blood cells," Dr. Shane says. When folic acid is in short supply, DNA synthesis slows, and cells lose their ability to divide and multiply. That has the potential to create major, bodywide problems. In the blood, for instance, it can cause anemia, a lack of red blood cells. In the intestines, it can create absorption problems. Folic acid deficiency can also be a factor in heart disease. In some cases, when your body is short on this nutrient, it produces abnormal cells. This condition is called dysplasia, and it can lead to cancer. Low folic acid levels during pregnancy can set the stage for birth defects.

SUPPLEMENT SNAPSHOT

▶Folic Acid

Also known as: Folate; folacin.

Daily Value: 400 micrograms.

May help: Prevent birth defects, including defects of the neural tube, cleft palate, and cleft lip; reverse precancerous cell changes (dysplasia) in the cervix, lungs, or colon; treat megaloblastic anemia, canker sores, depression, gout, and gingivitis. With vitamins B_6 and B_{12}, can also lower blood levels of homocysteine to reduce risk of heart attack and prevent intermittent claudication, phlebitis, Alzheimer's disease, angina, and high blood pressure.

Good food sources: Spinach, lentils, navy beans, pinto beans, fortified breads and cereals, and sunflower seeds. Heat and oxidation during cooking and storage can destroy as much as half of the folate in foods, so many food sources don't provide very much.

Who's at risk for deficiency: People who use the cholesterol-lowering drug cholestyramine (Questran); people with cancer; the elderly, especially if their diets are nutritionally deficient; pregnant women; people recovering from burns; those who have had blood loss, gastro-intestinal tract damage, chickenpox, or measles; alcoholics; and smokers.

Special instructions: Best taken on an empty stomach.

Cautions and possible side effects: Do not take doses above 1,000 micrograms a day without medical supervision. Large doses may increase your need for B_{12}.

Tired Blood

If folic acid intake is low enough for long enough, you'll develop mega-loblastic anemia. In this form of anemia, "your red blood cells are unable to fully mature, and if you look at them under a microscope, they're large and egg-shaped," Dr. Shane explains. Your body also produces fewer red blood cells than you need for good health. Normally, cells in the bone marrow crank out red blood cells at the rate of 200 million a minute, but in this case, there's just not enough folic acid to maintain this pace without producing a lot of duds.

Megaloblastic anemia is most likely to occur during pregnancy, when there is an increased requirement for growth, and in people taking drugs that deplete the body of folic acid, Dr. Shane says. "Most people who develop this sort of anemia have been low on folic acid for months. It is also a fairly common problem in the elderly," he adds.

Cancer Cop?

Folate's reputation as a nutrient that reduces your risk of developing cancer comes from studies that show that folate deficiency definitely increases your cancer risk. Here's how it works: Cancer results from an accu-mulation, over time, of damage to the DNA. Smoking, exposure to harmful chemicals, frequent exposure to x-rays, and certain viruses can damage a cell's genetic material. Add the injury of a folic acid shortage to any one of these insults, and "you are turning up the speed of the damage severalfold," explains Patrick Stover, PhD, professor of nutri-tional biochemistry and cell biology at Cornell University in Ithaca, New York.

Folic acid deficiency has been strongly linked to DNA damage in sev-eral studies. In one, researchers at the University of California at Berkeley found that even a mild deficiency caused a large increase in the amount of damaged DNA. Other studies have shown a link between folic acid defi-ciency and dysplasia in the cervix, colon, and lungs.

On the other hand, once cancer is established, cancer cells need folate just as much as normal cells do. "In fact, drugs that mimic the structure of folate and inhibit its function, such as methotrexate, are used to treat cer-tain cancers," says Dr. Stover.

Does that mean you should limit your folate intake if you have cancer? Not necessarily, Dr. Stover says. "The theory that taking large amounts of folic acid can increase cancer risk is highly contentious in the scientific arena, but the literature has some seriously flawed studies and the well-done studies show that high levels of folic acid intake neither prevent nor accelerate cancer," he explains. Lung cancer may be an exception, he says, so it may end up being one case where you do want to limit high-dose folate.

So the recommendation for people with cancer (as well as those trying to prevent it) is to get 400 micrograms a day, which is plenty for just about everyone. You'll get that amount by eating folic acid–fortified foods, such as enriched breads and cereals, pasta, rice, and cornmeal, and by eating naturally rich foods like dark leafy greens, citrus fruits, lentils, and dried beans. If you're taking a multi, chances are that has folate, too. But don't take an additional folate supplement with the intention of preventing cancer.

Healthy Heart Combo

What happens to that steak you devour? In your body, protein from the steak is broken down into bits—amino acids—that your body can disassemble even further, then reassemble to make some urgently needed new amino acids. The amino acids may be strung together again to form new proteins, so that steak may eventually help form cells in your nose. Folic acid helps that happen because it helps to metabolize—break down and reassemble—several amino acids.

In that role, folic acid deficiency may play a part in the development of heart disease. It is needed to transform homocysteine—an amino acid by-product that in high concentrations is toxic to the body—to a more useful form called methionine. "When you don't have enough folic acid, blood levels of homocysteine rise, and those higher levels are linked with an increased risk of heart disease and stroke," says John Pinto, PhD, associate professor of biochemistry at Weill Medical College of Cornell University and director of the nutrition research laboratory at Memorial Sloan-Kettering Cancer Center, both in New York City. "In fact," he says, "the connection seems to be as strong as, if not stronger than, the connection between high cholesterol and heart disease. So this isn't a mere curiosity. It's something to pay attention to."

High levels of homocysteine contribute to heart disease in a couple of nasty ways, Dr. Pinto says. They damage the cells lining the blood vessels, creating rough spots that attract cholesterol deposits. Plus, they cause blood to clot more readily at those rough spots. When that happens, the artery-clogging clots begin to set the stage for heart attack or stroke.

"One problem being investigated right now is how much folic acid you need to protect against heart disease," Dr. Pinto says. In one study, people who got 5 milligrams a day for 2 weeks had significant drops in homocysteine, especially those whose initial levels were high.

But don't take folate acid alone at this high dose to reduce homocysteine levels. A combination of three vitamins—folate, B_{12}, and B_6—is most effective at reducing homocysteine levels. A good dosage combination to start with is 50 to 100 milligrams of B_6 a day, in divided doses; 400 micrograms of folic acid; and 2,000 micrograms of B_{12}.

Building Better Babies

To "construct" a baby, a woman's body has to turn a single fertilized egg into billions of cells, all in 9 months. That takes a lot of DNA and RNA—and so it takes a lot of folic acid. "Requirements for folic acid increase in a pregnant woman, both because of the rapid rate of cell growth and division in the fetus and because the woman is making more cells herself," says Joseph Mulinare, MD, chief of the prevention branch at the birth defects division of the Centers for Disease Control and Prevention in Atlanta. During pregnancy, a woman's blood volume may increase by as much as 50 percent.

For years, pregnant women in the United States and other countries sometimes weren't getting enough folic acid, and the result was birth defects, especially spinal cord and brain problems called neural tube defects. These defects are initiated very early in fetal development—often before a woman knows she is pregnant. That's why, starting in 1998, the folic acid fortification of grains became mandatory in the United States and Canada. That increased folic acid intake by 100 to 200 micrograms a day and led to a dramatic reduction in neural tube defects.

Still, some women benefit from additional amounts from a multivitamin or prenatal supplement started about 3 months before they begin trying to conceive and continued for at least the first 3 months of pregnancy. Those who might benefit include women using birth control pills prior to conception and women who've had a previous pregnancy resulting in a neural tube defect. (They may have a higher-than-normal need for folate.) Amounts recommended range from 400 micrograms to 4 milligrams a day (for women with a previous neural tube defect), so it's best to talk with your doctor about the amount that's right for you.

gamma-linolenic acid

In the Middle Ages, people used borage, an herb with bright blue flowers, to treat heart disease and rheumatism and to reduce inflammation. They were on to something: Borage is a source of gamma-linolenic acid (GLA), a polyunsaturated fat with anti-inflammatory properties. Those properties are why today it's used to treat eczema, endometriosis, and premenstrual syndrome (PMS).

The three other GLA sources include evening primrose, black currants, and hemp seeds. But the human body also manufactures its own supply of GLA from linoleic acid, a nutrient that's abundant in vegetable oils and meats, according to Elson Haas, MD, director of the Preventive Medical Center of Marin in San Rafael, California, and author of *The Staying Healthy Shopper's Guide.*

GLA has fallen out of favor a bit because of the concern that the fatty acid could actually end up backfiring when it comes to your health. When converted in your body, GLA can go one of two ways: the healthy anti-inflammatory route or the not-so-great inflammatory route. GLA is also an omega-6 fatty acid. Most of us get more than enough omega-6 fatty acids in our diets (too much, in fact), and not enough omega-3s. We should have an omega-6 to omega-3 ratio of anywhere from 2:1 to 4:1, but the typical American diet is about 25:1, which leads to dangerous inflammation that can break down the body in various ways. That's why many experts have turned away from GLA to fish oil and fatty fish, since they are rich in omega-3s and have anti-inflammatory properties.

Possible Skin Saver

Still, proponents of GLA also believe the oil can help treat inflammatory skin disorders such as eczema, even though research has come up with conflicting evidence. (Two large studies have shown no benefit at all, but others have found improvement, particularly for patients with mild to moderate eczema.) The United Kingdom no longer allows GLA to be marketed as a treatment for eczema, but the National Institutes of Health's MedlinePlus gives it a "B"—meaning there is good scientific evidence that it is helpful for eczema and skin irritation. One thing is certain: If you use it, don't expect quick results. It can take months to see an improvement. Stick with evening primrose oil as a source of GLA. It outperforms borage oil, and hemp seed oil and black currant oil haven't been studied enough. Each 500-milligram capsule of evening primrose oil contains 45 milligrams of GLA. A typical dose of GLA is 200 to 250 milligrams a day, or five capsules.

SUPPLEMENT SNAPSHOT

▶Gamma-Linolenic Acid

Also known as: GLA.

May help: Eczema or dermatitis, fingernail problems, endometriosis, menstrual cramps, breast pain, premenstrual syndrome, and sunburn.

Special instructions: Take after a meal.

Cautions and possible side effects: Use organic, cold-pressed oil. Use in balance with omega-3s and only for 3 months or less to treat specific conditions. Do not use supplements without the supervision of a physician if you are taking aspirin or anticoagulants (blood thinners) regularly, have a seizure disorder, or are taking epilepsy medication such as phenothiazines. Do not take borage oil if you are pregnant or breast-feeding. May cause headaches, indigestion, nausea, and softening of stools.

garlic

No other medicinal herb is more universally recognized and consumed by people worldwide than garlic. It is valued in every major culture in the world as a food, condiment, culinary herb, and botanical medicine.

For at least 5,000 years, since the time of the Egyptian pharaohs and even before the earliest Chinese dynasties, people have used garlic as medicine. In central Europe in ancient and medieval times, peasants wore necklaces of garlic cloves to keep away vampires and other evils. It is used in China as a preventive for colds and a folk remedy for dysentery. "I find it fascinating that people have been aware of garlic's medicinal properties for thousands of years," says William Page-Echols, DO, an assistant clinical professor of family medicine who teaches alternative medicine at the Michigan State University College of Osteopathic Medicine in East Lansing. "People weren't just using it in flights of fancy. They knew it was beneficial."

The Taste of Medicine

In the last few decades, more than 1,000 scientific papers have been published on garlic and related herbs of the allium family. These studies provide strong—although not conclusive—scientific evidence that garlic has extraordinary medicinal powers.

Garlic seems to reduce blood pressure and cholesterol levels, dilate blood vessels, and thin the blood, all of which lower the risk of heart attack and stroke. It's believed to kill harmful bacteria in the stomach and protect against gastric and colorectal cancer. It appears to be a potent antioxidant and may boost the response of your immune system. It also works as an anti-inflammatory.

"When you think about the health problems that most people suffer from today, such as heart disease, cancer, and pain, they usually have as a component some type of inflammation," says Alison Lee, MD, a pain-management specialist and medical director of Barefoot Doctors, an alternative medicine practice in Ann Arbor, Michigan.

Across cultures, garlic has been used to treat colds, flu, sore throats, high cholesterol, high blood pressure, atherosclerosis (hardening of the arteries), digestive disorders, bladder infections, and liver and gallbladder problems.

"Garlic is an inexpensive, easy-to-obtain medicine," says Dr. Page-Echols. "You can incorporate it into your diet and get its benefits through food. Or, if you don't like the taste or odor of garlic, you can take it as a supplement."

A Healing Burn

The stinking rose, as garlic was called by the Greeks and Romans, is a member of the genus *Allium*, which also includes onions, leeks, shallots,

SUPPLEMENTSNAPSHOT

▶Garlic

Botanical name: *Allium sativum.*

Origin: May have originated in a west-central Asian desert; most garlic used today comes from widely cultivated modern hybrids.

May help: Heart disease, high blood pressure, infections, colds and flu, sore throat, high cholesterol, atherosclerosis, digestive disorders, diarrhea, bladder infections, liver problems, and gallbladder problems. May also help prevent stomach and colorectal cancer.

Special instructions: Try to get your quota of garlic from food, as it may be more easily absorbed into your system and it contains more active ingredients than garlic supplements do.

Cautions and possible side effects: Don't use garlic supplements if you're taking anticoagulants (blood thinners) or hypoglycemics (a type of diabetes drug). Do not take supplements if breastfeeding. Rarely, may cause allergic reactions. Can interfere with the therapeutic effect of some drugs, such as protease inhibitors and isoniazid (a tuberculosis drug). Use with caution if you have an infectious disease or an inflammatory condition of the stomach or intestines, as garlic can be irritating.

and chives. Allium, the ancient Latin name for garlic, is believed to come from an ancient Celtic word: *all*, meaning "hot" or "burning."

The volatile oil of garlic gives the herb its distinctive smell and taste. The oil contains more than 30 sulfur compounds, including allicin and a number of others that are biologically active.

The most important of these is allicin, which is produced only when you crush, bruise, or cut a garlic clove. As the membranes of the garlic cells break down, alliin, a sulfur-containing amino acid, comes into contact with an enzyme called alliinase. The resulting chemical reaction produces allicin, a pungent and strongly antibiotic compound.

Allicin is highly unstable and quickly degrades into a number of other chemical compounds. Some of these have therapeutic properties, but exactly how they work in the body has not been determined. Since the process begins with the formation of allicin, researchers believe the allicin content of garlic is the best indication of its medicinal value.

Killing Bad Bacteria

Louis Pasteur, who invented the process of milk pasteurization and developed the germ theory of disease, first demonstrated back in 1858 that allicin is a strong antibacterial. Before the advent of modern antibiotics in the 1930s, cuts and abrasions were treated by expressing garlic juice into a wound. On the Russian front in World War II, the Soviet army relied on garlic to treat the wounded when penicillin and sulfa drugs were not available.

This proven antibacterial action may have profound implications in the prevention of one of the world's most commonly fatal cancers: stomach cancer.

Scientists have found that *Helicobacter pylori,* a type of bacteria sometimes found in the stomach, appears to be involved in the development of stomach cancer and peptic ulcers, says Jonathan Sporn, MD, an oncologist and associate professor of medicine at the University of Connecticut Health Center in Farmington. There may be other factors as well, but the link to *H. pylori* is strong.

"We're not sure where these bacteria come from, but they're probably very common in the environment," explains Dr. Sporn. In fact, *H. pylori* infects half of the people on the planet and up to 90 percent of the populations of some developing countries.

In cultures with diets high in allium vegetables such as garlic and onions, the risk of stomach cancer is low, says Dr. Sporn. And in laboratory tests conducted at the Fred Hutchinson Cancer Research Center and University of Washington Medical Center in Seattle, scientists were able to kill *H. pylori* using a garlic extract. This study and others have found that garlic is toxic to many "bad" bacterial strains—even some that resist standard antibiotic treatment.

"It's very provocative evidence, and it fits with the folk wisdom surrounding the use of garlic," says Dr. Sporn. "These studies suggest that there may be something very valuable in garlic."

According to studies in India, garlic may actually benefit the good bacteria in the intestine, thereby improving digestion and boosting immunity in the gut. It has been used to reestablish good bacteria in the gut after an infection or antibiotic treatment.

Does all this mean that you should be eating garlic or taking garlic supplements every day? Perhaps, says Dr. Sporn. But how much? And how often? "That's the problem," he says. "Although we have evidence that garlic may be preventive against cancer, we don't have enough information yet to make any specific recommendations." However, in population studies where garlic has shown a preventive effect against colorectal and stomach cancers, people were eating anywhere from 3.5 to 29 grams of fresh or cooked garlic every week. A typical clove weighs about 3 grams, so that comes out to between 1 and just fewer than 10 cloves a week. Any good cook can figure out how to make that work.

Have a Heart for Garlic

Garlic may prevent two other major killers, heart disease and stroke, says Dr. Page-Echols. According to several studies, if you make garlic part of your diet or if you take it as a supplement, you may lower your risk of heart disease and atherosclerosis.

When fatty plaque builds up in arteries, blood flow to the heart and brain may be impeded. Clots can form, or chunks of plaque may break loose and form blockages. That sets the stage for a heart attack or stroke.

Garlic benefits the circulatory system in several ways. It lowers levels of cholesterol and triglycerides, another type of blood fat. It also has an antispasmodic action, meaning that it dilates blood vessels and increases blood flow to the heart and brain.

One especially important group of chemicals, called ajoenes, thin the blood and make clotting less likely. So even if you have plaque-filled arteries, the blood platelets are less likely to bunch up behind blockages. Essentially, they slide by a little more easily, says Dr. Page-Echols.

"Garlic can do a lot for your circulatory system. Just keeping the blood vessels more open can have a significant effect on hypertension. Your blood pressure drops," he says.

One study found that after just 4 weeks of taking garlic supplements, participants had a 5 to 6 percent reduction in total cholesterol. In another study, researchers at the University of California, Irvine, gave 40 men with elevated cholesterol levels either a combination garlic/fish-oil supplement or a look-alike, inactive capsule (a placebo). During the study, the men maintained their normal, Western-style diets and kept up their usual activities.

After 4 weeks, cholesterol levels in the group taking the supplements dropped by 11 percent. The placebo group showed no significant change. The researchers concluded that the combination of garlic and fish oil significantly reduces risk potential in people with elevated levels of cholesterol.

"The good thing is that garlic doesn't tamper with the good cholesterol, only the bad stuff," observes Dr. Page-Echols. "And for someone who wants to take a natural approach to taking care of their heart—in addition to better diet and more exercise—garlic can be very beneficial."

Spice Up Your Immune System

At least one component of garlic, alliin, is also an antioxidant. Some nutrients, such as selenium, vitamin C, vitamin E, and in particular alliin, scavenge free radicals—the free-roaming, unstable molecules that lead to cell damage and premature aging. Free radicals have also been implicated in the growth of tumors. In laboratory animals, garlic extracts have actually inhibited the growth of cancer cells.

Garlic is effective against bacterial, fungal, viral, and parasitic infections. The volatile oil is excreted by way of the lungs—hence garlic breath—and can fight infections in the upper airway. Some Chinese studies have shown that garlic has a beneficial effect in helping to battle colds and flu.

Because of garlic's antibacterial properties, it can help prevent secondary infections in people who have lowered immunity. An American study in 1989 found that protective natural killer cell activity was restored in some AIDS patients after they took garlic supplements for 6 weeks.

Fresh Is Best

Although some studies show that certain garlic supplements can have medicinal effects, the most consistent benefits seem to come from real garlic. Raw garlic is best, but lightly cooked garlic also retains many of its beneficial properties. Add some garlic during the last minute or two of cooking a stir-fry or some marinara, or even a minute or two before serving chicken soup. Use it raw in hummus, bean dips, and salad dressings.

If you want some of the benefits of garlic without eating it, supplements are available as tablets, capsules, and tinctures. Although oil-based garlic preparations are widely available, their effectiveness is questionable, since allicin is unstable in oil. Moreover, since allicin is formed only when the cells of garlic are crushed to create the enzyme reaction, dried garlic doesn't contain this important component. Therefore, there is concern that marketed garlic preparations may not have enough of the active ingredient allicin to be effective. And some odorless garlic preparations may contain no active ingredients at all.

Most clinical studies have used a standardized garlic powder extract containing 1.3 percent alliin, which is what you should look for in health food stores.

ginger

In ancient Rome, most spices were expensive because they were so scarce. Ginger was costly for just the opposite reason—because it was plentiful. It was so common and in such demand that the government taxed it.

After the fall of the Roman Empire, ginger almost disappeared from Europe, until Marco Polo rediscovered it in China and India in the 13th century. Once again, the European taste for spices made it a treasured and expensive ingredient. In 14th-century Britain, a pound of ginger could cost you an entire sheep.

Columbus was trying to find another way to bring ginger and other spices home when he stumbled upon North America, but he didn't find ginger in the New World. It wasn't until the English introduced it to the colonies that it became a popular spice in the Americas.

Once introduced, ginger didn't go away. Today, this lowly root enhances a wide variety of food and drink, from the flavoring in ginger ale to the thin-sliced pickled ginger that's served alongside sushi. For thousands of years, it's also been appreciated for its medicinal properties and employed by many cultures, including India's Ayurvedic medicine, traditional Chinese medicine, and Western herbalism. People have used ginger to treat indigestion, nausea, gout, flu, fever, headache, and flatulence.

Good for the Gut

The medicinal part of ginger is the rhizome, an underground stem that most people mistakenly refer to as a root. In Chinese and Ayurvedic medicine, the rhizome has a long-standing reputation as a digestive aid. It is ground up and used in numerous Chinese herbal prescriptions. Ayurvedic practitioners refer to ginger as the universal medicine because it aids the body's digestive function by relieving gas, bloating, and cramps, says Joseph Selvester, an Ayurvedic herbalist in Gainesville, Florida.

Western herbalists classify ginger as a carminative, an anti-inflammatory, and a diaphoretic, among other things. A carminative is an herbal remedy that settles the intestine and eases pain by removing gas from the digestive tract. Most herbs high in volatile oils have the ability to dispel gas and reduce bloating in the intestine, and ginger is rich in such oils.

As an anti-inflammatory, ginger is known to reduce the production of inflammatory compounds, which makes it useful for some types of headaches, for body aches caused by flu, and for arthritis.

A diaphoretic is capable of slightly raising body temperature and promoting sweating. "I use ginger for my patients who are unable to develop a fever to recover from a cold or flu," says Jill Stansbury, ND, assistant professor of botanical medicine, chair of the botanical medicine department at the National College of Naturopathic Medicine in Portland, Oregon, and a naturopathic doctor in Battle Ground, Washington. She recommends boiling sliced gingerroot in water, then adding honey and lemon to taste. "A cup or two of hot ginger tea, drunk while in a hot bath, can help induce a brief fever and speed recovery from an infection," she adds.

Lose the Woozies

If it's just an upset stomach or a woozy feeling that's unsettling your gut, you may want to turn to ginger. Two of the herb's active ingredients, gingerol and shogaol, help combat nausea, whether it's caused by flu,

SUPPLEMENTSNAPSHOT
_____

▶Ginger

Botanical name: *Zingiber officinale.*

Origin: Unknown; probably Southeast Asia; cultivated in India and China for thousands of years.

May help: Arthritis, indigestion, intermittent claudication, phlebitis, muscle soreness, heartburn, diarrhea, and nausea (including morning sickness and motion sickness).

Cautions and possible side effects: Fresh ginger is safe when used to season food. Do not use the dried root or powder if you have gallstones.

motion sickness, or the surging hormones of early pregnancy, says William Page-Echols, DO, an assistant clinical professor of family medicine who teaches alternative medicine at the Michigan State University College of Osteopathic Medicine in East Lansing.

Ginger appears to have no side effects, while many motion sickness drugs, such as dimenhydrinate (Dramamine), cause drowsiness. This makes it a safe alternative for pregnant women battling morning sickness. In a Danish study of pregnant women, 1,000 milligrams of ginger powder daily, divided into four doses, was effective. But you may need to experiment to find a dosage that works for you, says Dr. Page-Echols.

"It is safe to take during pregnancy, but as with any drug, I'd still recommend that you use it only when necessary or for short periods of time," he adds. Be sure to talk to your doctor first.

Motion sickness drugs act on the central nervous system, so some researchers believe that gingerol and shogaol work in the same way. Others believe that the medicinal action takes place in the stomach itself.

Saying No to Nausea

No one knows exactly how ginger helps to quell nausea, says Alison Lee, MD, a pain-management specialist and medical director of Barefoot Doctors, an alternative medicine practice in Ann Arbor, Michigan. You can't rule out some effect on the brain, she says, because a ginger tincture seems to work as well as a powdered supplement.

"Sometimes it just takes a drop or two on the tongue to stop nausea," she says. "It apparently gets into your bloodstream and inhibits the vomiting center in your brain."

If the mechanism isn't certain, the results are. A study involving 80 Danish naval cadets found that ginger is an effective treatment for seasickness. While the cadets were learning the ropes of seamanship aboard a training vessel in heavy seas, half the group was given 1,000 milligrams of ginger powder, while the other cadets received an inactive substance that looked the same (a placebo).

The cadets, ages 16 to 19, were good test cases because none had experience on the open seas, nor were any of them overly susceptible to becoming seasick. They were, so to speak, fresh fish. Over the following few hours, the ginger group had "remarkably" fewer symptoms of vertigo and nausea, according to the researchers. Ginger reduced vomiting and cold sweats better than the placebo did. The placebo group presumably spent more time retching over the side or running to the head. (That's ship talk for bathroom.)

Hot Spice for Heart and Joints

Ginger is good for your heart as well as your stomach. Among its other benefits, it seems to have a blood-thinning effect. In a study conducted in India, powdered ginger significantly reduced the clumping of blood platelets in people with coronary artery disease.

If platelets clump up, they can cause rough spots on artery walls, which then attract fat molecules that build up to form a dense, clogging substance called plaque. When enough plaque builds up, the arteries narrow, causing blockages that can lead to heart attack and stroke.

"The Chinese use dry ginger in many heart and kidney treatments, and in Ayurvedic medicine, ginger is considered a heart tonic," says Selvester.

In limited test-tube studies, ginger has also shown anti-inflammatory action. Research has shown that it can reduce pain and swelling in people with rheumatoid arthritis, osteoarthritis, and muscle pain.

Common over-the-counter anti-inflammatories like aspirin and ibuprofen work in a similar manner, but long-term use of anti-inflammatory drugs can have serious consequences. These drugs sometimes reduce the beneficial enzymes that maintain the protective mucous lining of the stomach. If that happens, the corrosive gastric juices that help digestion may irritate the stomach and cause an ulcer, says Dr. Page-Echols.

Easy Relief

Ginger appears to regulate two types of chemicals that are responsible for inflammation and to do it without the stomach-irritating side effects caused by anti-inflammatory medications.

Dr. Page-Echols recommends ginger—often in combination with the herb turmeric—to many elderly patients who have a history of using anti-inflammatories for chronic pain and arthritis. "They are at risk for developing bleeding ulcers from the typical drugs taken for inflammation," he says. "Ginger is easier on the system."

As with most herbal anti-inflammatories, if you take ginger for pain, it takes time to have the desired effect. You can't just pop a ginger supplement as you might an aspirin and get immediate relief, says Dr. Lee.

"Herbs do take time to work, but if you're in a situation where you have a chronic, recurring problem like arthritis, you need something that you can take often and safely," she says. "Eventually, the ginger will have an effect."

Food or Pill?

Ginger is readily available in several forms. Most pharmacies and health food stores sell ginger powder in pills or capsules. Look for an extract standardized to 5 percent gingerols when trying to treat arthritis or motion sickness, suggests Dr. Stansbury.

Candied ginger sticks are sold at many health food stores and may do in a pinch, especially for nausea, but they are probably less valuable for arthritic problems, says Dr. Stansbury. You can also incorporate ginger into your meals as a flavoring to help lower cholesterol. "Use fresh sliced or grated gingerroot in soups, stir-fries, rice, and salad dressings," she suggests.

Dr. Page-Echols recommends that his patients cook with ginger at least twice a week to help with arthritis, heart health, and general health. Many people in India use 8,000 to 10,000 milligrams of fresh ginger a day in cooking, he says. "A lot of people aren't accustomed to thinking of food as a medicine, but in this case, it really is. Ginger is something that most people have used in their food. I try to encourage them to use more and use it more often."

ginkgo

In 1945, a few months after the A-bomb leveled Hiroshima, the blackened, apparently lifeless stubs of ginkgo trees near ground zero sprouted new leaves. Although in its 200 million years on Earth, the ginkgo tree had never before encountered a nuclear blast, it was well equipped to survive the devastation.

Ginkgo is indifferent to fire, resists bug infestation, and thrives in dirty, polluted air; some individual trees have been known to live for up to 1,000 years. Such tenacity has made the ginkgo the oldest living tree species on Earth, a living fossil preserved from days when dinosaurs plodded the terrain.

Delaying Fossilhood

The medicinal compounds found in this ancient and remarkable tree may enable you to avoid turning into a fossil yourself—or at least keep you from doing so prematurely. A concentrated extract of ginkgo leaves can intensify blood circulation, avert heart attacks and strokes, rev up the brain, and even delay the progress of dementia and Alzheimer's disease. Thus, this mighty herb can help deter many of the afflictions associated with growing old.

Ginkgo biloba is *the* herb for an aging population, says Jennifer Brett, ND, a naturopathic doctor at the Wilton Naturopathic Center in Stratford, Connecticut. Most of Dr. Brett's older patients—those over 65—are taking supplements of ginkgo.

"People who are getting old worry about two things: Is my heart going to fail? Is my brain going to fail?" she explains. "In terms of prevention, this is an herb that people can take every day for the rest of their lives. It improves their general circulation and mental acuity."

In Europe, where botanical healing is common, many older people routinely take ginkgo extract to improve their mental fitness. It is the most widely prescribed herb in Germany and has been approved in that country as a treatment for dementias—afflictions (including the type caused by Alzheimer's disease) that are associated with loss of memory in older people.

It's in the Leaf

Ginkgo is native to China, where the fruit and seeds have been used for 4,000 years to treat everything from asthma to problems with frequent urination and nocturnal emissions. The seeds and fruit are highly toxic, always require careful preparation, and need to be given in carefully measured doses to avoid poisoning. The leaves were rarely used as a medicine until a few decades ago, when European researchers concentrated dried leaves into an extract and discovered their remarkable medicinal properties.

Working with the extract, the researchers isolated two groups of active chemicals: flavone glycosides and a unique set of terpenoids that the scientists called ginkgolides. Over the years, an extract of 24 percent flavone glycosides and 6 percent ginkgolides became the standard used in scientific studies. Today, this formula, known as EGb 761, is used throughout

SUPPLEMENT SNAPSHOT

▶ Ginkgo

Botanical name: *Ginkgo biloba.*

Origin: Native to China; the oldest living tree species on Earth.

May help: Age-related memory impairment, dementia, cognitive function, premenstrual syndrome, Raynaud's disease, vertigo, peripheral vascular disease, sexual dysfunction related to use of antidepressants, intermittent claudication, and diabetic neuropathy and retinopathy.

Cautions and possible side effects: Avoid ginkgo if you are taking anticoagulants (blood thinners), aspirin, or other nonsteroidal anti-inflammatory drugs, or antidepressant MAO inhibitor drugs such as phenelzine sulfate (Nardil) or tranylcypromine (Parnate). Taking more than 240 milligrams of concentrated extract may cause vomiting, diarrhea, or rash. Rarely, ginkgo may cause headache, stomachache, or other allergic reactions. Avoid ginkgo if you are pregnant.

Europe to treat heart disease, eye ailments, impotence due to low blood flow, tinnitus (ringing in the ears), poor circulation to the extremities, and head injuries and other brain-related conditions.

Although doctors and scientists don't fully understand how the chemicals in ginkgo work in the human body, the effects and benefits are pretty well known, says Alison Lee, MD, a pain-management specialist and medical director of Barefoot Doctors, an alternative medicine practice in Ann Arbor, Michigan. "Ginkgo is really an important herb because there's a lot of good research behind it," she says. "It works for many conditions."

The Blood Flow Balancer

Ginkgo is known as a vasoregulator herb, meaning it can either relax or contract blood vessels, and it seems to target the hair-thin capillaries that get blood, cell by cell, into every crevice in your body. It keeps capillaries dilated as they should be, and at the same time, contracts abnormally dilated capillaries. Ginkgo seems to restore the balance between prostacyclin, a biochemical that helps blood flow, and thromboxane A2, which promotes blood stickiness and clotting.

Dr. Brett routinely uses the herb to treat Raynaud's disease, a severe constriction of blood vessels in response to cold. Raynaud's sufferers literally can't get blood to their fingers and toes, she says, but with the active chemicals in ginkgo, the blood vessels expand, allowing more warming blood to flow to the extremities.

Dr. Brett also prescribes ginkgo to people with diabetes who have lost feeling in their feet due to inflamed nerves and high blood sugar levels. Ginkgo stabilizes the blood flow, and its glycosides have strong anti-inflammatory properties. "I use it for any circulatory disorder," she says. If you have diabetes and want to consider using ginkgo, discuss it with your doctor. Taking ginkgo can stimulate insulin secretion and speed up the breakdown of some diabetes drugs.

Thinning Action

Increasing blood flow isn't ginkgo's only action. The ginkgolides apparently thin the blood by counteracting the effects of platelet activating factor (PAF), a chemical that causes blood platelets to stick together and clot.

Clotting, as you might imagine, is pretty important when you've sliced yourself with the potato peeler. But PAF also forms clots when there's an irregularity in an artery, such as a chunk of fatty plaque sticking to the vessel wall, says Dr. Lee. "You want your platelets sticky when you get a wound, but you don't want them bunching up around plaque in a blood vessel," she explains. "That's going to create a blockage and reduce the flow of blood."

Thin blood will still clot, but it may take longer, says Dr. Lee. If you're already on an anticoagulant (blood-thinning) medication or taking aspirin to reduce your risk of heart attack or stroke, you should be very cautious about using ginkgo. "If you're already on a blood thinner, talk to your doctor," she cautions. "Two of my patients got nosebleeds after they started the ginkgo." There is also the possibility of bleeding within the brain.

Platelets are not the only blood cells modified by ginkgo, adds Dr. Lee. There's evidence that after several weeks, the herb eventually makes the membranes of red blood cells bend and stretch more easily. This effect may be important in increasing blood flow to the brain.

"If the membrane is more pliable, the cells can actually squeeze their way into tighter places, past blocked or partially blocked arteries and vessels," she says. "That may be very important in increasing blood flow, particularly in the small vessels in the brain."

Feed Your Head

The benefit of any increased blood flow is that your tissues and vital organs receive additional nutrients and oxygen. Increased blood flow to the brain has been shown to improve alertness, short-term memory, and the ability to concentrate. It may also relieve inner ear disorders such as vertigo and tinnitus, improve mood, and counteract depression.

Ginkgo not only feeds your head, it also improves the action of substances called neurotransmitters, which help carry signals between nerve cells. Influenced by the herb, these substances work more efficiently, so that messages travel from cell to cell more quickly. "This is an herb that can make you think better. It directly stimulates the brain," says Dr. Brett.

Ginkgo also apparently holds off or slows down the destructive consequences of an aging brain. Free radicals—the free-roaming, unstable molecules that invade cells and damage them—are natural metabolic by-products of aging. When free radicals cause damage in the brain, those cells quickly become inoperative. Substances in ginkgo help to scavenge free radicals and slow down the rate at which brain cells are damaged.

Some research in Europe and the United States has shown that ginkgo can be helpful to people who have age-related cognitive decline, dementia, and Alzheimer's disease. Unfortunately, a large-scale study in the United States found that it was not effective against Alzheimer's disease. But one study found that people with mild to moderately severe dementia who took 120 milligrams of ginkgo a day for a year appeared to stabilize or, in some cases, improve mental functioning. The researchers estimated that the ginkgo may have bought the patients a 6-month to 1-year delay in the disease. They note, however, that the treatment appears to work best in the early stages of the disease.

A Slow Process

For treating any condition, ginkgo takes time to build up in your system. You may have to take the herb for weeks before you begin noticing the benefits, says Dr. Lee. "I tell people to give it about 6 weeks," she says.

For long-term use, ginkgo is considered a relatively safe herb. Except at very high levels—more than 240 milligrams of concentrated extract—it usually produces no side effects, as long as you are not taking anticoagulant (blood-thinning) medication or taking aspirin.

Ginkgo is available in tablets and capsules, but the best way to take it is in tablets, says Dr. Lee. A standard dose is 120 milligrams a day. To avoid possible gastrointestinal discomfort, take one 40-milligram tablet three times a day.

At the drugstore or health food store, look for a supplement that contains 24 percent ginkgoflavonglycosides and 6 percent terpene lactones, says Dr. Brett. "Then you have the same concentration of the active ingredients that has been used in all the studies."

ginseng

If you drive through north-central Wisconsin on your way from Minneapolis to Green Bay, no doubt you'll notice some odd-looking farm fields along the way: 1- to 2-acre plots of knee-high, red-berried bushes growing beneath canopies of fabric.

You're in the ginseng capital of the United States. Those fabric canopies cut the light by about 80 percent, artificially reproducing the muted light of a hardwood forest, which was the original home of American ginseng.

Wild ginseng, once found east of the Mississippi River, is rather rare these days due to overharvesting. Cultivating the herb remains a difficult endeavor, but Wisconsin's cool weather and glacial soils, along with growing techniques that have been passed down through many generations, permit the region to produce 95 percent of America's ginseng crop. Most American ginseng root—the medicinal part of the plant—is exported to the Orient, where herbalists and doctors of traditional Chinese medicine value it as an overall body tonic or energy tonic.

American ginseng (*Panax quinquefolius*) is only one type. There are two other plants that are commonly called ginseng. Asian ginseng (*P. ginseng*) is also used in the Orient.

For over 2,000 years, Asian ginseng has been a mainstay of oriental medicine, used as a revitalizing agent for general weakness, lack of appetite, anemia, forgetfulness, and deficiency of the "vital energy" known as *chi*. But oriental doctors now often use American ginseng instead of the Asian species because it is said to be milder, less stimulating, and better suited for older patients and long-term use.

In recent years, many herbalists and herbal companies have begun using Siberian ginseng (*Eleutherococcus senticosus*), the third type. This plant isn't a true member of the ginseng family, but it's less expensive. Although it's a bit weaker than the true ginsengs, it has many of the same properties. Siberian ginseng is most often found as part of herbal formulas.

The medicinal properties and active ingredients of the three types are similar, and all can accurately be called energy herbs. Take them when you're fatigued, run-down, worn-out, or dealing with stress, suggests Alison Lee, MD, a pain-management specialist and medical director of Barefoot Doctors, an alternative medicine practice in Ann Arbor, Michigan.

Herbalists credit ginseng with elevating mood and reducing fatigue. It won't make you leap tall buildings or run a 4-minute mile, but it does seem to restore energy and improve performance—both physical and mental—says Julie Clemens, ND, a naturopathic doctor in Sagle, Idaho.

"I use it primarily as a tonic, mostly to improve people's vitality when they've been experiencing times of weakness," says Dr. Clemens. "That could be after the flu, after a funeral, or during times of great mental stress. I tell patients to use it for a short period of time, until they start feeling better."

Dr. Lee notes that the herb is not an instant stimulant. You might have to take it for a while before you begin to feel its effects.

SUPPLEMENT SNAPSHOT

▶Ginseng

Botanical names: *Panax quinquefolius* (American ginseng), *P. ginseng* (Asian ginseng), and *Eleutherococcus senticosus* (Siberian ginseng).

Origin: Grows only in eastern Asia and parts of North America; plants may be remnants of ancient forest that covered much of the Northern Hemisphere some 70 million years ago.

May help: Fibromyalgia, chronic fatigue syndrome, genital herpes, impotence, stress, muscle soreness, low immunity, and depression. May improve stamina, breathing, and coordination; normalize blood sugar levels; strengthen appetite; and increase alertness and reaction time.

Special instructions: Avoid coffee while taking.

Cautions and possible side effects: If you have a heart condition, high blood pressure, or an anxiety disorder, consult your doctor before taking ginseng. May cause insomnia, nervousness, diarrhea, headaches, and sometimes high blood pressure. Has been reported to cause menstrual bleeding in postmenopausal women.

The Friskiness Factor

Ginseng comes from the Chinese words *jen shen,* meaning "man root." The branches of the root resemble arms and legs, and the Chinese felt that the human appearance was a clue to its effectiveness as a whole-body tonic. Many Native Americans viewed the herb in the same way. The Penobscots believed that native ginseng increased female fertility, while the Fox of Wisconsin considered the plant a universal remedy. The plant genus, *Panax,* actually comes from the Greek word *panacea,* or cure-all.

There's some evidence that an active ingredient in ginseng, ginsenosides, might cause an increase in sexual activity, and the herb does have a reputation as an aphrodisiac. In the early 1800s, Appalachian folks gathered the plant in the wild to use when "old-timers used to go a'courting." As for the science behind the folklore, ginseng seems to cause the release of nitric oxide in blood vessels, which relaxes and dilates them. Increased nitric oxide release is the mechanism behind Viagra, the popular drug for erectile dysfunction.

Despite all of its folk use, ginseng never became a very important herb in American medicine, and it was never a favorite among old-time practitioners. One reason may be that ginseng really isn't a panacea, and many of the claims for it are exaggerated, says Tirun Gopal, MD, an obstetrician and gynecologist who practices holistic and Ayurvedic medicine in Allentown, Pennsylvania.

"Ginseng is one of the most abused herbal medications that I know of. If you look in any lay literature or magazine, it's still being touted as therapeutic for everything from cancer to an ingrown toenail," he says. "It certainly has its uses, but it is not a panacea."

Despite these reservations, though, there are still some things that ginseng seems to do quite well.

Adapting to Conditions

The Chinese think of ginseng as a normalizing or restorative agent. Western herbalists classify it as an adaptogen, an herb that has the ability to normalize function. It can be a stimulant, increasing alertness, reaction time, respiratory output, and motor coordination, or it can have a milder tonic action, lowering blood pressure, regulating blood sugar (glucose) levels, maintaining the immune system, and helping the body deal with the effects of stress.

"An adaptogen just sort of goes where it's needed, putting your body into a more balanced state," says William Page-Echols, DO, an assistant clinical professor of family medicine who teaches alternative medicine at the Michigan State University College of Osteopathic Medicine in East Lansing.

Ginseng's dual nature as both a calming influence and an energy booster can be traced to a group of active ingredients called panaxosides or ginsenosides. There are at least 13 types of ginsenosides in ginseng. Some stimulate the central nervous system, while others apparently act as pain relievers and tranquilizers, calming the stomach and nervous system.

Asian ginseng may be more stimulating than its American cousin because it contains a different balance of ginsenosides. No one is really sure, however, because there may be as many as 30 active ingredients in ginseng.

"I prefer American ginseng, because less stimulation is usually better," says Dr. Lee.

Energizing Agent

Ginseng has been used for thousands of years as a tonic to elevate mood and reduce fatigue. Some of the first scientific studies to gauge the herb's effectiveness included a study of mice that were able to swim longer distances after being given ginseng and a Russian study showing that soldiers who were given an extract of ginseng ran faster in a 3-kilometer race than those given a look-alike substance (a placebo).

Ginseng may give you an extra push in several ways. It temporarily increases the amount of oxygen uptake by the body and causes the muscles to use glycogen, the body's stored sugar, more efficiently, says Dr. Page-Echols. Also, ginseng augments the number of insulin receptors in the body, thus driving the sugar in foods into your cells, where it can be burned, he says.

"Not only does that give you more energy, it also lowers or regulates your blood sugar," says Dr. Page-Echols. "Ginseng improves the glucose balance in the body and improves its sensitivity to insulin." That's important to people who have high blood sugar, because insulin is the chemical released by the body to "escort" glucose into the cells, where it becomes a useful energy source.

A Finnish study found that newly diagnosed type 2 (non-insulin-dependent) diabetics who took 200 milligrams of ginseng extract daily for 8 weeks experienced improved blood glucose levels, enhanced mood, and better psychological and physical performance. When first diagnosed, these people were fatigued and depressed by their illness. Ginseng gave many of them the energy lift they needed to make lifestyle changes and cope better with their conditions, the researchers concluded.

Ginseng's stimulating properties have also been helpful in treating people with chronic fatigue syndrome. It can also help with depression when fatigue and stress are contributing factors.

Withstanding Stress

Adaptogens like ginseng have a unique capacity to strengthen the body's resistance to stress and limit damage caused by stress, says Dr. Lee.

Stress can make you irritable, weaken your immune system, and accentuate any pain or discomfort you may be feeling, she says. She sometimes prescribes ginseng to her chronic pain patients, especially if they work in stressful environments like noisy offices or construction sites or have high-pressure jobs. "Pain is a stress, too, so I use ginseng to help people tolerate pain and not be so run-down by it," says Dr. Lee.

Apparently, ginseng helps inhibit the output of chemicals and hormones that stress you out, says Dr. Page-Echols. An increased capacity to withstand stress keeps your immune system strong and makes you less susceptible to colds and other illnesses, he adds.

Ginseng also stimulates the immune system directly, increasing the function of natural killer cells and accelerating phagocytosis, the process in which white blood cells eat up invading bacteria or viruses. Although ginseng is not as powerful an herb as echinacea in this regard, it can help you fight off an infection, says Dr. Page-Echols.

"In the wintertime, some people take an immune stimulant, like echinacea or astragalus, daily, but you don't want to take the same one all the time because eventually, the herb loses its effect," says Dr. Page-Echols. "You can use ginseng as a substitute for a couple of weeks."

Spotting the Disguises

Each one of the ginsengs—American, Asian (Panax), and Siberian—is slightly different in its effects, and most herbal experts in the United States prefer to use American or Panax, because Siberian ginseng is often adulterated. Finding ginseng at your health food store is easy, but finding a quality product is a bit more difficult.

Dr. Page-Echols recommends looking for a tincture or capsules standardized to 7 percent ginsenosides. Most clinical studies of ginseng use this standard, and the supplement gives you some assurance that you're getting the real thing, he says. A good product will say on the label what kind of ginseng it contains, and that it is "whole root."

goldenseal

At the beginning of the 20th century, between the demise of old folk remedies and the emergence of professional medicine, came the hucksters of patent medicines—an odd breed of shady entrepreneurs, self-appointed doctors, and bona fide quacks.

One of the most successful was Dr. Roy Pierce, a physician who made a mint hawking Dr. Pierce's Golden Medical Discovery: The Only Guaranteed Liver, Blood, and Lung Remedy.

Dr. Pierce, who created an entire line of popular patent medicines, never discovered anything beyond the power of mass advertising and the public's gullibility in believing in a so-called magic elixir. His "discovery" consisted mostly of alcohol and sugars, but it did get its distinctive amber color from goldenseal, a medicinal herb long used by Native Americans.

Bacteria Batterer

The Cherokees used the roots and rhizomes of the plant to treat skin diseases and relieve sore eyes. Today, goldenseal is still used as an external wash for canker sores and skin wounds, but most people take it internally, usually in capsule form, to soothe inflamed mucous membranes, stop or slow down infections, and stimulate digestion, says Jennifer Brett, ND, a naturopathic doctor at the Wilton Naturopathic Center in Stratford, Connecticut. It is frequently recommended for ulcers in the upper intestine and especially advocated for respiratory infections, she says.

"It seems to be really effective for upper respiratory infections like sore throats and sinus infections," says Dr. Brett. "It has the ability to stimulate your immune system and slow down the rate at which bacteria invade your cells and tissues."

If used early, goldenseal is effective against nearly any kind of infection, from a sore throat to a cut on the hand, says Dr. Brett. Its antibacterial and antiseptic properties can help fight off bacteria. While that doesn't mean that goldenseal should be used in place of an antibiotic when one is needed, "it can help keep an infection from spreading long enough so that your immune system can take care of it," she says. "If the infection has really set in, though, you may need more help than goldenseal can give you."

Goldenseal can make the symptoms of an infection less bothersome. It's especially effective in reducing phlegm and drying up secretions from inflamed mucous membranes, the tissues that make up the inner lining of the body, explains Dr. Brett.

When you have irritated sinuses or a sore throat from postnasal drip, the herb can bring great relief, Dr. Brett says. "It works best when you can get the goldenseal right on the infection. I tell people to gargle with a tea of goldenseal when they have a sore throat."

Tastes like Medicine

In olden days, people generally put goldenseal root into water and brewed a tea, but it was a bitter tonic to swallow. Even rinsing out your mouth with goldenseal can be a memorably unpleasant experience. Herbalists classify it as a potent, bitter, astringent herb, and it simply tastes

SUPPLEMENT SNAPSHOT

▶Goldenseal

Botanical name: *Hydrastis canadensis.*

Origin: United States; was introduced to European settlers by Native Americans.

May help: Upper respiratory infections, inflamed mucous membranes, diverticulitis, colds and flu, heartburn, diarrhea, canker sores, chronic fatigue syndrome, urinary tract infections, and skin infections; also used for ulcers and as a digestive stimulant.

Cautions and possible side effects: Do not take while pregnant. Do not use if you have high blood pressure or an autoimmune disease such as multiple sclerosis or lupus or if you are allergic to plants in the daisy family, such as chamomile and marigold. Do not take for more than 1 week.

terrible, says Alison Lee, MD, a pain-management specialist and medical director of Barefoot Doctors, an alternative medicine practice in Ann Arbor, Michigan.

Traditionally, bitter herbs were used as stomach medicines, and goldenseal has a well-deserved reputation for stimulating the digestive system to secrete more bile and salivary and gastric juices, says Dr. Brett.

Whenever you produce more digestive juices, you also produce more digestive enzymes, which aid in digestion and can normalize bowel movements, she says. She often prescribes goldenseal as a cure for diarrhea caused by either a bacterial or viral infection.

"It's also a good treatment for stomach ulcers. Since we now know that most ulcers are caused by bacteria, it makes sense that it would be effective," she adds.

Flush the Toxins

Goldenseal has long been touted as a blood purifier, an herb that normalizes liver function. Some herbalists believe that the blood and liver can become congested with toxins when there's too much poison in the body for the liver and endocrine system to process, metabolize, and purify, says Dr. Lee.

By stimulating the digestive system, a bitter herb like goldenseal can increase the actions of the liver and spleen, pump out more bile from the gallbladder, and, in the process, expel more toxins through sweating and the excretion of waste. "It's a way to clean out the system. That's what bitters are said to do," says Dr. Lee.

Seeking Out Goldenseal

Many health food stores and drugstores carry goldenseal capsules and tinctures. Look for a standardized extract that concentrates berberine, the active ingredient, suggests Dr. Lee.

In comparison with other herbs with similar infection-fighting actions, such as echinacea and astragalus, goldenseal is expensive. Today, it is rare in the wild because of overcollecting. In fact, Dr. Lee cautions against its overuse because the plant is becoming endangered. Herb growers are just beginning to domesticate and cultivate it.

gotu kola

Commonly called Indian pennywort, gotu kola grows abundantly in the wetlands of India, Sri Lanka, and other parts of the Southern Hemisphere. When people in Sri Lanka observed elephants feeding extensively on the slender, creeping plant, they suspected that the herb was responsible for the elephants' long life span—up to 75 years. A Sri Lankan proverb advises, "Two leaves a day will keep old age away."

If this elephant tale sounds fanciful, consider the legend of Li Ching Yun, a Chinese herbalist who supposedly lived to be 256 years old because he regularly consumed gotu kola.

These stories clearly show one thing—people on the Indian subcontinent and in the surrounding region plainly believed that gotu kola promoted longevity and a healthier life.

Clear Thinking

Medicinal use of gotu kola comes from the Chinese and Indian (Ayurvedic) herbal traditions. The herb normalizes the nervous system, improving mental activity and well-being, says Priscilla Evans, ND, a naturopathic doctor at the Community Wholistic Health Center in Chapel Hill, North Carolina.

Gotu kola appears to have steroidlike properties, and in a number of studies, it also improved circulation. Either action could have a beneficial effect on the chemistry of the brain, says Dr. Evans. "We're not really clear about the herb's mechanism in the body, but we know it relaxes people and increases their mental clarity," she says.

Naturopathic doctors frequently mix gotu kola into their herbal formulas to help their patients relieve stress and rejuvenate their minds and bodies, says Irene Catania, ND, a naturopathic doctor and homeopathic practitioner in Ho-Ho-Kus, New Jersey. Gotu kola tends to balance out the function of the adrenal glands, which secrete hormones in response to stress, she says.

"When you're exhausted or burnt out, your adrenals are often fatigued," says Dr. Catania. "Gotu kola is a nice rejuvenating herb." Studies have also shown that gotu kola works as a botanical treatment for high blood pressure, varicose veins, burns, and circulatory problems. In Ayurvedic medicine, it was a popular treatment for healing skin ulcers and treating leprosy.

A Wound Healer

In Sri Lanka, people eat the leaves in salads or use them to brew a medicinal tea. The entire plant, however, has healing properties.

The most active compounds in the herb are triterpenes and saponin glycosides. The glycosides are particularly important. Animal studies have shown that two kinds of glycosides, taken in large doses, have a sedative or calming quality, while another type has anti-inflammatory properties. A fourth type seems to stimulate wound healing.

When researchers injected gotu kola extract into animals, they found that one of the glycosides seemed to increase the development and maintenance of blood vessels in connective tissue. That mechanism relates directly to its healing properties, because any time more blood is delivered to the site of a wound, the healing process is enhanced, says Dr. Catania.

In addition to helping the blood arrive where it's needed, gotu kola is like a food or balm for the connective tissues, says Dr. Catania. It contains many important raw materials, such as flavonoids, that help build healthy tissues.

SUPPLEMENT SNAPSHOT

▶Gotu Kola

Botanical name: *Centella asiatica.*

Origin: India, Sri Lanka, and other countries in the Southern Hemisphere.

May help: Varicose veins, poor circulation, wounds, scarring, keloids, stress-related high blood pressure, exhaustion, and burnout.

Special instructions: Take on an empty stomach.

Cautions and possible side effects: Do not take if you are pregnant or breastfeeding. Talk to your doctor if you are thinking of taking it for an extended period of time. Rarely, may cause rash or headache.

"Although you get some of these building blocks in your food, they're more concentrated in the herb," says Dr. Catania. "Gotu kola helps the structure of connective tissues develop normally."

Dr. Catania recommends gotu kola for people with skin conditions and for those who are about to have surgery or are recovering from an injury. It's also helpful for anyone who tends to heal poorly, a condition sometimes caused by diabetes.

Making Scars Scarce

Because gotu kola works well for skin conditions, it can be helpful in the treatment of cellulite and keloids, used topically or orally, says Dr. Evans.

Cellulite is caused by a hardening of connective tissue cells below the skin's surface. Gotu kola seems to be able to reduce or slow down this process.

"But you can't just take a few capsules of gotu kola and expect cellulite to go away," Dr. Evans warns. "The herb is beneficial because it has a general strengthening and toning effect on connective tissue. It should be just one part of a therapy that includes diet, exercise, and massage."

For keloids, gotu kola's action is much more direct. Keloids are raised, irregularly shaped, progressively growing scars. They form when healing fails to proceed as it should, resulting in an excessive formation of collagen. In other words, the scar continues to grow until it eventually turns into a type of benign tumor.

Gotu kola makes scars mature faster by enhancing the later stages of the healing process. In a study, researchers applied a topical extract of gotu kola to 139 patients with keloids or hypertrophic scars—scars in which the cells had grown dramatically in size. After 2 to 18 months of treatment, 82 percent of the study participants showed signs of improved healing as a result of using gotu kola.

Vein Vitality

Beneath the skin, gotu kola has long been an important herbal therapy for varicose veins. These lumpy purple veins form when the blood vessel walls weaken and blood flow is sluggish, particularly in the legs. Tiny valves within the veins no longer work efficiently, so instead of flowing steadily upward toward the heart, blood slips down through the weakened valves. As a result, the veins bulge and swell with stagnated blood.

Gotu kola strengthens the epithelium, the layer of cells that line the outside and inside of blood vessels and arteries, says Dr. Evans. It also strengthens the connective tissue sheath surrounding the vein, which makes it beneficial for preventing varicose veins.

"Gotu kola is an ideal tonic for the elderly," says Dr. Evans. Older people, she notes, are more likely to have problems with weakened blood vessels, particularly their veins. Also, it may take longer for their skin to heal after cuts, scratches, bruises, or similar injuries. Gotu kola helps with both of these problems—plus, it helps to improve mental clarity.

Gotu kola isn't difficult to find in health food stores, and it's also available in some drugstores. It's sold as a tincture, in capsules, and in bulk herb form. For topical use, look for a cream containing 1 percent gotu kola.

green tea

Drinking green tea is a soothing ritual for many people, as it has been for hundreds of years. It's said to nourish the body and mind and to provide a calming lift. But there's more to it than just taking the opportunity to slow down and sip a refreshing, hot cup of tea.

Research shows that there are lots of compounds in green tea that provide health protection. A class of flavonoids called catechins gets a good deal of the attention because of their anticancer possibilities. And drop for drop (or tea leaf for tea leaf) there's no better source of catechins in the human diet than tea. But what makes green tea so special is that even in the tea world, it is a catechin powerhouse—green tea contains about three times the quantity of catechins found in black tea. Green tea is less processed than black tea, and it's the fermentation process used to make black tea that reduces some of its catechin content.

Some of the catechins found in green tea are epigallocatechin gallate (EGCG), epigallocatechin (EGC), epicatechin gallate (ECG), and epicatechin (EC.) "These seem to be responsible for many of the proposed benefits of green tea, but there are many other constituents in green tea that may provide additional health benefits," says Chung S. Yang, PhD, director of the Rutgers University Center for Cancer Prevention Research, in Piscataway, New Jersey.

A Cup for Cancer Prevention

"In animal models, green tea does a remarkable job of preventing cancer—that is, of preventing tumors and reducing the size of tumors," says Jeffrey Blumberg, PhD, director of the USDA's Human Nutrition Research Center on Aging at Tufts University, in Boston. "In humans, however, it is not as potent."

In population studies, where people who drink green tea are compared with those who don't, green tea drinkers tend to have a reduced risk for gastrointestinal cancer, especially esophageal, stomach, bladder, liver, and colorectal cancer. They also have a reduced risk for skin cancer and for lung cancer, at least among nonsmokers.

When it comes to clinical trials, "there is data showing that biomarkers of cancer risk are reduced," Dr. Blumberg says. "That's a good indicator of how green tea may help to prevent cancer, but it's not the same as showing a reduction in the incidence of cancer." The few studies that have shown an actual reduction in cancer development have looked at oral leukoplakias, precancerous lesions in the mouth. Green tea, used as an oral rinse or paste, helps this precancerous lesion to change back to normal, healthy tissue.

How does it work? Researchers found that green tea may block receptors on the cancer cell surface and affect cell growth. But green tea also has indirect effects, as evidenced by lung cancer prevention, Dr. Yang says. For

SUPPLEMENT SNAPSHOT

▶Green tea, green tea extract

May help: Stroke, cardiovascular disease, cancer, cognitive function, genital warts (used topically), skin damage from sunburn, bone and teeth mineralization.

Special instructions: Drinking green tea appears to be safer and may provide stronger benefits than taking green tea extract or capsules. A commonly recommended dose of green tea is based on the amount typically consumed in Asian countries, which is 2 or 3 cups per day, providing 300 to 400 milligrams of polyphenols. Adding milk to tea reduces its effectiveness because milk binds to catechins and makes them unabsorbable. (Plant-based milks such as soy or almond don't have this effect, however.) Adding lemon or another citrus juice increases catechin absorption.

Cautions and possible side effects: Very high amounts of green tea components can interact with drugs that affect blood clotting, such as aspirin, and change the way the body metabolizes certain medications. High doses of green tea extract have caused liver damage, as shown by elevated liver enzymes. There is some concern that EGCG, concentrated in green tea extract, might decrease activity of folic acid.

one thing, it can affect signaling pathways—the messages a cell uses to control its functions. Green tea helps to "upregulate" or crank up antioxidant and other defense mechanisms in cells so that they are better able to fight inflammation and promote apoptosis—that is, programmed cell death when cells are in danger of becoming cancerous.

That might be one reason it seems to provide some protection from breast cancer. In one study, women with Stage I or II breast cancer who drank 3 or more cups of green tea daily had a reduced risk of breast cancer recurrence. In another study, women who consumed 2 or more cups of tea daily had a 46 percent lower risk of ovarian cancer compared to women who didn't regularly consume tea. And green tea taken as a drink or used as a topical preparation seems to reduce cervical dysplasia, a precancerous condition caused by human papillomavirus infection.

A Potential Stroke Fighter

There is also strong evidence that green tea can help prevent heart disease and stroke, says Dr. Blumberg.

In general, polyphenols tend to have a protective effect on blood vessels, and green tea is no exception, Dr. Blumberg says. In studies, green tea has been shown to improve blood vessel reactivity, reduce the oxidation of LDL cholesterol that leads to fatty buildup in arteries, and reduce both arterial stiffness and blood pressure.

In human studies, the strongest evidence for protection is for strokes. A large-scale population study in Japan suggested that consuming 3 or more cups of green tea a day reduced stroke risk by 20 percent. It also significantly decreased the risk of death from cardiovascular disease, or any cause, compared to drinking less than 1 cup daily. This association appears to be related to a decreased risk for cerebral infarction—that is, a stroke caused by a blood clot.

You Can Think Clearly Now

Green tea also contains an interesting amino acid called L-theanine. "L-theanine has been shown not only to improve deep sleep, but also to help people maintain a calm alertness during the day," says Jacob Teitelbaum, MD, author of *From Fatigued to Fantastic* and director of the Fibromyalgia and Fatigue Centers, a national group of clinics. L-theanine may help the brain form a calming compound called gamma-aminobutyric acid (GABA), Dr. Teitelbaum says. He uses it in his patients with fibromyalgia or chronic fatigue to reduce anxiety without causing "brain fog."

Green tea may protect the brain in other ways as well, perhaps by helping to maintain blood flow or improving glucose uptake. One study found that elderly Japanese people who consumed more than 2 cups of green tea each day had a 50 percent lower chance of having cognitive impairment, in comparison to those who drank fewer than 2 cups a day. And a study of 4,800 people in the United States found that people who consumed tea had 37 percent less decline compared to the non–tea drinkers. Those who drank tea one to four times a week had the biggest drop in risk.

Build Up Teeth and Bones

Some research suggests that drinking green tea for at least 10 years increases bone mineral density. Exactly how it may affect bone isn't known, but one possibility is that tea leaves contain fluoride, which may help slow osteoporosis. Tea also contains flavonoids and phytoestrogens, two compounds that may improve bone mineral density or mineral absorption. That natural fluoride in green tea also helps prevent cavities and strengthens tooth enamel. Plus, a chewable candy that contains green tea extract has been found to kill dental plaque–causing bacteria and reduce gum inflammation.

Take Tea and See?

Researchers who are studying the various components of green tea suggest using it as a tea rather than taking it as capsules or an extract. The reason: The tea version has more evidence to back it up, and it may actually have more benefits in your mouth and throat because it comes into contact with your cells. Plus, no one gets toxic from drinking a lot of green tea—up to 10 cups a day, Dr. Yang says.

"When you are sipping green tea throughout the day, you are taking in small amounts at a time," he says. "If you take many capsules at a time, you may overload your liver with more catechins than it can handle." There have been more than 10 reports of liver toxicity associated with green tea extracts, mostly from people using it to lose weight and deciding that if one tablet is good, more is better, Dr. Yang says. "That is not the case," he warns.

Experts also say it is difficult to pinpoint a beneficial dose. However, the commonly used dose of green tea is based on the amount typically consumed in Asian countries, which is 2 or 3 cups per day, providing 300 to 400 milligrams of polyphenols, Dr. Yang says.

iron

Considering how much iron surrounds us (it's the fourth most abundant element on Earth) and how little we need in our bodies (less than a teaspoon), it's surprising that iron deficiency is the most common nutritional shortcoming both in the United States and worldwide.

Iron problems may hit infants, especially between the ages of 6 months and 2 years, if they're weaned from breast milk (which contains sufficient iron) to cow's milk (which doesn't). For them, iron-fortified formula and cereals are the solution.

Adults also need iron, and sometimes, we just plain come up short. A woman's iron needs are especially great. During her childbearing years, she needs one-and-a-half times as much iron as a man does. Liver and red meat—both loaded with iron—are considered health foods in parts of the world where meat is scarce, and that's just what they are to tired women and irritable, listless babies. The form of iron found in meat is also more easily absorbed than iron from, say, vegetables or soy.

Men rarely become iron-deficient unless they've lost blood. Because getting too much can increase a man's risk for other conditions, doctors say that men should not take supplements unless a deficiency is diagnosed.

Show Me the Oxygen

It takes only about 30 seconds, maybe a minute at most, for us to realize how vital oxygen is to our well-being. Stop breathing, and in 10 minutes or so, you're dead. Every cell in your body requires oxygen to make the energy that keeps it going.

Iron delivers the oxygen. "It's kind of like the breeze that fans the flames," explains Janet Hunt, PhD, RD, a researcher with the USDA Human Nutrition Research Center in Grand Forks, North Dakota.

This mineral looms large in oxygen delivery because it's a vital part of hemoglobin, a protein that's found in red blood cells. Each hemoglobin molecule can carry four molecules of oxygen. A particular kind of iron, called heme iron, plays an integral role in this process of toting oxygen molecules from the lungs to other parts of the body. As red blood cells pass through the lungs, the heme iron, which is indirectly bound to the hemoglobin in a special way, readily picks up oxygen. Then, as the red blood cells pass through other tissues in the body, they release their oxygen freight wherever it's needed.

Iron is also a crucial part of another protein, myoglobin, which is found in muscles. Myoglobin picks up and stores additional oxygen for use

SUPPLEMENTSNAPSHOT

▶Iron

Supplement forms: Ferrous gluconate, ferrous sulfate, and ferrous glycinate.

Daily Value: 18 milligrams.

May help: Iron-deficiency anemia, heavy menstrual bleeding, and canker sores.

Good food sources: Lean beef, dark chicken meat, shellfish, and iron-fortified cereal products.

Who's at risk for deficiency: Children; teenagers, especially teenage girls; premenopausal women; pregnant women; and vegetarians.

Special instructions: For maximum absorption, take on an empty stomach; if indigestion occurs, take with food. A meal containing 25 to 30 milligrams of vitamin C can enhance absorption by as much as 85 percent. Avoid using over-the-counter preparations such as enteric-coated tablets or capsules containing slow-release granules. Don't take iron at the same time as calcium supplements, prescription medications to reduce stomach acid, or antacids, and don't wash down your iron tablet with tea. All can significantly decrease absorption.

Cautions and possible side effects: It's best not to take supplements unless you are a woman with heavy menstrual bleeding or have been diagnosed with low iron or anemia. May cause constipation. For people with hemochromatosis, taking iron supplements can be dangerous.

when muscles have to go at it long and hard. When you're low on iron, your capacity for exercise is reduced because your myoglobin can't transport enough oxygen to the muscles for the long haul.

The Energy Hand-Off

True, oxygen is needed for a cell's energy production, but iron plays another vital role in the energy-producing process as part of a cell's energy "assembly line."

In a cell's power plant, called the mitochondria, a set of proteins, some containing iron, are lined up in a bucket brigade called the electron transport chain. "These proteins transfer electrons from energy-yielding nutrients to oxygen, forming water and carbon dioxide, and in the process of respiration make a molecule called ATP, a cell's basic energy currency," says Paul Saltman, PhD, professor of biology at the University of California at San Diego. "Without enough iron, a cell's capacity to produce energy drops way off."

Iron also helps to oxidize compounds. It takes away electrons, a process that generates free-roaming, unstable molecules called free radicals, which damage cells. In a way, this puts iron in head-to-head competition with vitamin E, which is well known as an antioxidant that helps neutralize free radicals and prevent electron pilfering. "One is not necessarily better than the other," Dr. Saltman says. In fact, both processes are necessary for life, and they tend to balance each other out.

Iron is found in many enzymes, so it plays a role in the enzyme activity that affects your cells. And this mineral is in the production line that leads to the making of amino acids, hormones, and neurotransmitters. It's on-site when beta-carotene is converted to the active form of vitamin A. It plays a walk-on part in the production of collagen, one of the body's major structural proteins. In the liver and intestines, iron also does essential emergency work, converting harmful toxins into safer compounds that can be more easily excreted.

Fighting Microbes, Helping Enzymes

Given iron's role in energy production and protein synthesis, it only makes sense that a shortage may decrease our resistance to infection. "We

Strange Cravings? Check Your Iron

It's not unusual to have a hankering for chocolate brownies, ripe watermelon, or a nice, juicy steak. But what if it's laundry starch, glue, or Styrofoam cups that you find yourself snacking on?

Doctors have a word for this bizarre disorder. It's called pica, a name that comes from the same Latin root as magpie, a bird known for its indiscriminate appetite. Over the years, doctors have reported cases of people with pica eating many unpalatable items including dirt, chalk, clay, library paste, paint chips, paper, cardboard, ice chips, and Styrofoam.

In one case, a 22-year-old woman showed up in the emergency room with undigested pieces of tube socks in her stomach. She had begun chewing socks to relieve the stress of moving away from her family. Unfortunately, instead of moving right along, the remains of the socks wadded up in her stomach, forming a painful, indigestible ball.

"Pica is a strange mix of the physical—usually an iron deficiency—influenced by psychological and even social settings," says William H. Crosby, MD, a retired hematologist in Joplin, Missouri, who has studied pica for many years. The condition tends to occur in pregnant women, who are often low in iron, and in some babies. The babies affected tend to be

fight off infection by building up our armies of immunity—our white blood cells—and that takes lots of energy and protein," Dr. Saltman explains. Iron helps produce both.

Inside certain immune cells, iron plays an additional microbe-zapping role. Immune cells called macrophages, which can engulf and digest bacteria, rely on iron-containing enzymes. These enzymes are kept safely away from other parts of the cell inside special sacs. When they are released, they break down the bacteria that the macrophages engulf, Dr. Saltman says. "That whole system would be compromised in the case of iron deficiency."

Good for the Brain and Body

In addition to helping out macrophages, iron plays an important role in physical and mental functions. It is a crucial component of an enzyme, "milkaholics," meaning that they drink milk to the exclusion of other foods, thus lowering their intake of iron. No one knows why iron deficiency would cause such strange behavior, but often, when the deficiency is corrected with iron supplements, eating habits return to normal, Dr. Crosby says. Even the woman with a taste for socks got back to normal with iron supplementation.

Sometimes, people who are iron-deficient compulsively chew ice or gum or eat crunchy, salty, or sour foods such as potato chips, pickles, or unripe fruit, Dr. Crosby says. The name for this is food pica, which is the most common type in the United States.

Rather than put up with this behavior, see a doctor to be tested for iron deficiency and to get supplemental iron if necessary, Dr. Crosby says. A common problem with food pica is that people are ashamed about compulsively eating ice or other unusual items. "Don't let shame stop you from seeking a diagnosis," he says. "A good doctor will realize that this disorder can have an easily treated physical cause." People with pica are often amazed at how easily their compulsive behavior stops once they begin treatment, he says.

amine oxidase, that helps to produce three neurotransmitters: dopamine, serotonin, and norepinephrine. These brain chemicals are involved in dozens of different functions, including movement, intellectual performance, waking, sleeping, and emotional states like excitement, grief, happiness, and depression. No wonder iron deficiency has been strongly linked with changes in behavior and mood.

In adults, the symptoms are likely to be trouble concentrating, listlessness, and perhaps some irritability and trouble sleeping, Dr. Saltman says. Those problems get better when iron levels are restored.

Children who are iron-deficient may develop permanent problems. "There's growing evidence that children can have permanent brain damage if they are iron-deficient during critical times in brain development," Dr. Saltman says.

People with iron deficiency may have another problem as well—an impaired ability to maintain body temperature in a cold environment. In other words, they just can't get warm. "In this case, the lack of iron may be stopping the thyroid gland from functioning properly," Dr. Hunt says. That's because the thyroid controls the body's metabolism—its ability to burn calories for energy and for heat.

Your body must have iron on hand to be able to incorporate another essential nutrient, iodine, into molecules of thyroxine, the main thyroid hormone. Iodine activates thyroxine, letting it do its job of revving up your metabolism and letting you burn some calories as heat. No iron means no heat.

Coming Up Short?

Iron supplements used to be considered fairly safe for just about anyone, but now researchers have some reservations. High iron levels have been associated with a slightly increased risk of cancer and heart disease, probably because excess iron can cause cell damage. Plus, about 1 in every 300 people has an inherited disorder called hemochromatosis, which can cause a buildup of iron in your liver, spleen, heart, and other organs. This can be dangerous if you get lots of iron in your diet or from supplements, says James D. Cook, MD, a hematologist and professor of medicine at the University of Kansas Medical Center in Kansas City. A blood test can reveal whether you have this condition.

Frequently, diets that are low in iron—like the diets of some vegetarians—are also low in copper, says Dr. Saltman. Be sure that there is some copper in your multivitamin/mineral supplement.

If you're a woman who is still menstruating, it's safe to take a daily supplement with up to 18 milligrams (the Daily Value) of iron, says Dr. Cook. If you think that you may be really short on iron, though, you should have your blood levels checked by a doctor. People who are consistently deficient in iron, as shown by blood tests, need to take much higher amounts initially to restore normal levels. After you reach a normal level, which is easily determined by a quick blood test, your doctor may say it's okay to slack off on supplementation. Anyone else—older women, men, children, and regular blood donors—should take supplemental iron only on a doctor's advice.

vitamin K

Consider blood. It has the remarkable ability to remain liquid even though it's loaded with all sorts of solid stuff—red and white blood cells, protein, vitamins, minerals, even gobs of fat from the last cheeseburger you ate. But blood can also become solid within seconds when a blood vessel breaks. That particular ability can spell the difference between life and death if you're seriously injured—and it requires vitamin K.

This vitamin got its name from the Danish researchers who discovered it. The "K" stands for "koagulation," the Danish spelling of "coagulation."

Your body needs vitamin K to make several blood proteins involved in clotting, including the most important, prothrombin. When bleeding starts, these proteins go through a quick series of changes that ends with a blood clot, says John Suttie, PhD, professor of biochemistry at the University of Wisconsin in Madison. If your body ran short of vitamin K, your blood would clot very slowly, and you might develop many symptoms that indicate this deficiency—easy bruising, frequent nosebleeds, or cuts that won't quit bleeding.

Potential Bone Builder

You need vitamin K to make two proteins found in bone. Without it, the bones produce an abnormal form of these proteins that can't bind to the minerals that normally form bone.

One Japanese study suggests that low vitamin K levels play a role in the breakdown of bone after menopause. Some researchers contend that postmenopausal women are at risk for a low-level vitamin K deficiency that the traditional blood-clotting test would not detect. "However," Dr. Suttie says, "much more needs to be learned about vitamin K's function in bone before we know for sure whether it plays a role in diseases such as osteoporosis."

Eat the Garnish

Most people get enough of this vitamin from their diets. The average intake is 80 micrograms or so per day, which is the Daily Value. Some researchers think the Daily Value is too low, though, and that a healthier intake would be 100 micrograms per day.

Good sources include leafy green vegetables such as parsley, spinach, watercress, turnip greens, kale, and broccoli. Vitamin K is also produced in the intestines by bacteria, but it's likely that these bugs in our guts don't produce all that much, Dr. Suttie says.

Vitamin K deficiency is not common, he says. People who are most likely to be deficient probably don't eat leafy green vegetables, or they have medical problems that interfere with fat absorption.

"People who are in the hospital for one reason or another are also at an increased risk for problems," Dr. Suttie says. That's because they may

SUPPLEMENT SNAPSHOT

▶ Vitamin K

Daily Value: 80 micrograms.

May help: Bleeding problems associated with vitamin K deficiency. Helps calcium bind to protein during new bone formation, so helps harden new bone.

Good food sources: Broccoli, kale, parsley, spinach, turnip greens, and watercress.

Who's at risk for deficiency: Newborns; people taking anticoagulants (blood thinners), long-term antibiotic therapy, or sulfa drugs; people who eat no green vegetables; and those who have problems with dietary fat absorption.

Special instructions: For best absorption, take a K-containing multivitamin with a meal that contains some fat. There is no need to take supplements unless prescribed by your doctor.

Cautions and possible side effects: Don't assume that easy bruising or bleeding is being caused by a vitamin K deficiency; see a doctor if you have these symptoms. If you are taking the anticoagulant warfarin (Coumadin), do not take vitamin K without medical supervision.

not have eaten anything for a while, and a deficiency can occur relatively fast—within a few days. There's an added risk of vitamin K–related complications for people who are taking anticoagulant (blood-thinning) drugs such as warfarin (Coumadin), which block the action of vitamin K. Other causes of depletion are antibiotics or sulfa drugs that can wipe out bacteria in the intestines, making even this small supply unavailable.

Do You Need Special K?

Luckily, doctors check blood-clotting times in people who are taking anticoagulants or who appear to have bleeding problems. Any problems that might occur are easily corrected with an injection of vitamin K, which some infants get after they are born.

Doctors sometimes tell their patients who are taking anticoagulants not to eat anything that contains vitamin K, but that's not the best advice, Dr. Suttie says. "They should continue to eat the way they did before they started taking the drug and try to keep their intake pretty much the same from week to week," he says. This helps to stabilize the dose of anticoagulant.

Vitamin K is found in some multivitamins and in single supplements. If it's in a multivitamin, you'll find it listed on the label.

Large doses of vitamin E—on the order of 2,200 international units (IU) a day—can reduce the absorption of vitamin K in the intestines, according to Dr. Suttie. "People who eat normal amounts of vitamin K–rich foods, however, can safely take 400 IU of vitamin E every day for long periods of time," he says.

magnesium

Magnesium doesn't get the kind of celebrity endorsements that calcium does, but it should. What other nutrient can claim chocolate as one of its better sources?

A real workhorse in the body, magnesium is essential for some 325-plus biochemical reactions, more than any other nutrient. Many of those tasks are basic and indispensable.

"Its function is so broad that it touches on almost all physiological systems, all the way from energy generation inside cells to the interaction of nerve impulses and muscles in the heart," says Henry Lukaski, PhD, research leader for mineral nutrient functions at the USDA Human Nutrition Research Center in Grand Forks, North Dakota.

Getting enough magnesium has been hailed as an all-around protective measure. In research discussions, this mineral has been tentatively linked with protection from heart arrhythmia (irregular heartbeat), high blood pressure, migraine headaches, and heart attacks.

Energy Everywhere

Magnesium is needed so that the body can produce energy from any food we eat—carbohydrate, protein, or fat. It works in the mitochondria, the energy-generating powerhouses inside cells. There it plays an essential role in producing the body's basic energy currency. "Magnesium is needed for a cell to make ATP, the molecules that contain the energy, and then to break these molecules down to release the energy," explains Dr. Lukaski.

That's important, because our bodies produce a large number of ongoing chemical reactions, none of which can take place without ATP. We need ATP all the time, to move nutrients and other substances in and out of cells; to break down molecules and rearrange them into new molecules, such as protein or hormones; and to make muscles and nerves

244

work. Without magnesium helping to make ATP, that energetic activity would be reduced to zero.

In fact, Dr. Lukaski found that female volunteers who consumed 150 milligrams of magnesium a day—which is less than half the Daily

▶Magnesium

Supplement forms: Magnesium lactate, magnesium orotate, magnesium glycinate, magnesium gluconate, magnesium oxide, and magnesium hydroxide.

Daily Value: 400 milligrams.

May help: Heart arrhythmia, migraine headaches, angina, restless legs syndrome, Raynaud's disease, asthma, binge-eating disorder, osteoporosis, and pregnancy-induced high blood pressure; also used for chronic fatigue syndrome, fibromyalgia, intermittent claudication, celiac disease, menstrual cramps, PMS, tinnitus, mitral valve prolapse, kidney stones, diabetes, insomnia, endometriosis, leg cramps, and high blood pressure.

Good food sources: Wheat germ; unmilled grains such as whole wheat and brown rice; pumpkin, sunflower, and other seeds; cocoa; chocolate; unblanched almonds and filberts; rice bran; beans; lentils; tofu; spinach; Swiss chard; halibut; and mackerel.

Who's at risk for deficiency: People with uncontrolled diabetes, who lose magnesium through their urine; alcoholics; people taking "loop" or non-potassium-sparing diuretics; people who seldom eat magnesium-rich foods; and those under severe physical and emotional stress.

Special instructions: Take a form of magnesium, such as magnesium lactate, orotate, glycinate, or gluconate, that is easily absorbed and least likely to cause diarrhea. Magnesium oxide and hydroxide are more likely to cause diarrhea at higher dosages and are not well absorbed.

Cautions and possible side effects: Do not take a supplement of more than 350 milligrams a day without medical supervision. Consult your doctor before taking if you have heart disease or arrhythmia, impaired kidney function, high blood pressure, or migraine headaches, or if you are taking diuretics. May cause diarrhea.

Value but is the amount consumed by most women age 50 and older—soon began to slow down. After only 2 months on a low-magnesium diet, they were asked to ride a stationary bicycle at a moderate pace. On the low-magnesium regimen, volunteers used 15 percent more oxygen and had heart rates an average of 10 beats a minute faster than when they were getting higher doses of 350 milligrams a day.

"This means that people who are low in magnesium use more energy and have a greater strain on their hearts," Dr. Lukaski says. "They can't exercise as long or as hard and they get tired faster. It may even limit their ability to work or to do daily activities."

There's more besides magnesium involved in energy production, but one thing's for sure: If magnesium is in short supply, your tail will soon be dragging.

Making Muscles Work

Together with calcium, magnesium is involved in making sure that muscles work properly. "It's the ratio of calcium to magnesium that's important," explains Burton M. Altura, PhD, professor of physiology and medicine at the State University of New York (SUNY) Health Science Center in Brooklyn.

Magnesium is important for muscles to be able to relax, while calcium helps them contract. Too little magnesium in relation to calcium (or low levels of both) can make muscles cramp more easily and may make some muscles, like the smooth muscles that wrap around big blood vessels, stay somewhat contracted, Dr. Altura explains. Magnesium deficiency can make muscles go into spasms easily. When you're short on magnesium, the waste products of metabolism, such as lactic acid, are harder to flush out, so you may get tired, burning, sore muscles.

Supplemental magnesium often helps people with migraine headaches or high blood pressure if they're low in magnesium, Dr. Altura says. Since magnesium can also relax muscles in airways in the lungs, it sometimes helps people with asthma breathe easier, he adds. Magnesium even helps some forms of angina—spasms of the coronary arteries that can cause chest pain.

Magnesium is also needed for the body to be able to construct its basic building materials, including protein, carbohydrates, fat, and nucleic acids, a cell's genetic material. In some cases, magnesium simply provides the energy needed for the body to link together the molecules of amino acids that make up a protein or the fatty acids that make up fat and cell membranes. At other times, it helps change the shapes of molecules so that they can bind together. In the case of genetic material, magnesium molecules bind to the "backbone" of the famous double-stranded DNA helix, helping to stabilize its structure and maintain order. This is important because each cell uses DNA as the blueprint for reproducing itself or parts of itself. Body maintenance and repair depend on accurate DNA blueprints.

Healthy Heartthrobs

Certain minerals play important roles in maintaining your heart's proper rhythm. These include potassium, magnesium, sodium, chloride, and calcium. Here again, a proper ratio is important.

When magnesium levels in the heart are low, people can develop certain types of heart arrhythmias, some of them potentially very dangerous, says Carla Sueta, MD, PhD, assistant professor of medicine and cardiology at the University of North Carolina at Chapel Hill School of Medicine.

One type of potential arrhythmia problem affects the upper chamber, or atrium, of the heart. Another type, called ventricular arrhythmia, involves the lower heart chambers. In studies, intravenous magnesium reduced the incidence of death from several types of ventricular arrhythmia. "In fact, intravenous therapy with magnesium is now considered standard therapy for two types of ventricular arrhythmia," Dr. Sueta says.

Too little magnesium can also induce something called refractory potassium deficiency. Unfortunately, you can't correct a refractory deficiency simply by taking more potassium. But by getting more magnesium, you may ensure that this kind of deficiency never occurs in the first place.

Heart patients—and their doctors—need to pay heed to magnesium. Studies have shown that 65 to 75 percent of all people in intensive care units and 5 to 11 percent of people in general care sections of hospitals are deficient in magnesium. Also, magnesium deficiency can be caused by the very drugs meant to help heart problems. Some types of diuretics cause the body to excrete both magnesium and potassium, as does the heart-stimulating drug digitalis.

Overreactive Rodents

Years ago, German researchers dubbed magnesium a natural tranquilizer because it seemed to soothe jangled nerves. In people who are low in magnesium, it may do exactly that.

Magnesium is essential to the regulation of central nervous system functions, explains James Penland, PhD, head research psychologist at the USDA research center in North Dakota. Animals—and humans—low in magnesium have more "excitable" nervous systems that make them tend to overreact to stimulation. Rats, for instance, will jump in their cages at the sound of a closing door.

The human equivalent of the jumpy rat may experience symptoms of shakiness, insomnia, irritability, and anxiety, Dr. Penland says. He's found changes in brain waves in women who get a low dose of 115 milligrams a day of magnesium. "Even when they have their eyes closed, their brain waves indicate a state of enhanced vigilance, or hyperreactivity," he explains. In other words, their brains just can't relax completely.

Certainly, if you wake up several times during the night, if you're irritable or seem jumpy during the day, or if you are experiencing tremors or shakiness and you know you're not getting much magnesium, it's worth discussing with your doctor, Dr. Penland says. Taking 200 to 300 milligrams a day as a supplement is safe for most people. If you're severely deficient, though, you may need more than that amount, or you may require injections. If that is the case, you'll obviously need medical supervision.

Free-Radical Chaser

The less magnesium you consume, the greater your chances of developing atherosclerosis—clogged, inflamed arteries that cause heart disease and heart attacks. A magnesium deficiency promotes the generation of free radicals, the free-roaming, unstable molecules that can harm cells, including those cells lining arteries. When your arteries are roughed up by these renegades, it sets the stage for cholesterol deposits, explains Dr. Altura.

Magnesium deficiency also promotes heart disease by making it easier for harmful LDL cholesterol to be oxidized and for hearts to be overloaded with calcium. Both are steps in the development of heart disease, says Dr. Altura.

Today, we get less magnesium in our diets than people were getting about a century ago. Back in 1910, the average was about 450 milligrams a day of magnesium, mostly provided by unprocessed foods and especially by whole grains. Nowadays, most people get less than 300 milligrams a day. Men average 185 to 250; women average 172 to 235. This raises a real concern that people who may have chronic magnesium deficiencies could be at greater risk for migraine headaches, heart disease, or high blood pressure, Dr. Altura says.

DV Delivery

If you're otherwise healthy but have reason to believe that you've been shortchanging yourself on magnesium, you can reach 400 milligrams a day (the Daily Value) fairly easily by eating magnesium-rich foods. Alternatively, you can figure out about how much you normally get in your diet and then supplement to get yourself up into the 400-milligram range, Dr. Altura says.

If you're ill, however—if you have heart arrhythmia, kidney problems, high blood pressure, or migraine headaches—you should discuss magnesium supplementation with your doctor, Dr. Altura says. You may be so low in magnesium that you need quite a bit to get you back to normal. You may need extended treatment with oral supplements, and some people require injections.

To help determine true magnesium status, get a blood test that measures ionized magnesium, the active form of magnesium in the blood. Some specialists are now able to perform the test, according to Dr. Altura. If you're concerned about a possible magnesium deficiency, ask your doctor about this test. Serum magnesium, which is the test doctors usually order, will only detect magnesium deficiency when it is severe.

melatonin

Astronauts orbiting the Earth see a new sunrise every 90 minutes. While that may be an awesome spectacle, it really does a number on their internal body clocks.

The human body clock relies on the complex interplay of certain chemicals (especially hormones) and your sensory organs (especially your eyes). In any 24-hour period, there's likely to be a time when your body says, "I'm sleepy, I need rest." That's when you should head for bed.

If that cycle is interrupted, however, you're likely to lose sleep. Orbiting astronauts, bothered by the frequent sunrises, are plagued by insomnia. They average only 5 to 6 hours of shut-eye for every day in space. That's why NASA decided to study whether the hormone melatonin was "the right stuff" to help them sleep. And it was. It helped shift their internal clocks so they could both sleep better and work better on the Space Shuttle.

Melatonin is produced by the pineal gland, a little cone-shaped structure in the brain that releases the hormone into the bloodstream. Darkness stimulates the pineal gland and causes it to produce more melatonin, which is why some call it the "hormone of darkness." Light puts the brakes on production, but both light and dark seem necessary for this gland to function properly.

During a normal night, production of melatonin peaks during the darkest hours—between 2:00 and 4:00 a.m. After that, production starts to decline, and it's essentially switched off when you wake up. The longer the night, the more melatonin will be secreted.

Under the Influence

Although we all have some melatonin in our systems, the amount doesn't remain constant during our lifetimes. Between the ages of 1 and 3, we have the highest levels. As we age, we produce and secrete less. When melatonin levels get too low, we sleep less, which might be one reason why so many people over age 65 suffer from chronic insomnia.

Melatonin is also present in some plant and animal foods, although in very small amounts. Bananas have it, but you'd have to eat 40 at one sitting to get 1 milligram of melatonin. Supplements are the only source of significant concentrations.

When scientists isolated this hormone of darkness, they naturally began to wonder whether it could change sleep patterns. Today, melatonin is widely available as a supplement, and while it does seem to have other properties and is used in cancer treatment, the most widely accepted use is for sleep-related problems.

When taken in proper doses at the appropriate time of day, this hormone can indeed increase sleepiness and help you fall asleep, says Irina Zhdanova, MD, PhD, principal research scientist for the brain and cognitive sciences department at the Massachusetts Institute of Technology in Cambridge. Studies have shown that people who take melatonin may fall asleep faster, are less susceptible to awakening during the night, and feel that their sleep is more restful.

Supplementing with melatonin is not like taking a sleeping pill, however. Instead, it nudges you toward sleep by promoting general relaxation.

SUPPLEMENT SNAPSHOT

▶Melatonin

May help: Insomnia; jet lag; seasonal affective disorder; depression and chronic fatigue syndrome associated with sleep problems; delayed sleep phase syndrome (a type of insomnia). It may also improve treatment outcomes in some forms of cancer.

Special instructions: As a sleep aid, take a half-hour before bedtime. As part of cancer therapy, discuss with your doctor.

Cautions and possible side effects: Take no more than 3 milligrams daily unless you have medical supervision. Melatonin may worsen symptoms of depression, so do not take it unless you're under the supervision of a doctor. Do not take if you are pregnant or trying to conceive. Use in children only with medical supervision. May cause headaches, morning dizziness, daytime sleepiness, or upset stomach.

Changing the Clocks

Whether you're traveling east from San Francisco to Boston or west from Los Angeles to Singapore, you're probably going to lose some sleep. You are also likely to suffer other symptoms of jet lag, such as headache, irritability, and poor concentration.

Supplementing with melatonin appears to alleviate these symptoms. It fights jet lag in two ways, says Dr. Zhdanova. First, it helps you fall asleep. Second, it can reset your body clock, either forward or back, to help you adapt to a new time zone.

When you take melatonin in the afternoon, it tends to advance the body clock. In other words, if you take it at 3:00 or 4:00 p.m., you're likely to feel ready for bed earlier than you usually would. When you take it in the early morning—say, 3:00 or 4:00 a.m.—it delays the body clock so you're willing to stay awake longer than you normally would.

Because of these effects, melatonin has been studied as a sleep aid for shift workers, including those who rotate between day and night shifts. Most of us find it hard to stay alert at night, even if we sleep during the day. Night workers have an especially tough time and seldom adapt completely because they don't get the time cues they need from daylight.

The question of whether melatonin can help shift workers is not an easy one to answer, says Dr. Zhdanova. Individuals respond differently to melatonin. Even if they time it to help them adjust to new work schedules, it may actually make some workers more groggy and less alert as they move from a day shift to a night shift, then back again.

Can Melatonin Slow Cancer?

Researchers began to look at melatonin as a cancer treatment after they realized that some chemotherapy treatments worked better and had less toxicity when administered at certain times of the day, says David Blask, MD, PhD, a professor and head of the Laboratory of Chrono-Neuroendocrine-Oncology at Tulane University, in New Orleans. "The basic idea is to use melatonin to optimize circadian rhythms and create a situation where chemotherapy would work more efficaciously and with less toxicity," he says.

Italian researchers have done about 40 small human studies using standard chemotherapy treatments with and without added melatonin. "Those studies are promising," Dr. Blask says. "They showed stabilization and some partial regression, but very few complete regressions," he says. Melatonin increased 1-year and even up to 5-year survival rates by at least 50 percent. It's been used in studies involving lung, liver, pancreas, colon, breast, and brain cancer.

Since melatonin is considered nontoxic and people with cancer have trouble sleeping anyway, doctors generally go along with it when their patients want it, Dr. Blask says. Most of these studies simply used 20 milligrams of melatonin at bedtime.

A Little Melatonin Goes a Long Way

Dosages vary depending on what you are using melatonin for. For insomnia or jet lag, 0.3 to 5 milligrams is generally recommended. For use in cancer treatment, go a bit higher: 20 milligrams a day.

Just as important as the dose is what time of day you take the supplement. For jet lag and insomnia, take it in the evening because melatonin has the ability to advance the circadian rhythm. For cancer, researchers believe that evening doses are also best since melatonin is most effective in the evening.

Although it's available over the counter in health food stores and drugstores in the United States, melatonin is now regulated as a medication in Canada and in some European countries.

milk thistle

Poisons enter your body whenever you smoke cigarettes, drink alcohol, work with solvents and paints, take medications to combat pain, or walk down a city street breathing the exhaust of cars and buses. Even if you live in the country, hundreds of miles from an industrial hub, you probably breathe air laced with some of the 851 million pounds of toxic chemicals that are released into the environment each year.

What keeps these poisons from overwhelming your body is your liver. The liver breaks down toxins in the bloodstream and turns them into less harmful substances that are eventually flushed from your system. Your liver is the great detoxifier, and it has the capacity to serve you well for a lifetime.

When your liver becomes damaged by toxins, however, milk thistle, a plant with a long history of use as a liver tonic, may be helpful. This herb has been used to treat inflammation of the liver, hepatitis, mushroom and chemical poisoning, and liver damage from alcohol abuse or long-term use of certain medications.

"Milk thistle strengthens your liver and reduces the damage from environmental irritants like pesticides," says Jennifer Brett, ND, a naturopathic doctor at the Wilton Naturopathic Center in Stratford, Connecticut.

The Liver's Bodyguard

Milk thistle is native to the Mediterranean but now grows wild in North America, especially California and the eastern United States. Although it was used for centuries in Europe as a liver tonic, by the beginning of the 20th century, its value was nearly forgotten.

Some years ago, German scientists began investigating the chemical properties of the milk thistle fruit and discovered a concentrated group of flavonoid compounds called silymarin. Flavonoids in general are an important group of antioxidants that devour free radicals, the free-roaming, unstable molecules that rage through the body, harm healthy cells, and accelerate aging.

Silymarin is actually a group of flavonoids that function as an anti-hepatotoxic, meaning that it acts directly on the liver to protect it from poisons. It mounts the defenses on two fronts. First, it binds to the membranes of liver cells and creates a tough shield so that toxins have a more difficult time penetrating the cell walls. If toxins do make it into the cells and cause damage, silymarin stimulates the liver to speed up production of beneficial enzymes and proteins as part of a healing restoration.

"Silymarin is an antioxidant that acts very specifically on liver tissue. It also increases the activity of glutathione, the body's own antioxidant," says Alison Lee, MD, a pain-management specialist and medical director of Barefoot Doctors, an alternative medicine practice in Ann Arbor, Michigan.

More Life for the Liver

The human liver has a remarkable natural capacity to regenerate itself after being damaged, and studies of people who have liver problems show that milk thistle can actually help a damaged liver grow new cells.

"Milk thistle enhances the liver's own healing process," says Dr. Lee. "It can be used both for short-term acute liver injury, like that resulting from exposure to a virus or mushroom poisoning, and for long-term, chronic problems such as cirrhosis, as well."

SUPPLEMENTSNAPSHOT

▶Milk Thistle

Botanical name: *Silybum marianum.*

Origin: Native to the Mediterranean.

May help: Hepatitis, cirrhosis, liver inflammation, and liver damage caused by alcohol abuse, long-term use of medications, and chemical exposure; endometriosis; diabetes, and Parkinson's disease.

Special instructions: For maximum absorption, take with food.

Cautions and possible side effects: Generally regarded as safe; may cause loose stools.

Swedish doctors have successfully used an active component of milk thistle intravenously as an antidote for mushroom poisoning following accidental ingestion. But that doesn't mean that you can try to self-treat with milk thistle if you may have mushroom poisoning. See a doctor immediately.

The herb is commonly prescribed in Europe for a variety of liver conditions, including cirrhosis and hepatitis. It has sometimes been used as a digestive stimulant to encourage the release of bile, a fluid produced by the liver that plays an essential role in digestion.

In new research, milk thistle also seems to help people with diabetes. One study showed that people with type 2 diabetes who took 200 milligrams of the herb three times a day for 4 months in combination with conventional treatment had lower fasting blood glucose, lower hemoglobin A1C (a marker of long-term glucose control), lower total cholesterol and LDL or "bad" cholesterol, and lower triglycerides compared to those who took a placebo pill. Some other research suggests that the same dose reduces insulin resistance in people who have both diabetes and alcohol-related cirrhosis of the liver.

A Tonic for Toxicity

Who should take milk thistle, and how often? Most people would benefit from a daily supplement, according to Dr. Brett. She believes that Americans are routinely exposed to many toxins and that we should use it as a preventive. "It will not do you any harm and probably a lot of good, considering how toxic our society is," she says.

Milk thistle is most often sold in capsules or tablets. So far, Dr. Lee adds, there's no evidence to suggest any problems with taking the herb over the long term, which suggests that it's safe to take regularly as a preventive. Certainly, people who are regularly exposed to environmental hazards—such as painters, anyone who works around chemicals, folks who live in areas of heavy industrial pollution, and people recovering from alcohol abuse—are good candidates for milk thistle, she says. "That doesn't mean, though, that you can take milk thistle and just drink all you want. It doesn't work that way," she warns.

Dr. Lee often prescribes milk thistle to her new acupuncture patients, people who have been taking drugs for years to control inflammation or pain from chronic conditions. Many pain-relieving drugs—even common over-the-counter medications like acetaminophen—can be damaging to the liver with long-term use, she says. Milk thistle helps detoxify her patients' livers and helps while they are being weaned from medications, she says.

"If somebody is taking a lot of medications, their liver may not be as responsive as it might be," she adds. "I wouldn't recommend milk thistle for everyone. First, I do a simple blood test to determine liver function. If the test reveals a problem, I might recommend it."

Most clinical studies of milk thistle's effectiveness have used a specific extract standardized to 70 to 80 percent silymarin. In the United States, this formulation is found in the brand-name product Thisilyn, made by Nature's Way. Dosages vary. For cirrhosis, 420 milligrams is suggested. For chronic active hepatitis, a special milk thistle extract, silibinin (brand name: Silipide) has been found to be useful in doses of 240 milligrams.

Tea is not a good way to take milk thistle, as the active ingredients are not very active in water. Some brands of milk thistle are made superpotent by enhancing the body's ability to absorb and use them. For instance, one brand, Silipide (trade name Siliphos), a complex of silymarin and phosphatidylcholine (an emulsifier containing lecithin), is about 10 times more bioavailable than silymarin. A holistic doctor can help you select a brand, and dosage, that is right for you.

Milk thistle can interact with some drugs, so it's best to check for interactions with any drugs you are taking before you start using it.

nettle

When Roman soldiers invaded the dank climate of Great Britain, they kept warm by rubbing their chilled arms and legs with nettle, a common weed found along the trails. The hairy spines covering the plant released histamines and formic acid that caused their skin to burn and itch, but the soldiers from Mediterranean climes preferred the irritation to the chill.

As far back as biblical times, people throughout Europe practiced urtication, the practice of flogging or swatting themselves with nettle. They believed that by thus injecting irritating chemicals into their skin, they could ease rheumatism and arthritis pain.

Because the histamines in nettle limit the body's response to pollen and other irritating substances, nettle was also a favored treatment for asthma and allergies. The astringent or constricting quality of the roots and leaves led to its use to stop diarrhea, dysentery, and bleeding.

Old-time herbalists favored nettle for its diuretic action and prescribed it for many urinary tract conditions. Today, several companies in Europe manufacture a nettle extract to combat urine retention caused by an enlarged prostate.

"It was used for a long time as a detoxifying agent, helping to flush the body," says Debra Gibson, ND, a naturopathic doctor in Woodbury, Connecticut. "A lot of folks drank nettle tea in the springtime when hay fever season came on. It was a spring tonic."

A Worldwide Weed

The common or stinging nettle is a perennial plant and common weed that grows in temperate climates throughout the world. It stands 2 to 3 feet high and has dark green, serrated leaves and small, inconspicuous flowers.

Young shoots of nettle are edible when cooked. They contain about the same amounts of beta-carotene and vitamin C as spinach and other greens. Other parts of the plant are used for healing.

In North America, nettle was a popular plant medicine with mainstream physicians throughout the 19th century and into the 20th. A popular medical textbook published in 1928 mentions that people used it to reduce inflammation from sprains and arthritis. Since then, scientists have learned that nettle contains about 20 different chemicals, including lectins, phenols, sterols, lignans, and histamines.

Histamines, which occur naturally in the body, are the culprits behind allergic reactions, says Stanley W. Beyrle, ND, a naturopathic doctor at the Kansas Clinic of Traditional Medicine in Wichita. When you are exposed to allergens—substances that cause allergic reactions—your body releases histamines, which in turn cause hives, constrict bronchial vessels, and inflame your skin.

The histamines in nettle attach to histamine receptor sites in your cells and keep your body's histamines from attaching to those cells during an allergic reaction. Nettle's action is very similar to that of pharmaceutical antihistamine drugs, says Dr. Beyrle.

"What's important here is that the plant histamines have a less sensitive trigger than the body's histamines. Although they attach to the receptor sites, they are so weak that they rarely cause any allergic reaction in the person," he says.

Allergic reactions to nettle itself are rare but not unheard of. Although it is a very benign herb, touching the plant may cause skin irritation similar to an allergic reaction, notes Dr. Gibson.

SUPPLEMENT SNAPSHOT

▶Nettle

Botanical name: *Urtica dioica;* also known as stinging nettle.

Origin: Found in temperate zones throughout the world; cultivated in Europe.

May help: Allergies, rhinitis, urinary problems, asthma, diarrhea, dysentery, hemorrhage, gout, hair loss, and prostate problems.

Special instructions: For maximum absorption, take with food.

Cautions and possible side effects: Rarely, may aggravate allergy symptoms; if you have allergies, take only one dose a day for the first few days and discontinue use if you notice allergy symptoms. May cause stomach pain.

"People with extreme mold sensitivity should be cautious when using nettle teas, since the leaves may harbor molds that would be ingested," she says. "This is less likely to be a problem with capsules containing the freeze-dried herb or with tinctures." If you have allergies, take only one dose a day for the first few days to avoid aggravating symptoms.

Nettle may help people who have a tendency toward rhinitis, an inflammation of the mucous membranes in the nose that can be brought on by colds, dust, and allergies. Initially, nettle can prevent rhinitis by stifling allergic reactions, but its strong anti-inflammatory properties make it a kind of balm for red, swollen tissues.

In a study of 69 people in Portland, Oregon, researchers found that a freeze-dried extract of the herb was better than a similar but inactive substance (a placebo) at improving the symptoms associated with rhinitis. Some chemicals in the plant also seem to inhibit a destructive enzyme that's released into tissues during the inflammation.

Turning On the Flow

It's only been within the last 20 years—and mainly in Europe—that nettle root has been employed in the treatment of benign prostatic hyperplasia (BPH). BPH is a noncancerous enlargement of the prostate gland that constricts the urethra, the tube that leads from the bladder to the penis. Some men with this condition have problems with frequent urination, but they may also have trouble urinating when they have a strong urge. This can be particularly disruptive at night, when the urge to go is like a frustrating alarm clock.

No one is really certain how nettle helps. It's thought that the herb may limit the amount of testosterone, the male sex hormone, circulating in the blood, or it may inhibit an enzyme, aromatase, that leads to the formation of testosterone. BPH is caused mainly by an overabundance of testosterone, says Dr. Gibson.

Whatever the mechanism, German health authorities have concluded that nettle root extract is an effective treatment for urinary problems caused by BPH, but only when the prostate is slightly to moderately enlarged.

A French study found that men who had to get up several times a night to urinate found significant relief after taking an extract of nettle. Every 8 hours, researchers gave a dilute extract of nettle root to 67 patients over

60 years old. The men with the mildest problems found significant relief in just 3 to 6 weeks.

The results were less encouraging for men with more severe cases, as it took a few more weeks before any effect was noticed. Nevertheless, many of the subjects had fewer nighttime awakenings to urinate. The herb did not shrink the prostate but apparently reduced inflammation and swelling. For BPH, stinging nettle is most often used along with another prostate helper, saw palmetto, which helps shrink the prostate.

Commission E, a team of physicians, toxicologists, pharmacologists, and other specialists established by the German government to study herbal medicines, determined that nettle is also a good supportive therapy for inflammatory diseases of the lower urinary tract. All of these scientific conclusions fit with the traditional use of nettle as a diuretic, notes Dr. Beyrle. "This is really one of the great herbs for increasing the secretion of urine," he says. "I've also used it to treat chronic inflammation of the bladder." For best results, make sure to drink plenty of water while taking nettle.

Freeze-Dried Is Best

Nettle comes as a tincture, capsules, and dried root, from which you can brew a tea. "To get the full benefit of nettle, you really need a freeze-dried extract," says Dr. Beyrle. The freeze-dried preparation is made from nettle that is processed soon after harvesting, he says. Slow drying and processing remove many of the active ingredients. A typical dosage for nasal allergies is 300 milligrams, three times a day, of stinging nettle leaf extract. People with osteoarthritis frequently apply fresh nettle leaves over their aching joints.

niacin

Try to survive on a corn-based diet and you run the risk of getting pellagra, a disease caused by niacin deficiency.

Corn lacks niacin. Years ago, people in the South who depended on corn grits as a diet staple suffered from this bodywide disease that leads to dermatitis, diarrhea, and depression. It can even lead to death, if deprivation continues long enough.

Today, nearly everyone gets sufficient niacin. Meat, poultry, and fish are rich in this B vitamin, and it's also added to flour and other cereal products to help ensure that our needs are met. Pellagra, for the most part, is a thing of the past.

Like most of the other B vitamins, niacin assists enzymes, the catalysts that help spark chemical reactions. An all-around booster shot for enzymes, it helps many of them do their jobs properly.

Niacin is also a major player in the process of breaking down food into a form of energy that the cells in our bodies can either use or store for future use. Niacin-dependent enzymes help "package" this energy and then release it in an orderly fashion as it's needed.

The niacin-dependent enzymes also play important roles in the body's handling of fat and cholesterol and the production of many biochemicals, including some hormones.

Confusingly, niacin has several different chemical structures, which also have different names. One of the forms prescribed by doctors is nicotinic acid. A second form is called niacinamide—also known as nicotinamide. And there's yet a third form—different from the other two—called inositol hexaniacinate.

Some forms are recommended for certain conditions but not for others. Niacinamide, for instance, is used to treat osteoarthritis and rheumatoid arthritis. Other forms may be selectively prescribed in large doses to treat high cholesterol and Raynaud's disease, a circulatory problem that causes cold hands and feet.

Clobbering Cholesterol

Large doses of nicotinic acid and inositol hexaniacinate do a good job of lowering cholesterol, possibly by affecting liver function.

Niacin also raises "good" HDL cholesterol. In fact, it does this better than any drug on the market. Several studies also show that regular doses of niacin can reduce the risk of death from heart disease. It is thus considered a good treatment choice when someone needs more than diet to control cholesterol, says Martin Milner, ND, a naturopathic doctor who

SUPPLEMENTSNAPSHOT

▶Niacin

Supplement forms: Nicotinic acid, niacinamide (nicotinamide), and inositol hexaniacinate; also known as vitamin B_3.

Daily Value: 20 milligrams.

May help: Niacin and inositol hexaniacinate may help high cholesterol and Raynaud's disease; niacinamide may help osteoarthritis, rheumatoid arthritis, and diabetes.

Good food sources: Meat, milk, eggs, fish, poultry, peanuts, and enriched breads and cereals. Coffee and tea also contain appreciable amounts.

Who's at risk for deficiency: Alcoholics and people taking isoniazid (Laniazid) for long periods of time.

Special instructions: Take with food to minimize side effects whenever you're taking high doses.

Cautions and possible side effects: Do not take more than 35 milligrams a day of any form without medical supervision; do not take more than 35 milligrams a day if you have a history of gout, liver damage, peptic ulcers, gallbladder disease, or heart rhythm disturbances. Taking niacin in addition to certain cholesterol-lowering drugs (statin drugs) increases risk of liver damage. High doses can cause drops in blood pressure and can raise blood sugar in people with diabetes. May cause flushing and allergic reactions. Sustained release niacin can be hepatotoxic, so do not use it if you have liver disease.

teaches at the National College of Naturopathic Medicine in Portland and Bastyr University in Kenmore, Washington.

This is one treatment, however, for which knowledgeable medical supervision is a top priority. In the large doses needed to lower cholesterol—1,500 to 3,000 milligrams a day—niacin can cause liver problems. In fact, problems can start with doses as low as 500 milligrams, although some effects might not show up for years.

Anyone who is taking high doses must have regular blood tests to measure three essential liver enzymes, says Dr. Milner. You may find timed-release forms of niacin on your drugstore shelf, but immediate-release niacin is less likely to cause liver damage.

Dr. Milner uses inositol hexaniacinate (Niacinol) because studies show that it is also less likely than the timed-release form to cause liver damage. There's also less chance of this form causing niacin flush, the characteristic reddening of the skin and itching that some people experience after taking niacin. Even though it's readily available from naturopathic doctors and at some health food stores, it's not something that you should try without regular monitoring by your physician, Dr. Milner says.

With inositol hexaniacinate, the doctor might start you on a dose of 1,500 milligrams. If you take regular niacin, your doctor will begin with a much lower dose and increase it gradually over a period of weeks to help minimize flushing, says Dr. Milner.

Helping Vessels and Joints

Niacin can help people with Raynaud's disease for reasons that are related to the way it causes blood vessels to expand. For someone with Raynaud's, the blood vessels in the hands essentially clamp down, cutting off a warming blood supply. When it's severe, the hands literally turn white with cold.

Because niacin helps blood vessels expand, it seems to be just what the doctor ordered for Raynaud's. Some doctors, usually naturopaths, do prescribe it for this condition. "Niacin's ability to dilate the superficial blood vessels of the skin, mostly around the chest and face but also in the hands, helps to stop bouts of Raynaud's," Dr. Milner says.

The rationale for using niacinamide for arthritis is based mostly on the work of William Kaufman, MD, PhD, a doctor who pioneered nutritional therapy for people with the joint inflammation caused by this disease.

Some naturopathic doctors recommend up to 500 milligrams twice a day. "This form acts differently in the body than niacin does," Dr. Milner says. "It's thought to improve certain functions in the cells. It does seem to be safe at these amounts, though."

pantothenic acid

Pantos is a Greek word that means "everywhere"—an appropriate prefix for the name of a vitamin that's found in most foods.

It's fortunate that this B vitamin is so plentiful, because it's very important to our bodies. "It is involved in many different metabolic pathways, including the conversion of food to energy, the synthesis of important hormones, and the body's utilization of body fat and cholesterol," says Won O. Song, PhD, RD, professor of nutrition at Michigan State University in East Lansing.

This vitamin helps to convert carbohydrates and fats to energy and to break down and reassemble fats into new forms, some of which are used to make important hormones. It acts as a matchmaker between proteins and fatty acids, combining them into molecules called lipoproteins, which in turn make up the membranes that enclose our cells.

Pantothenic acid also plays an important role in making hemoglobin, the protein found in red blood cells that transports oxygen throughout our bodies. It helps our bodies detoxify a virtual Love Canal's–worth of nasty chemicals, and at high doses it could prove useful for chronic diseases such as rheumatoid arthritis and chronic fatigue syndrome.

Good—And Good for You

Pantothenic acid is an essential component of a substance called coenzyme A (CoA). Enzymes are like spark plugs, helping to jump-start the chemical reactions that go on continuously in our bodies and allowing us to turn food into energy and produce the tissues that hold us together.

CoA plays an extremely broad role, especially in the production of energy. It helps to transport blood sugar, fatty acids, and even protein as these compounds are combined or converted to different forms. Our bodies also use it to detoxify many of the harmful man-made compounds found in herbicides, insecticides, and drugs, says Dr. Song.

Apart from its role in CoA production, pantothenic acid has some benefits on its own. Research suggests that it and pantethine, a form of the vitamin, may be therapeutic for some diseases.

In doses of 900 milligrams a day, pantethine has been shown in studies to significantly reduce cholesterol and triglycerides. This is important because high levels of either can lead to atherosclerosis (hardening of the arteries) and blockages in the blood vessels. Pantethine apparently inhibits the body's production of cholesterol while accelerating the use of fat as an energy source. Plain old pantothenic acid has no such effect, Dr. Song says.

Also in studies, pantothenic acid in the form of calcium pantothenate (50 to 2,000 milligrams a day) has been used to reduce the stiffness and pain of rheumatoid arthritis.

Acidic Action

Pantothenic acid is sometimes considered an antistress vitamin by doctors of alternative medicine because of its important role in the function of the adrenal glands, which produce hormones that help our bodies respond to stress. In studies in which people were made deficient in pantothenic

SUPPLEMENT SNAPSHOT

▶Pantothenic Acid

Supplement forms: Calcium pantothenate and pantethine; also known as vitamin B_5.

Daily Value: 10 milligrams.

May help: Stress, rheumatoid arthritis, osteoarthritis, chronic fatigue syndrome, menopausal discomforts, and high cholesterol and triglycerides.

Good food sources: Meat, fish, poultry, unprocessed whole grains, fortified cereals, legumes, peanuts, mushrooms, soy flour, and split peas.

Who's at risk for deficiency: Deficiency is thought to be rare, but people with serious drinking problems, older people on restricted diets, and people taking cholesterol-lowering drugs may be at risk; also, some people may simply need more than normal.

Cautions and possible side effects: Generally regarded as safe.

acid by feeding them something that interfered with its use in the body, symptoms of listlessness and fatigue developed after about 9 weeks.

Deficiencies have been known to produce other problems, as well. Possible symptoms include a burning sensation in the feet, depression, fatigue, insomnia, vomiting, and muscle cramping or weakness. Since pantothenic acid is so widely available in foods, such deficiencies are seldom seen, but studies indicate that some people in the United States aren't getting enough. The Daily Value is 10 milligrams, and studies have shown that the average intake for most Americans is 5 to 10 milligrams a day.

Since up to 50 percent of the pantothenic acid in foods is lost in processing or cooking, the best sources are unprocessed whole grains, fortified cereals, and supplements. When sold as a supplement, pantothenic acid is sometimes labeled as vitamin B_5. Other forms include calcium pantothenate and pantethine.

phytonutrients

Despite the complicated sound of this word, there's no mystery to it. *Phyto-* simply means "plant," and phytonutrient supplements contain nutrients derived from plants.

Each of those nutrients is thought to have some sort of health benefit. Some can help reduce inflammation and aid digestion. Others may help protect your arteries from plaque, the sticky stuff that can clog up blood vessels and raise your risk of heart attack or stroke. Still others can help reduce cell damage.

Once isolated from the plant material, phytonutrients can be recombined in various ways. A phytonutrient such as isoflavone, for instance, may be isolated and concentrated from soybeans, then put into a pill. Add some lycopene from tomatoes, some beta-carotene from carrots, and a few anthocyanins from red cabbage, and you have a sort of vegetable soup in a pill that may, at least in theory, give you a few of the many health benefits of a real vegetable soup.

A Surfeit of Nutrients

Sometimes, there are so many nutrients included in a supplement that the soup is almost a stew. One well-known vitamin manufacturer, for example, makes a supplement called the MaxiLife Phytonutrient Protector. The greenish yellow, grassy-smelling capsules contain beta- and alpha-carotene, lutein, zeaxanthin, lycopene, citrus bioflavonoids, quercetin, bilberry extract, pine bark extract, red cabbage extract, red wine concentrate, grape skin extract, elderberry extract, green tea extract, soy isoflavone concentrate, citrus terpene extract, broccoli extract, garlic, rosemary extract, and turmeric extract.

Many of these food components have some potential value, at least when they are consumed as part of your diet. Rosemary, for instance, is a strong antioxidant that helps to protect cells from the kind of speeded-up aging and cell damage that can be caused by free-roaming, unstable molecules called free radicals. In fact, it works so well that rosemary oil extract is used as a food preservative.

Another phytonutrient source, turmeric, is a yellow spice that's often used in Indian cooking. It can help reduce inflammation and aid digestion.

But aren't you only getting a pill-size amount of the nutrient in a pill? Well, actually, a lot can be packed into that pill. It is possible to isolate and then concentrate certain components from foods—such as isoflavones from soybeans—and come up with a pill that contains as many isoflavones as a serving of tofu.

What the Labels Leave Out

It's hard to tell just by looking at the label of a supplement whether you're getting a substantial amount of a phytonutrient or just a smidgen. "Right now, it is very difficult to evaluate such products," says Ronald Prior, PhD, a research scientist at the Jean Mayer USDA Human Nutrition Research Center on Aging at Tufts University in Boston.

SUPPLEMENT SNAPSHOT

▶Phytonutrients

Individual names: Isoflavone, lycopene, carotenes, anthocyanins, lutein, and zeaxanthin, among others.

May help: Cancer, heart disease, stroke, restless legs syndrome, and macular degeneration.

Good food sources: Dark leafy greens, berries of all sorts, grapes, red wine, tea, citrus fruits, cruciferous vegetables such as red cabbage, red onions, deep orange vegetables, herbs, spices, garlic, and tomatoes.

Special instructions: Take with food.

Cautions and possible side effects: Don't take more than the recommended dosage. Never consider supplements to be a substitute for food; the best variety and quantities of phytonutrients are found in a diet that's rich in fruits and vegetables.

Since there's no standardization of such products, the only thing you can count on when shopping for phytonutrient supplements is a lot of inconsistency. Even though, based on their labels, products seem similar, the potency of each product is different.

"You can't knock all these products," concludes Dr. Prior. "Some are good and some are not so good. Right now, though, there's no way for the consumer to really tell which ones are good just from reading the labels."

One product's daily dose offers 100 milligrams of soy isoflavone concentrate. That's about the amount found in 1½ cups of tofu. It also has 25,000 international units (IU) of beta-carotene, which helps resist cell damage and may reduce the risk of some kinds of cancer. You'd get only half that much in a 9-inch carrot. With the supplement providing an additional 100 milligrams of citrus bioflavonoid complex—another cell-protecting cancer fighter—you'll get about the same amount that you'd find in one or two Valencia oranges.

That same supplement product, however, contains only 5 milligrams of lycopene, the red pigment in tomatoes that's linked with a reduction in prostate cancer. By comparison, ½ cup of tomato sauce has 22 milligrams.

Even paying top dollar doesn't ensure quality, Dr. Prior has found. "Some of the better products that we have evaluated are also the cheapest," he says.

Picking the Phytos

How can you make the best selection from the variety of phytonutrient products on the market?

You might think that the more, the better, but unfortunately the quantity of phytonutrients doesn't determine the quality of the supplement. Three sources of flavonoids listed on a label, for instance, might seem impressive. But that number is small compared to the approximately 4,000 different flavonoids in all of the different fruits and vegetables, Dr. Prior notes.

The best policy is to select a major store brand or a product from a major manufacturer. Either supplier has more to lose if it's revealed that a product doesn't deliver what it promises.

Avoid products that simply say "broccoli" or "parsley" in their list of ingredients. It means that you are getting only a costly, microscopic, freeze-dried serving of that vegetable. Instead, look for products whose labels say that they contain standardized extracts of a phytonutrient. It's no guarantee, but it at least suggests some initial quality control, Dr. Prior says.

Also, look for a mixture of those phytonutrients with the strongest evidence of health benefits. These include mixed carotenoids (just beta-carotene is not enough), including lycopene, suggests Andrew Weil, MD, director of the Center for Integrative Medicine at the University of Arizona, in Tucson, and author of *Eight Weeks to Optimum Health*. Or look for a supplement that includes substantial amounts of a particular phytonutrient you want, he says.

If you're concerned about prostate cancer, for instance, look for lycopene. If you're worried about macular degeneration, a common cause of deteriorating vision in older people, look for capsules that contain lutein and zeaxanthin, the two phytonutrients that, in dietary studies, seem to be most strongly linked with a reduced risk of this condition.

Whatever phytonutrients you take, it's important to keep in mind that they are not substitutes for real fruits and vegetables. More and more evidence suggests that there does seem to be something beneficial about getting nutrients in the whole food package as opposed to just taking supplements. You still need to consume (in other words, eat!) the natural sources of these health-conferring compounds.

potassium

If you have a family history of stroke or have had a stroke yourself, if you have high blood pressure or need to prevent it, and especially if you take diuretics to control high blood pressure, you'll want to learn all you can about potassium. It could save your life.

Potassium is one of those essential nutrients that's found pretty much everywhere in your body. It's especially concentrated inside cells. There, it helps maintain the proper balance of fluid and other electrolytes, such as sodium and chloride, which allow a cell to act like a tiny battery with its own electrical charge. The ability to generate an electrical charge is what lets cells do their work: If they're in muscles, they can contract and relax; if they're in nerves, they can fire off signals; and if they're in glands, they can secrete hormones.

The electrical charge also lets cells move things in and out through their membranes, activate enzymes involved in chemical reactions, and maintain proper pH (acid-base balance) within the cell walls. "Potassium plays a very basic and vital role in practically all aspects of cell activity," says Louis Tobian, MD, professor of medicine at the University of Minnesota Medical School in Minneapolis.

Potassium does a balancing act with sodium, which is one reason that it's so vital in maintaining proper blood pressure, Dr. Tobian explains. It works with sodium but also helps to keep it in check. During nerve transmission and muscle contraction, potassium and sodium briefly trade places across the cell membrane. Then they swap again, returning to their original positions and ready for action.

Proper Pressure

There's growing evidence that the more potassium you get in your diet, the less likely you are to develop high blood pressure. One reason for this probably has to do with potassium's interaction with sodium, says David

B. Young, PhD, professor of physiology and biophysics at the University of Mississippi Medical Center in Jackson. "The more potassium you get in your diet, the greater your ability to excrete sodium in your urine," he says.

Think of sodium as a water magnet. "When you excrete sodium, you also excrete water," says Dr. Young. "Excreting water reduces your blood volume, which in turn reduces your blood pressure. Thus, potassium achieves the same goal as a diuretic."

Potassium also inhibits the release of a hormone called renin from the kidneys. Renin activates another hormone, called angiotensin, which throws the switch on a kind of internal suction pump. When angiotensin is activated, your blood vessels constrict and your kidneys start to retain sodium. Both of these actions bump up blood pressure. "Having low renin levels is good in terms of lowering blood pressure," Dr. Young says.

Some popular blood pressure medications such as captopril (Capoten) and enalapril maleate (Vasotec) work along similar lines by interfering

SUPPLEMENT SNAPSHOT

▶Potassium

Daily Value: 3,500 milligrams.

May help: High blood pressure, stroke, leg cramps, and heart arrhythmia.

Good food sources: Baked potatoes, spinach (raw, microwaved, or steamed, for highest potassium content), dried apricots, dried prunes, cantaloupes, honeydew melons, adzuki beans, avocadoes, watermelon, acorn squash, and bananas.

Who's at risk for deficiency: People taking non-potassium-sparing diuretics such as furosemide (Lasix), digitalis, or steroids; those who don't eat fruits or vegetables, are heavy drinkers, have prolonged vomiting or diarrhea, overuse laxatives, or have eating disorders.

Cautions and possible side effects: Appears to be safe at any amount in foods, even up to 11,000 milligrams a day. But when taking supplements, do not take more than 5,000 milligrams without medical supervision. Large-dose supplements are available only by prescription; do not take without medical supervision. Excessive potassium can upset the balance of other minerals in the body and cause potentially fatal heart and kidney problems.

directly with angiotensin. "Possibly, you could use potassium to get some of the same effects that these drugs provide," Dr. Young says. In fact, that's the approach that some doctors take.

Independent of its effect on blood pressure, high potassium intake also seems to have a protective effect on the kidneys, Dr. Young says. In animal studies, a high-potassium diet has been shown to help prevent thickening of the small arteries that feed blood to this pair of vital, blood-cleaning, urine-producing organs.

Keeping the Beat

A normal heartbeat may seem simple, but it's a highly coordinated event, directed by the sequential firing of nerves that signal each chamber of the heart. When all goes well, the lower chambers and the upper chambers work in sequence, pumping blood to the lungs and the rest of the body.

When things go awry, the nerve signals may be delayed, or the nerves may fire more often than necessary. The chambers may not pump in proper sequence. The end result is that the heart pumps blood less efficiently. In fact, instead of pumping, it may go into a kind of quivery state, or arrhythmia, called fibrillation. This condition can be fatal if it's not quickly corrected.

You need potassium for the muscles of the heart to stay strong, Dr. Young says. Even moderate potassium depletion weakens the heart muscle. Most people whose hearts are affected by low potassium already have some sort of heart damage, such as an enlarged heart or damage to the heart muscle from a heart attack. Then, if their potassium levels decrease, their risk for arrhythmia rises. That's why most heart doctors monitor their patients' blood levels of potassium.

Stop a Stroke

Because they can maintain low blood pressure and help your heart beat normally (which reduces your chances of developing blood clots), a potassium-rich diet and possibly even supplements have the potential to reduce your chances of having a stroke. In a study from the Harvard School of Public Health, doctors analyzed data from food question-naires completed by nearly 44,000 healthy men ages 45 to 75. The study's conclusions were based on two groups: men in a high-potassium group who consumed nine servings of fruits and vegetables a day and men with diets that were lower in potassium, who ate only four servings of fruits and vegetables a day.

During the 8 years of follow-up, doctors found that men in the first group had a 38 percent lower risk of stroke than men in the low-potassium group. Remarkably, the greatest benefit was seen among men who had a history of high blood pressure and who were taking potassium supplements along with diuretics. Their risk was slashed by a whopping 64 percent.

Even if you can't seem to get your blood pressure down all that much, potassium still offers protection, Dr. Young says. In the arteries, for instance, it helps stop the buildup of cholesterol-laden plaque. "We believe it does this by interfering somehow with the action of certain immune cells, called macrophages, that attack LDL in the blood vessel wall," Dr. Young says.

Potassium also decreases the sensitivity of platelets—the parts of the blood that clot—to things that activate them and make them sticky. It also prevents the overgrowth of smooth muscle cells in blood vessels. This is important because thickened and stiffened blood vessels are more prone to blockages. "In several types of animals, we know that if we give extra potassium, we can prevent lesions in the arteries, and we can prevent blockages that occur after arteries have been reopened with a procedure such as balloon angioplasty," Dr. Young says.

Potato Chips versus Oranges

If you were to have a severe case of potassium deficiency, you might experience symptoms of muscle weakness, confusion, and heart irregularities. Most of us will never have that problem, however, because our bodies carefully regulate potassium levels.

"People don't develop severe potassium deficiencies unless they have some sort of endocrine or kidney problem, and then they are pretty sick for a number of reasons," Dr. Young says. While some diuretic drugs can seriously deplete the body of potassium, doctors monitor blood levels of potassium in people taking diuretics and supply extra potassium if necessary.

It's likely that a fair number of people in the United States are on the same kind of low-potassium, high-sodium diet that can cause high blood pressure and heart disease in animals, Dr. Tobian says. Many people just don't get their share of potassium-rich fruits and vegetables, and because of safety concerns, potassium isn't found in adequate amounts in multivitamin/mineral supplements.

While potassium from foods has not been associated with any ill effects, the same can't be said for potassium supplements. "You can kill yourself if you take too much potassium," Dr. Tobian says.

Prescription supplements do offer more potassium, but amounts need to be carefully monitored with blood tests, Dr. Tobian says. People might need prescription potassium supplements if they are taking diuretics that deplete potassium. For his patients with high blood pressure, those who have had strokes, and those who have family histories of stroke, Dr. Tobian combines a potassium-rich diet with supplements if necessary.

probiotics

Did you know that you have more bacteria and other microorganisms in and on your body than you have cells? That you wouldn't be able to live long without the little critters that cohabit with you? That antibiotics can wipe out not only the bad bugs, but the good ones, as well? That those good bugs are star players in your immune system? That's why these super small guys are called probiotics: They're "pros" at keeping you healthy.

Probiotics have been around for as long as we have, but in the last 20 years or so, research has revealed new findings that have only enhanced their reputation. In our intestines, probiotics provide a live barrier to infection. *Bifidobacteria* appear to be the most important microorganisms for this, and they literally park themselves on intestinal cells and won't budge for any bad bugs that come along. The list of bugs they can resist includes salmonella, *Heliobacter, Clostridium difficile, Pseudomonas,* and others.

They also produce lactic acid, which wards off other bugs. *Bifidobacteria* come in a variety of "strains" and belong to a large family of lactic acid–producing bacteria. These bacteria are found in live-culture yogurt and other fermented dairy products and include *Lactobacillus acidophilus,* the "original" yogurt bacteria known for calming GI upsets. In fact, the *lactobacillus* species in yogurt can stimulate the production of mucin, a slippery, protective coating secreted by intestinal goblet cells, which improves the intestinal environment.

Probiotics do other good things, too. They help us break down and absorb nutrients from foods. They even make some vitamins themselves, like vitamin K. They help nourish the cells lining our intestines, and they help break down fatty acids. They help to prevent food allergies in infants and adults. They help to prevent sepsis, a potentially fatal bodywide infection that can happen in seriously ill and immune-compromised people as an infection moves from the gut and into the bloodstream.

Friends of Your Immune System

Probiotics are considered to be "immunomodulators." That is, they both enhance the body's natural immunity and keep it from getting out of control, as it does with autoimmune diseases such as inflammatory bowel disease, says Tamara Trebilcock, ND, a specialist in integrative medicine in Santa Monica, California.

There is also some evidence that *Bifidobacteria* and other probiotics might help protect against cancer. *Bifidobacteria* decrease fecal enzymes such as beta-glucuronidase, beta-glucosidase, nitroreductase, and urease. These enzymes are involved in the activation of some chemicals that

SUPPLEMENT SNAPSHOT

▶ Probiotics

Scientific names: *Bifidobacteria, Lactobacillus, Saccharomyces boulardii, Streptococcus,* and many others.

May help: Vaginal yeast, vaginal bacterial and protozoal infections, urinary tract infections, bacterial overgrowth in the intestines, lactose intolerance, diarrhea, fibromyalgia, autoimmune diseases (such as inflammatory bowel disease, rheumatoid arthritis, and lupus), irritable bowel syndrome, high cholesterol, indigestion, constipation, gas, and respiratory infections.

Good food sources: Fermented milk products, including yogurt and kefir. High temperatures destroy probiotics, so fermented milk products are not good sources if they've been warmed.

Special instructions: Take with food that includes some soluble fiber, like that found in oatmeal or artichokes, to provide the probiotics with some nourishment. A minimum of 10 billion colony-forming units (CFU) per dose is needed to establish sustained growth in the intestines.

Cautions and possible side effects: If you have any serious gastrointestinal problems that require medical attention, check with your doctor before taking. Some prescription probiotic products, such as VSL#3, are pharmaceutical grade and are a good choice for people with inflammatory bowel disease because they are less likely to contain unwanted microorganisms that could cause additional problems.

promote the mutation of DNA and the development of cancer in cells lining the intestines. *Bifidobacteria* might also fight cancer by altering the way colon cells function, helping them to produce biochemicals that fight off cancer-promoting toxins, Dr. Trebilcock says.

Probiotics can also help women ward off not only vaginal yeast infections, but also other chronic low-grade infections, such as bacterial vaginosis (usually *Gardnerella* or *Mobiluncus*) or trichomoniasis—all conditions that are hard to get rid of, even after drug treatment. Probiotics can help prevent a recurrence because, taken orally and used vaginally, they can make the vagina inhospitable to these organisms.

Probiotics cut the risk of developing pneumonia in ventilator-assisted patients and show promise for the prevention of asthma, both by stimulating immunity and by helping to prevent aspiration of bad bugs from the stomach into the airways.

Different Strains for Different Folks

Researchers are still figuring out just how many strains of probiotics there are. Current count: more than 400. About 15 have been pretty well studied, Dr. Trebilcock says. In our digestive tract, there are two main *Lactobacillus* bacteria (*L. acidophilus* and *L. rhamnosus*), two main *Bifidobacteria* (*B. bifidum* and *B. lactis,* which used to be called *infantis*), and *Saccharomyces boulardii,* a good yeast. These are also the main forms found in probiotic products.

Different strains of probiotics do different things and act in different ways, and that's why treating yourself effectively takes more than just going to the health food store and picking up the first bottle that catches your eye, Dr. Trebilcock says.

If you are looking for something to take to prevent traveler's diarrhea, you just need *Bifidum* and *Lactobacillus,* Dr. Trebilcock says.

To prevent problems while taking antibiotics (which kill off the good bacteria as well as the bad), she recommends first using Proboulardi, to stimulate GI immunity, then using UltraFlora Plus DF from Metagenics to replenish beneficial microflora. (This is a 3:1 blend of *Bifido* to *Lactobacillus,* with a high number of CFU.) "You are taking 16 billion colony-forming units, twice a day, 4 hours away from antibiotic use, and then taking the same amounts for 30 days afterward," she says.

What about Yogurt?

Supplements aren't the only sources of probiotics. You can also get them from foods such as live-culture yogurt and other cultured milk products, as well as from naturally fermented foods such as sauerkraut and pickles. (However, most commercial products are not naturally fermented and contain no probiotics.)

Although probiotic supplements can be a predictable, concentrated source of probiotics, yogurt can have its own good things going for it, providing it's made right. Yogurt is made using one or more of a variety of probiotics, including *Lactobacillus acidophilus, Lactobacillus rhamnosus, Lactobacillus bulgaricus, Enterococcus faecium, Streptococcus thermophilus,* and others.

These bacteria provide the action that modulates the immune system and improves lactose tolerance. They partly digest milk, creating forms of calcium that are easily absorbed.

Two forms of probiotics used to create yogurt, *L. bulgaricus* and *S. thermophilus,* are thought not to easily survive the acid environment of the stomach. That's why more acid-resistant forms, such as *Lactobacillus,* are sometimes added to yogurt. Different manufacturers add different probiotics, and even prebiotics (soluble fibers, such as inulin, that help establish colonies), so check labels.

Other components of yogurt, such as whey protein, short peptides, and conjugated linoleic acid, are not usually found in probiotic supplements and may contribute to yogurt's immune-enhancing effects.

If you have a serious problem such as inflammatory bowel disease, or you have had colon cancer, see an integrative medicine doctor who can do a stool analysis and figure out what probiotics you need and whether you have an overgrowth of bad bacteria or yeast in your intestines, Dr. Trebilcock says. "If someone has ulcerative colitis, I am going to give them *Lactobacillus salivarius,* which has been found to be very effective at reducing inflammatory cytokines," she says. "*Lactobacillus planetarium* (grown on soy) has been found to reduce colorectal risk and to put Crohn's disease into remission, so I also use that with patients who have that concern," she adds.

How to Choose the Best Kind

Here's some additional advice to help you choose your supplement, from Dr. Trebilcock.

• Don't buy unrefrigerated brands, and don't bother with enteric-coated products. "I haven't found either to be as effective as refrigerated, noncoated brands," she says. Use capsules, not powders, unless you are unable to swallow capsules.

• Choose a product that has the strains of bacteria listed, has the strains of bacteria you specifically want, and has about 10 billion CFU of each.

• Check the expiration date. A good product will always have that.

• If you buy something online, request expedited shipping so that the product is less likely to be mishandled (exposed to heat).

• Store it right. Keep it in the refrigerator after you buy it, with the lid tightly closed. Heat, light, humidity, and oxygen can rob supplements of their live bacteria, although some top brands will retain potency for about 90 days without refrigeration.

red yeast rice

It doesn't sound all that appetizing to use a yeast that grows on fermented, soupy rice. But red yeast rice is cultivated in China both as a food and as a medicine. If you're a Chinese food fan, you've probably eaten it: The food version of red yeast rice is used mostly as coloring for Peking duck.

Medically, red yeast rice has been used in China for centuries to treat poor circulation and to improve conditions related to the heart. With the rise of cholesterol-lowering statins (and the subsequent rise of statin side effects), the popularity of red yeast rice as a natural cholesterol reducer has also shot up.

Red yeast rice—the real stuff, that is, and we'll get to that in a minute—does lower cholesterol. It contains a number of cholesterol-lowering substances, including monacolin K, which is identical to the cholesterol-lowering drug lovastatin. This has caused a bit of a rub with the FDA, since they state that monacolin K is a drug, yet red yeast rice is a supplement. Because of this, the FDA required one manufacturer, Pharmanex, to remove all but trace amounts of monacolin K from its product, Cholestin, saying that it is an unapproved drug and not a dietary supplement.

Many other red yeast rice products with varying amounts of monacolin K remain on the market, but it is very hard to figure out what's what, says David Becker, MD, of Chestnut Hill, Pennsylvania, one of the few American cardiologists doing research with red yeast rice. "It really is buyer beware," Dr. Becker says. "The FDA ruling doesn't make a lot of sense for this product, because the monacolins are there naturally and always have been." The ruling does nothing to help consumers make an informed choice about what to buy, either, he says.

It's in There

Even though the focus has been on monacolin K, red yeast rice contains about 10 similar monacolin compounds, and all are thought to help reduce cholesterol. In the case of monacolin K, it competitively inhibits an enzyme, 3-hydroxy-3-methylglutaryl-coenzyme A (HMG-CoA) reductase, which is needed for the body to produce cholesterol. Despite the insinuation of a few years back that dietary cholesterol was the main cause of elevated levels, we now know that your body is actually the bigger producer of cholesterol. Therefore, blocking cholesterol production in your own body can do a lot to keep your levels in a safe range.

There's even more stuff in red yeast rice that can help lower cholesterol and maintain cardiovascular health, says David Molony, DOM, PhD, a doctor of traditional Chinese medicine in Catasauqua, Pennsylvania. Red yeast rice also contains sterols, including beta-sitosterol. This plant form of cholesterol blocks the absorption of cholesterol in the gut. It also contains campesterol, stigmasterol, and sapogenin, a kind of plant hormone. All of these appear to have anti-inflammatory, anticlotting effects. And it contains even more anti-inflammatory compounds, such as isoflavones and isoflavone glycosides, as well as monounsaturated fatty acids.

SUPPLEMENT SNAPSHOT

▶Red Yeast Rice

Botanical name: *Monascus purpureus.*

Also known as: Xue Zhi Kang, hong qu.

Origin: China. Now cultivated in laboratories around the world.

Cautions and possible side effects: Although it seems to cause fewer side effects than most statin drugs, red yeast rice still has the potential to cause similar side effects: muscle pain, liver toxicity, and, rarely, rhabdomyolysis (the rapid breakdown of muscle tissue). Red yeast rice that has not been fermented correctly has the potential to contain citrinin, a compound that is toxic to the kidneys. Do not take red yeast rice without the same kind of medical supervision and liver enzymes tests you would get if you were taking statin drugs. Be aware that over-the-counter brands of red yeast rice contain widely varying amounts of monacolins, and some do contain citrinin. It's best to work with a health-care professional who can help you select an effective, safe red yeast rice product and monitor your health while you take it.

"It's strong stuff," Dr. Molony says. "With my patients, I tend to use it along with other treatments for a period of time until we get heart and circulation problems improved, and then, stop using it. I don't have people on it all the time."

Red Yeast Rice versus the Big Guys

Research is showing that red yeast rice is as up to the job as its pharmaceutical counterparts. A study from China showed that red yeast rice lowered the risk for heart disease by about 30 percent after an average of 4.5 years of use. It also decreased the need for bypass surgery, lowered triglycerides, and raised beneficial HDL, and it did so without any adverse effects.

Research conducted in the United States showed that people who were intolerant of statin drugs due to muscle pain were able to tolerate red yeast rice. They took 1,800 milligrams of red yeast rice twice a day for 24 weeks and had an average decrease in LDL cholesterol of 35 mg/dl, which is comparable to statin drugs.

Dr. Becker, the study's main investigator, noted that participants' tolerance of red yeast rice was better than expected. "Usually, about half the people who are intolerant of one statin drug are also intolerant when they switch to a different one," he says. "But people who switched to red yeast rice were able to tolerate it better. Only three people (about 10 percent) on red yeast rice dropped out of the study because of muscle pain."

Another recent study found that red yeast rice was comparable to pravastatin, a fairly well-tolerated statin drug. The people in the study taking red yeast rice attained slightly lower cholesterol than the group taking pravastatin, and both groups tolerated the treatment well, Dr. Becker says. "I believe that red yeast rice, if properly regulated to control for potential contaminants and regulate consistency between different manufacturers, might represent an option for these difficult-to-treat patients," he says.

Buying an Effective Product Can Be Difficult

Because of the lack of control over amounts of active ingredients and the possibility for contamination, it's hard for the average consumer to just go out there and buy a red yeast rice product, Dr. Becker says. Brands such as Cholestin and Traditional Supplements Red Yeast Rice have been used in clinical trials.

Health care professionals like doctors of traditional Chinese medicine and licensed naturopathic doctors—and even some cardiologists—may use professional brands of higher quality, too. Beware of products made in China, where oversight is lax.

Dr. Becker suggests several precautions if you're going to use red yeast rice to lower cholesterol or you're planning to switch from a statin drug you're currently taking.

• Talk to your doctor before going off any medication and switching to a supplement.

• Don't take both red yeast rice and a statin drug without medical supervision. You'll be double-dosing yourself.

• Take 100 to 200 milligrams of CoQ_{10} each day, to prevent the depletion of this important energy-producing biochemical. Both statins and red yeast rice interfere with the body's production of CoQ_{10}.

• Get your liver enzymes checked about 6 weeks after starting red yeast rice, and then every 6 months thereafter, for as long as you take it.

• Consider also taking additional phytosterols to further reduce LDL cholesterol.

• Dosages ranging from 600 to 1,800 milligrams twice a day have been shown to be effective. Don't take more than 1,800 milligrams twice a day; taking more doesn't lower cholesterol further.

• Support your efforts with a healthy lifestyle: Exercise for 30 minutes a day, reduce saturated and trans fats, drink green tea or take a green tea supplement, eat garlic or take garlic supplements, eat fish or take fish-oil supplements, and eat plenty of leafy greens and fresh fruit.

• Tell your doctor if you experience side effects. You'll have to stay off red yeast rice for about 6 weeks to see if the symptoms go away, confirming that the supplement caused the symptoms you've experienced.

riboflavin

If you take a multivitamin that contains riboflavin, you may have noticed that your urine takes on a yellow-green glow soon after you pop the supplement. Whenever an excess of this B vitamin is excreted, you're likely to see that mysterious glow.

Riboflavin does more than produce psychedelic urine, however. It is a key player in the body's production of energy from fat, carbohydrates, and protein. It also helps our bodies produce glutathione, which acts as an antioxidant by protecting us from the cellular damage that can lead to cancer and heart disease.

Riboflavin is also needed to help several other B vitamins go about their work. It changes vitamin B_6 into a form that the body can use, and it helps change the amino acid tryptophan into niacin, another essential B vitamin. "Even though we often focus on riboflavin's role in energy metabolism, it plays several other important roles throughout the body," says Donald McCormick, PhD, chairman of the department of biochemistry at Emory University in Atlanta.

Energy Relay

Like many of the other B vitamins, riboflavin helps us generate energy. Inside the mitochondria, a cell's tiny powerhouse, riboflavin acts as a kind of shuttle bus. It helps to move electrons derived from the foods we eat along a pathway called the electron transport chain. As the electrons are passed along, they release energy.

The energy is used to make a molecule called ATP that acts as the cell's basic energy currency. It is used extensively throughout our bodies any time energy is needed—to move muscles, make protein, and digest food. When it's in short supply, all body functions slow down, and we feel less energetic.

In addition, riboflavin seems to have the power to control migraines. While it's unlikely to rival aspirin as a headache stopper, researchers have noted that people with an inherited disorder that includes migraine headaches showed improvement with the supplement. "These people have fewer, less severe headaches when they get additional riboflavin," says Marc Lenaerts, MD, a neurologist at the University of Oklahoma Health Sciences Center in Oklahoma City.

Given the results of these studies, "we decided to study the effects of additional riboflavin in people with 'normal' migraines," Dr. Lenaerts says. Their first study with migraine sufferers showed a 68 percent reduction in headache symptoms among people who took riboflavin. Another study 4 years later included a second group that was given an inactive substance (a placebo) instead of riboflavin; it was more carefully controlled to account for a possible placebo effect. It showed 37 percent fewer migraines, plus less nausea and vomiting, in people who took 400 milligrams of riboflavin a day as one daily dose.

SUPPLEMENT SNAPSHOT

▶Riboflavin

Supplement form: Riboflavin-5-phosphate; also known as vitamin B_2.

Daily Value: 1.7 milligrams.

May help: Migraine headaches, cataracts, and sickle-cell disease.

Good food sources: Eggs, lean meat, milk, broccoli, and enriched breads and cereals.

Who's at risk for deficiency: The elderly, who tend to eat fewer riboflavin-containing foods; people who are exercising and dieting; people who don't drink milk; alcoholics; those who are undergoing dialysis or taking diuretics, antibiotics, or barbiturates; and people with intestinal problems that interfere with absorption.

Special instructions: Since riboflavin is destroyed by light, buy milk in cardboard containers. A translucent plastic jug of milk sitting in a lighted dairy case for just one day can lose up to 70 percent of its riboflavin.

Cautions and possible side effects: May cause photosensitivity at high dosages (more than a few milligrams a day).

"This improvement is similar to what can be achieved using conventional preventive migraine drugs," Dr. Lenaerts says. He's hoping to do more studies to confirm this benefit of riboflavin for migraine sufferers and to determine if a lower dose might be just as helpful.

Free Radical Rounder-Upper

Riboflavin also helps our bodies make glutathione, a free radical scavenger that's produced by cells. Some people simply can't produce glutathione because of an inherited abnormality, and they have a marked increase in cell damage. Red blood cells break down more easily, while white blood cells and nerves are also affected. With more riboflavin to support the production of glutathione, it seems reasonable to assume that people would experience less cellular damage.

Animal research has led some scientists to believe that people who are deficient in riboflavin are more likely to develop cataracts, because glutathione helps to protect the eyes from damage by sunlight.

In one study on animal tissue, researchers found that riboflavin can help protect tissues from damage from oxygen that occurs when blood flow stops, then starts again. That stop-start pattern is exactly what develops when someone has a heart attack or stroke.

People with sickle-cell disease, in which misshapen cells occasionally clog blood vessels, may also benefit from additional riboflavin. In one study, people with sickle cell disease who were given 5 milligrams of supplemental riboflavin twice a day for 8 weeks showed significant improvements in their health profiles.

Who Needs More?

The Daily Value for riboflavin is 1.7 milligrams, and most people get all that and more from the foods they eat, Dr. McCormick says. The majority of people who seem to benefit from extra riboflavin, such as those with migraine headaches, may be relatively riboflavin-deficient because of the way their cells work, not because their food sources are letting them down, says Dr. Lenaerts.

Some people don't get enough riboflavin and other B vitamins simply because they don't eat well. These include alcoholics, elderly people who don't eat enough calories, and people who have sworn off dairy products, eggs, or meat. The lack of dairy foods is particularly telling, since most people get about half of their daily riboflavin from milk and milk products. Vegans (strict vegetarians) can obtain ample riboflavin in their diets, especially if they include dark green vegetables. They can also get additional riboflavin from nutritional yeast, which is another good source.

People with intestinal problems that interfere with absorption and people undergoing dialysis may also show symptoms of riboflavin deficiency.

Long-term use of some antibiotics can increase riboflavin excretion, and a class of psychiatric drugs called phenothiazines, which includes Thorazine, can interfere with the body's ability to use riboflavin, Dr. McCormick says. People who are taking these drugs may need supplementation.

Classic deficiency symptoms include cracks and redness at the corners of the mouth; a painful, smooth, purplish red tongue; inflamed eyelids and sensitivity to light; and an unsightly skin rash called seborrheic dermatitis.

Shortages of other B vitamins can also cause these symptoms, and riboflavin deficiency can cause shortages of other B vitamins, notably B_6. If you suspect that you have a riboflavin deficiency, it's best to make sure that you're getting enough of all the B vitamins, Dr. McCormick says. If you do have a deficiency, your doctor may advise you to take supplements, he adds.

You need to be careful not to overdo it, however, since taking too much has the potential to cause photosensitivity. "If your body is saturated with riboflavin and you're sitting out in the sun, there is the possibility of injury to your skin or eyes," Dr. McCormick says.

saw palmetto

If you've read anything about saw palmetto in the popular press, you probably know that it has come to be known as a "guy herb." The guys most likely to want it are primarily middle-aged or older men who find that they're answering nature's call two or three times a night.

Typically, that call of nature ends up being an almost-false alarm: Even when it feels like a waterfall is about to pour forth, the result is more of a trickle. This problem is often a sign of benign prostatic hyperplasia (BPH), a noncancerous enlargement of the prostate gland that constricts the ure-thra, the tube that leads from the bladder to the penis. Picture what happens to your lawn sprinkler when you step on the garden hose, and you have a good idea of the problem.

Many men who take saw palmetto find that the herb shrinks the pros-tate and releases the squeeze so that urine flows normally, says Woodson Merrell, MD, a specialist in alternative and complementary medicine and assistant clinical professor of medicine at the Columbia University College of Physicians and Surgeons in New York City.

How well saw palmetto works is still controversial because it may not be strong enough by itself to make a significant difference for some men, says Dr. Merrell. "It may be effective for moderate cases of BPH or when the prostate is just beginning to enlarge, however."

Purging the Pipes

Saw palmetto is a low, scrubby palm that grows in sandy soil in the southern United States, from South Carolina to Florida.

The Seminoles of the Everglades ate the berries for food, but it's not known if they valued the plant as a medicine. European settlers in the region used it as a diuretic to flush excess water from the body. In 1849, one herbal practitioner referred to the herb's "purgative property, often producing a copious evacuation."

Herbalists of that era also touted saw palmetto's anticatarrhal properties, meaning that it seemed to relieve phlegm-producing conditions like colds and flu. The herb was used as an expectorant in some cough formulas.

Women took it to relieve painful periods and regulate the menstrual cycle. It has also been used for pelvic inflammatory disease and similar conditions.

Saw palmetto is known to stimulate the production of prolactin, a female hormone that, among other things, promotes breast enlargement and milk production in breastfeeding women, and prostate growth in men, says Tirun Gopal, MD, an obstetrician and gynecologist who practices holistic and Ayurvedic medicine in Allentown, Pennsylvania. "There also are some claims that saw palmetto can be used for infertility when the problem is the absence of ovulation," he says.

Perhaps that is where the herb got a reputation as an aphrodisiac and a tonic to increase sexual energy and revive low libido in both sexes. Some research demonstrates that a compound in saw palmetto has aphrodisiac effects. Ironically, some herbalists have been known to use saw palmetto to treat honeymoon cystitis, bladder irritation that results from excessive sexual activity.

A Drug No More

Sexual matters aside, saw palmetto was widely and routinely used in the early decades of the 20th century to treat urinary tract ailments, particularly

---

SUPPLEMENT SNAPSHOT

▶Saw Palmetto

Botanical name: *Serenoa repens*.

Origin: Southern United States.

May help: Prostate problems, bladder irritation, menstrual problems, and pelvic inflammatory disease.

Cautions and possible side effects: If you have prostate problems, see your doctor for a diagnosis before using. Use saw palmetto in addition to, not instead of, conventional medical interventions.

chronic cystitis, an inflammation of the bladder. From 1906 to 1950, it was officially listed as a drug in the United States, and it was prescribed both here and in Europe as a treatment for gonorrhea.

After World War II, saw palmetto fell out of favor in the United States, but research continued in Europe. Scientists found that patients who consumed an extract of the berries had increased urine volume, a decrease in frequent urination, and more ease of urination.

As with many botanical medicines, it's difficult to identify exactly what active ingredients are working in saw palmetto. Scientists believe that it has steroidlike properties. In the case of BPH, it interrupts a critical chemical process, says William Page-Echols, DO, an assistant clinical professor of family medicine who teaches alternative medicine at the Michigan State University College of Osteopathic Medicine in East Lansing.

BPH occurs when testosterone, the male sex hormone, is converted by an enzyme to a more potent hormone that causes cells and tissues to grow and proliferate. That growth is perfectly fine when the male sexual organs are developing, but later in life, when the organs are fully developed, the continued cell growth becomes a liability. Taken daily, saw palmetto inhibits the enzyme so the hormone conversion doesn't occur, says Dr. Page-Echols. Finasteride (Proscar), the prescription drug most often prescribed in the United States for BPH, causes much the same action, he adds.

Saw palmetto doesn't seem to affect overall prostate size, but it does shrink the inner lining, called the epithelium. It also has anti-inflammatory actions and inhibits overgrowth of prostate cells. Plus, it seems to help reduce spasms in the prostate.

Gentle and Effective

Researchers have compared the effectiveness of saw palmetto with that of other drugs prescribed for BPH. Although results were somewhat mixed, tests showed that the herb produces fewer side effects than prescription drugs. Finasteride, for example, sometimes causes headaches, erection problems, loss of libido, and decreased ejaculation volume.

The German Federal Ministry of Health has determined that people experience few side effects from saw palmetto berries. In one 3-year study, less than 2 percent of men taking an alcohol-based extract of the herb quit the study because of side effects. More than 80 percent of the men felt that the herb helped and improved their quality of life.

"When your medication is causing you to have decreased interest in sex and decreased capabilities, saw palmetto may be an important alternative to try," says Dr. Page-Echols. "A lot of men have come into my office asking about it. They've heard about it from friends."

Where to See Saw

When Dr. Page-Echols suggests saw palmetto, he usually advises using it in combination with zinc and plant-based medicines such as flower pollen. It's also available in capsule and tincture form.

Since saw palmetto isn't standardized for any active ingredient and analysis of products shows a wide variation in their chemical compositions, your best bet is to look for a product made solely from the berries and manufactured by a well-known company, says Dr. Merrell. Most clinical studies have used a liposterolic extract of saw palmetto berry containing 80 to 90 percent free fatty acids. This formulation is similar to several over-the-counter brands: Super Saw Palmetto (by Enzymatic Therapy), Saw Palmetto (by Centrum), and Standardized Saw Palmetto Extract (by Nature's Way), among others.

Also, remember that, like many herbs, saw palmetto has a fairly mild action. It may take 2 months or more before it starts to work. Plus, there is no proof that saw palmetto reduces your risk of getting prostate cancer.

"Don't just start taking the herb without seeing your doctor," Dr. Merrell warns. "You shouldn't assume that your symptoms are due to BPH. Make sure that you have a benign condition first, then try the herb."

selenium

If you've heard anything about this essential trace mineral, it's probably been news that's related to cancer prevention. Studies from around the world suggest that where selenium intake is very low—usually because of selenium-poor soil—cancer rates tend to be higher than normal.

Selenium has been associated with reduced cancer risk since the late 1960s, but findings were slow to be popularized because of exaggerated concerns about the potential for toxicity. It's true that selenium can be toxic in high amounts, but the mineral actually has one of the strongest bodies of literature supporting its role as an anticancer agent.

A study done at the University of Arizona hints at selenium's potential. It was designed to look for a change in the rates of skin cancer and included more than 1,000 people (with an average age of 63) with a history of skin cancer. The participants were divided into two groups and were followed for 6 years. For about 4 years, one group received 200 micrograms daily of selenium from high-selenium yeast, which contains a special form of the mineral. The other group got inactive look-alike pills (placebos). When the study ended, the members of the group that had gotten the selenium had a 37 percent reduction in cancer risk. They also had a 50 percent reduction in cancer deaths.

Surprisingly, there was no reduction in the incidence of skin cancer. Instead, there were 63 percent fewer cases of prostate cancer, 58 percent fewer colon and rectal cancers, and 45 percent fewer lung cancers in the selenium-taking group.

Like vitamins C and E, selenium helps to prevent damage throughout the body from free-roaming, unstable molecules called free radicals. "Selenium's role in the body is complex, however, and not yet fully understood," says Orville Levander, PhD, a research leader at the USDA Beltsville Human Nutrition Research Center in Maryland. "There are probably a dozen or so different selenium-containing proteins in the body," he says. "Some have antioxidant activity, and some apparently have other roles."

In addition to possibly helping to prevent cancer, selenium seems to inhibit certain viral infections. It also interacts with iodine to activate thyroxine, the thyroid gland's main hormone, and it promotes the infection-fighting abilities of certain immune cells.

Kind to Your Heart and Cells

Selenium is an indispensable part of a free radical–quenching enzyme called glutathione peroxidase, which, when teamed with another kind of selenium-containing enzyme, can help protect us from heart disease. We don't know exactly why selenium has this protective effect. Possibly, these enzymes offer protection by maintaining the essential fats that form a shield around cells in the artery walls, suggests Vladimir Badmaev, MD, PhD, vice president of scientific and medical affairs for Sabinsa, a corporation in Piscataway, New Jersey, that makes selenium supplements. Without the selenium needed, Dr. Badmaev speculates, this shield could be damaged by free radicals, causing the arteries to collect plaque.

SUPPLEMENT SNAPSHOT

▶Selenium

Supplement forms: Selenomethionine, sodium selenite, and high-selenium yeast.

Daily Value: 70 micrograms.

May help: Cancer, heart disease, angina, cataracts, hair loss, lupus, and HIV; may limit spread of chronic infections.

Good food sources: Lobster, clams, crab, cooked oysters, and Brazil nuts.

Who's at risk for deficiency: People who get most of their food from selenium-poor soil. Deficiency is rare in countries where food is transported or imported and where diets include meat and shellfish.

Cautions and possible side effects: Don't take more than 200 micrograms in supplement form; higher amounts may cause fragile, thickened nails; stomach pain; diarrhea; loss of sensation in the hands and feet; fatigue; and irritability. Doses of about 800 micrograms have been known to cause tissue damage.

Some research indicates that selenium may prevent cancer by inhibiting tumor growth and inducing a kind of suicide (called apoptosis) in malignant cells. In tumor cells grown in the laboratory, selenium stimulates programmed cell death, which is a very late effect in the cancer process.

Other selenium-dependent enzymes can disarm a veritable toxic waste–dump's worth of harmful substances, including drugs; chemicals such as the herbicide paraquat; and toxic metals such as mercury, cadmium, and arsenic.

Virus Fighter

Researchers first became interested in selenium's role in viral infections when their attention was drawn to one area of China where the soil is low in selenium. People living in that low-selenium neighborhood were much more likely than normal to die of a form of heart disease called Keshan disease, which is characterized by cardiomyopathy, or weakening of the heart muscle. It is thought to be a result of a viral infection that occurs when a selenium deficiency causes a normally harmless virus to change into a deadly strain, Dr. Levander says.

Researchers know that in selenium-deficient animals, the harmless virus can mutate into a virulent form capable of causing heart damage and death. "In studies where the virus was removed from the selenium-deficient animals and injected into animals that were getting sufficient selenium, it remained in its deadly, mutated form," Dr. Levander says.

Several viruses are known to interact with selenium, according to Will Taylor, PhD, an AIDS researcher and associate professor at the College of Pharmacy at the University of Georgia in Athens. "The rate of progression from HIV to AIDS, for instance, has been strongly correlated with selenium status," he says.

In a study at the University of Miami, people with HIV who were deficient in selenium were 20 times more likely to die from AIDS within 6 months than people with normal selenium levels. Other viruses potentially linked with the mineral include hepatitis C and measles, Dr. Taylor says. No studies have been done on the effect of supplements, however.

Selenium apparently is used initially by viruses to help establish themselves in the body, so a viral infection can deplete the mineral. Later, however, during a long period when many chronic viral infections don't create symptoms, selenium appears to act as a kind of viral birth control. It seems to restrict rather than encourage the spread of the virus.

Don't Take Too Much

The Daily Value for selenium is 70 micrograms, and people in the United States get an average of a little more than 100 micrograms of selenium a day. Food sources of selenium include crab, liver, fish, poultry, and whole wheat.

If you're taking a selenium supplement, says Dr. Levander, you'll want to use one that doesn't put your total selenium for the day much above 350 micrograms (for a 150-pound person). "We don't have good information on when selenium becomes toxic, but taking no more than 200 micrograms a day as a supplement seems to be within reason for most people if they choose to supplement," Dr. Levander says.

thiamin

To understand what thiamin does in your body, consider the word that describes thiamin deficiency: beriberi. This East Asian word means, literally, "I can't, I can't," and people with beriberi can't do a lot. They're tired, weak, and uninterested in things, especially food. They may have numb or burning feet, leg cramps, and sometimes even mental confusion and an enlarged heart.

Recurrent canker sores may also be a tip-off to thiamin deficiency. A study by Israeli researchers found that 70 percent of people with recurrent canker sores had low blood levels of thiamin, compared to only 4 percent of people who did not have canker sores.

Like the other B vitamins, thiamin is involved in energy metabolism. "That means it helps you to derive energy from the calories you get from food," explains Joanne Curran-Celentano, PhD, RD, associate professor of nutrition and food sciences at the University of New Hampshire in Durham. "It helps to break down the molecules in foods and either rearrange them into a form your body can use for energy or store them for later use as energy."

Thiamin interacts with several enzymes—the biochemical spark plugs that get chemical reactions going in your body. "Several of the enzymes involved in the process of breaking down carbohydrates for energy require thiamin," Dr. Curran-Celentano explains. The fatigue associated with thiamin deficiency is, figuratively, the equivalent of a clogged carburetor. You may have a full tank, but none of the gasoline is being burned to run the engine.

Have Diabetes? Take Note

Deficiency of several B vitamins, including thiamin, has been associated with type 2 diabetes. Adequate thiamin is essential to warding off diabetes because thiamin helps keep blood sugar from sticking to proteins and fats, a harmful process that literally gunks up your body. Research also shows that high sugar levels cause more damage when blood thiamin levels are low. Conversely, supplementing with thiamin reduces sugar damage. In one study, adding thiamin to a cell culture reduced sugar-related damage by an impressive 80 percent.

Brain Gain

Thiamin's ability to make energy available for the body has ramifications for the brain, too. "If you dramatically reduce thiamin intake, you reduce the ability of the brain to use glucose (blood sugar). If you reduce that, you have impaired mental function," says Gary Gibson, PhD, professor of neuroscience at the Burke Medical Research Institute of Weill Medical College of Cornell University in White Plains, New York. Unlike other body parts, which can switch to other fuels if they need to, the brain prefers to use glucose exclusively, Dr. Gibson explains.

Thiamin is also very important in the synthesis of critical neurotransmitters in the brain, including one involved in memory and performance—

SUPPLEMENT SNAPSHOT

▶Thiamin

Also known as: Vitamin B_1.

Daily Value: 1.5 milligrams. A therapeutic dose, such as is used to help treat diabetes, may be 50 milligrams a day or higher.

May help: Beriberi, diabetes, alcoholic brain disease and neuropathy, and canker sores.

Good food sources: Baker's and brewer's yeast, lean pork and ham, legumes, nuts, and whole-grain or enriched breads and cereals.

Who's at risk for deficiency: Alcoholics, diabetics, people with HIV, people with intestinal absorption problems, and the elderly.

Special instructions: For best absorption, don't take with alcohol, tea, or coffee.

Cautions and possible side effects: No known problems from oral doses.

acetylcholine. "We know that thiamin-deficient animals don't make much acetylcholine and that this lowers their ability to remember and respond," Dr. Gibson says. "So we believe that high levels of acetylcholine are important for proper brain function."

Just how much of a role thiamin plays in human mental performance has yet to be determined. In one study, though, young women with no signs of deficiency who took 50 milligrams of thiamin a day for 2 months reported feeling more clear-headed, composed, and energetic than those who weren't getting the supplements. Those taking the extra thiamin also had faster reaction times on tests than those without supplementation.

In other studies, thiamin deficiency has been found to cause mood changes, vague feelings of uneasiness, fear, disorderly thinking, and other signs of mental depression. All of these are symptoms that researchers say often affect memory, Dr. Gibson says.

Thiamin deficiency clearly plays a role in the mental deterioration associated with alcoholism, since alcohol causes thiamin to be excreted faster, and many alcoholics don't get much of the vitamin because they eat poorly. Some alcoholics develop a condition called Wernicke-Korsakoff syndrome, which is characterized by the inability to form new memories, poorly organized retrieval of old memories, apathy, and emotional blandness.

Thiamin supplementation corrects this condition if it's caught before permanent nerve damage occurs. When someone who abuses alcohol is admitted to the hospital, he or she is usually given supplemental thiamin in large doses, to help reduce the possibility of seizures associated with alcohol withdrawal. In the United States, thiamin is one of the vitamins found in fortified flour and cereals, so deficiency is not common, Dr. Curran-Celentano says.

The Daily Value is 1.5 milligrams. Men typically get about 1.75 milligrams, and women typically get 1.05 milligrams. Deficiency is most likely to occur in people who abuse alcohol or who live mostly on empty calories, such as soda and sweets. Others who may develop deficiency-related health problems include older people in nursing homes and hospitals, people who are very ill, and strict dieters.

valerian

The old adage that if it tastes bad, it must be good for you is true for valerian, an herb that's been used through the centuries to calm nervous jitters and bring on sleep.

Modern herbalists call it the gym-sock herb because the medicinal parts of the plant—the dried roots or rhizomes—smell really rank. One 18th-century herbalist likened it to the urine of cats, so you can imagine that an herbal tea of valerian root is a less-than-exquisite sipping experience. Because of its strong smell, valerian is most commonly taken as pills or a tincture.

Nevertheless, "valerian is a wonderful herb for relaxing the body, both the mind and the muscles," says Jill Stansbury, ND, assistant professor of botanical medicine and chair of the botanical medicine department at the National College of Naturopathic Medicine in Portland, Oregon.

A Centuries-Old Cure

Valerian is a perennial plant that reaches a height of 5 feet and grows wild throughout Europe and parts of Asia. In many countries, it is cultivated for medicinal purposes. The plant's unmistakable odor emerges only during the drying process.

Herbalists in Europe have known about its calming properties for centuries. The ancient Greeks and Romans called it wild nard, but by the 9th century, it appeared in written records as valerian. It was recommended as a treatment for hysteria and emotional disorders. By the 1700s, physicians were recommending valerian for numerous complaints, from living too luxuriously to having an ailment known as "the vapors."

Valerian is classified as a mild tranquilizer. It's also considered an antispasmodic, meaning that it eases muscle spasms or cramps in the body, and it has been used to relieve menstrual cramps and premenstrual syndrome. In the 1800s, a physician wrote that it had a "remarkable effect in quieting the nervous agitation which prevents sleep in delicate and irritable females."

A Balm That Calms

A number of scientific studies have shown that valerian has a sedative effect on the brain and also relaxes digestive tract muscles that clench under stress. In herbal medicine today, it's primarily used for insomnia, mild anxiety, panic attacks, and tension in the body. The herb hastens sleep, improves sleep quality, and reduces nighttime awakenings. In England, dozens of over-the-counter sleep aids contain valerian. In the United States, you'll have no problem finding it in most drugstores and health food stores.

"It's a mild herbal relaxant. You take it when you're feeling stressed or when something is bothering you and keeping you awake," says Woodson Merrell, MD, a specialist in alternative and complementary medicine and assistant clinical professor of medicine at the Columbia University College of Physicians and Surgeons in New York City. "It won't knock you out, but it can relax you enough so you can fall asleep."

Valerian isn't for long-term use, Dr. Merrell warns. If you have recurring insomnia, you should see your doctor for a sleep evaluation. You may have sleep apnea, and taking something that promotes sleep when you're not breathing right isn't a good idea. If you're just a bit tense or restless at

SUPPLEMENT SNAPSHOT

▶Valerian

Botanical name: *Valeriana officinalis.*

Origin: Europe and Asia.

May help: Anxiety, insomnia, menstrual cramps, tension headaches, sleep problems associated with chronic fatigue syndrome, muscle cramps, and muscle spasms.

Cautions and possible side effects: Do not use with prescription medications such as diazepam (Valium) or amitriptyline (Elavil), or with alcohol. Don't use valerian if you experience heart palpitations or nervousness after taking it.

bedtime, however, it may be just the thing. "It tends to make you less nervous, and sometimes, that's all you need," Dr. Merrell says.

Mild and Nonaddictive

Its mild tranquilizing power has made valerian a popular treatment for anxiety; in Europe, it is often prescribed for that purpose. Unlike diazepam (Valium) and alprazolam (Xanax), the drugs often prescribed for anxiety in the United States, valerian has few side effects.

Some people confuse valerian and Valium, believing that their similar names imply that they are somehow related. They are not. Valium is a synthetic drug, a member of the benzodiazepine family, while valerian is derived from a plant.

There is a connection, however. The herb and the drug seem to affect the brain in a similar fashion, binding to the same receptors. The differences are that valerian appears to be nonaddictive, and its effects tend to be milder than those of Valium.

Unlike some pharmaceuticals, valerian doesn't interfere with the deepest part of the sleep cycle, called REM or dream sleep. There's no hangover or grogginess the next day and little chance of dependency, says William Page-Echols, DO, an assistant clinical professor of family medicine who teaches alternative medicine at the Michigan State University College of Osteopathic Medicine in East Lansing.

"There's far less risk of building up a tolerance to valerian or becoming dependent on it," says Dr. Page-Echols. "In some cases of mild anxiety, people would do just as well taking a little valerian as opposed to a prescription drug."

If you're already taking sedatives or antidepressants, however, speak with your physician before taking valerian or trying to switch solely to the herb. Not everyone reacts to it in the same way, warns Dr. Merrell. "Valerian affects some people quite strongly. It really sedates them. For others, it's just the opposite: They actually become agitated after taking it. In general, though, the herb has few side effects."

Still a Mystery

Although researchers have been studying valerian for many years to determine the effective ingredient, they have discovered that many chemicals contribute to its actions. The plant contains a volatile oil, which includes valeric acid and valerenal, and alkaloids known as valepotriates.

Scientists do know that valerian alkaloids seem to lower blood pressure, and there is some evidence from animal studies that valeric acid and valerenal may be most responsible for the herb's sedating qualities. That's why, in the drugstore or health food store, you're likely to see valerian supplements and tinctures standardized to a specific percentage of essential oils or valeric acid. That's only a best guess, however. It may be that several ingredients are involved or that the ingredients act synergistically, interacting with each other to create the herb's calming properties. Many sleep products that contain valerian also contain other sleep-inducing herbs, such as lemon balm and hops.

Many herbalists contend that herbs work best in their whole forms and disagree with the notion that there is one best, most active compound in any plant. "Plants are wondrous and perfect combinations of numerous substances—some flashy active constituents and scores of enzymes, vitamins, minerals, and other compounds that all work in harmony with one another," Dr. Stansbury notes.

zinc

Scan a list of the health problems associated with poor zinc intake, and you'll get an immediate sense of this essential mineral's wide and varied roles in the body.

When children lack zinc in their diets, researchers have found, they tend to grow more slowly than normal, and their sexual maturity is delayed. Zinc deprivation has also been linked to poor appetite, decreased resistance to infection, slow wound healing, infertility, and low hormone levels, especially in men. Some people with zinc deficiency experience hair loss, skin and nail problems, taste and smell difficulties, night blindness, and ulcers on the surface of the eyes, among other ailments.

The deficiency doesn't have to be drastic for some of these problems to appear. "The body's immune system seems particularly sensitive to zinc status," says Philip Reeves, PhD, research chemist with the USDA Human Nutrition Research Center in Grand Forks, North Dakota. "Even a mild deficiency can cause immunity problems, and a severe deficiency can have devastating effects."

Zinc is needed by more than 300 enzymes, the spark plugs that get chemical reactions going in our bodies. It's found in every organ and every tissue—anywhere there is protein—because it is needed for the process of making protein.

Producing Protein

Since protein is needed to make tissues such as skin and muscles, it's no surprise that a zinc shortage leads to slow wound healing, skin breakdown, or muscle loss. Additionally, it is used for immune cells that fight infection; hormones that regulate growth, appetite, and sex drive; neurotransmitters that allow our various body parts to communicate with one another; and even the pigments in the backs of our eyes that allow us to see.

Zinc's role in protein processing is varied. In some cases, proteins called zinc fingers reach out and grab specific parts of DNA so that it can begin the process of making other proteins. Zinc also helps to retrieve and copy the "recipe"—the amino acid sequence—for a particular protein from the cell's genetic material.

Zinc also participates when a cell needs to produce a copy of its genes as it prepares to divide. "Some enzymes that string together the bits that

SUPPLEMENTSNAPSHOT

▶Zinc

Daily Value: 15 milligrams.

May help: Age-related macular degeneration, cataracts, male infertility associated with low hormone levels, hair loss, wound healing, impotence, prostate problems, dermatitis, canker sores, gingivitis, bedsores, loss of appetite, low immunity, loss of ability to taste and smell, genital herpes, binge-eating disorder, osteoarthritis, HIV and other viral infections, and inflammatory conditions such as lupus and rheumatoid arthritis. Zinc throat lozenges may help treat colds.

Good food sources: Cooked oysters, clams, crab, red meat, poultry, fish, and beans.

Who's at risk for deficiency: Pregnant women; infants; elderly people who don't eat well; vegetarians; people taking stomach acid inhibitors such as Pepcid, Prilosec, or Zantac; people with diabetes; and alcoholics.

Special instructions: Take with food to reduce stomach irritation, but avoid taking with a lot of high-fiber foods, since fiber interferes with absorption. Calcium also interferes, so separate calcium intake from zinc intake by about 4 hours. Absorption can also be compromised by large amounts of iron; for best results, do not get more than 30 milligrams of iron daily from food and supplements. Since large amounts of zinc impair copper absorption, get 1 milligram of copper for every 10 milligrams of zinc.

Cautions and possible side effects: Do not take more than 20 milligrams a day of zinc (and no more than 2 milligrams a day of copper) unless directed by your physician. Too much zinc suppresses immunity and delays wound healing.

make up the long chains of DNA and RNA are zinc-dependent," Dr. Reeves says. "When these enzymes don't work correctly, a cell's genetic material isn't made." When there's a lack of genetic material, he points out, there's a general slowdown in growth and tissue maintenance because new cells aren't being produced. There is a drop-off in the production of immune system cells and a breakdown in muscle and skin tissue.

Antioxidant Protection

Zinc is needed to make an important antioxidant enzyme called copper-zinc superoxide dismutase. Like vitamins E and C—other antioxidants that your body needs—this enzyme helps neutralize free radicals, the free-roaming, unstable molecules that can cause a chain reaction of damage throughout your body. "Superoxide dismutase is found in every cell in the body, but it's especially concentrated in the liver and kidneys, where it helps to neutralize toxins before they have a chance to cause problems," Dr. Reeves says.

Your lungs also get the support of this enzyme, which they need because they're constantly exposed to potentially damaging oxygen. Your eyes, too, get some protection from superoxide dismutase, as it helps shield them from the effects of ultraviolet light.

Zinc also helps to stabilize the structure of cell membranes, says Dr. Reeves. That's an important role because the membranes that surround cells act as a kind of security system. When they are intact and working right, they help to carefully regulate what goes in and out of a cell. Needed nutrients go in, and wastes go out.

"Zinc-dependent enzymes help to protect both proteins and fats in the membrane from being damaged by oxygen," Dr. Reeves observes.

If a cell's normally fluidlike membrane is damaged, though, it becomes rigid, interfering with the necessary flow of nutrients and wastes into and out of the cell. Specific receptor sites and transport systems—a cell's loading platforms—don't work. "The receptor sites for insulin, for instance, are one type that may be protected by zinc," Dr. Reeves says.

Are You Getting Enough?

Our bodies try to conserve zinc if we're not eating much, and we absorb more zinc from foods when it's available. "The absence of evidence of deficiency suggests that most people in the United States do get enough zinc, even if they're not always getting the Daily Value," says Janet Hunt, PhD, RD, also with the USDA research center in North Dakota. In the United States, people average about 10 milligrams a day of zinc, which is two-thirds of the Daily Value of 15 milligrams. Most of that comes from meat, fish, and poultry.

So who's most likely to be short on zinc? Vegetarians who aren't getting enough good nonmeat sources of zinc, such as beans; older people who simply aren't eating enough food; and people on diets that short-change them on numerous nutrients. Severe zinc deficiency is also a well-known complication of alcohol abuse. Stomach acid is needed to absorb zinc, which is why people who take strong acid-inhibiting drugs such as Pepcid, Prilosec, or Zantac may slowly become zinc-deficient.

If you're taking a zinc supplement, you don't need to worry about the form of zinc in the tablet, Dr. Hunt says. Most commercial forms are readily absorbed and utilized.

Mingling Your Metals

Zinc can interfere with copper absorption at amounts as low as 20 milligrams a day, so you should get 1 milligram of copper for every 10 milligrams of zinc that you take in through diet or supplements. Most people don't need to take more than 15 milligrams of supplemental zinc and 1.5 milligrams of copper a day, Dr. Hunt says. These amounts of zinc and copper are available in many multivitamin/mineral supplements.

Large amounts of iron can interfere with your ability to absorb zinc, so if you are taking supplemental iron to correct iron-deficiency anemia, you should take it a few hours before or after you take any zinc supplements, Dr. Hunt says.

3
fighting disease with supplements

alzheimer's disease and age-related memory loss

Your brain is a vital organ, and like the other vital organs in your body, it can be damaged by poor diet, stress, exposure to toxins, and aging.

Just like your heart, your brain won't work as well if cholesterol deposits or high blood pressure damages the arteries that supply its blood. In fact, a study from the Netherlands found that the same high-saturated-fat diet that raises your risk of having a heart attack or stroke also makes you more prone to developing age-related memory impairment and Alzheimer's disease.

"What works for the heart, works for the brain, with some modifications," says Dharma Singh Khalsa, MD, president and medical director of the Alzheimer's Prevention Foundation in Tucson and coauthor of *Brain Longevity*. That's why many of the nutritional supplements recommended to shield your brain from age-related memory impairment also offer protection from heart disease. But there are also some that specifically target your brain cells and neurotransmitter function.

In fact, there are a number of ways that you may be able to slow the progression, Dr. Khalsa says. "What works best is a synergistic approach, using a number of different ways to protect your brain," he says.

Lifestyle Matters

As crazy as life may be, experts agree that it's important to get a handle on stress to protect gray matter. Chronic, long-term stress may be the main cause of memory problems in people under age 40, Dr. Khalsa says. "The main stress hormone, cortisol, actually damages brain cells. In fact, it damages the same cells that control the amount of cortisol secreted, creating a vicious cycle of stress hormone–caused brain cell damage," he says. Over time, it gets harder for your body to calm itself down.

Two of the best ways to counteract stress are to get regular exercise and get quality sleep. In fact, exercise may be truly the best way to protect

313

your brain. Research consistently shows that older people who get regular exercise, such as walking, are less likely to experience age-related memory loss and other declines in mental function, and exercise may actually increase their number of brain cells. In one study from the University of California, San Francisco, researchers found that for every extra mile a person walked per week, there was a 13 percent decrease in the chances of cognitive decline. "You don't need to be running marathons," says Kristine Yaffe, MD, a neurologist involved in the study. "The exciting thing is there was a 'dose' relationship that showed that even a little is good, but more is better." Research also shows that people who exercise throughout their lives have better brain function as they get older.

The Brain's Food

Besides lifestyle, nutritional supplements and herbs can help prevent or slow cognitive decline. Some of them help prevent the breakdown of important messenger chemicals called neurotransmitters, says Dr. Khalsa. Other supplements actually stimulate the production of neurotransmitters. In his own practice, Dr. Khalsa uses a mix that targets the many different mechanisms involved in brain protection.

For them to really work, you also need to start early—ideally, before you ever even show a symptom. People should be on a "brain health" program their entire lives, Dr. Khalsa says.

If you want to protect your brain from age-related cognitive decline, and possibly from Alzheimer's disease, here's what complementary medical doctors (those who use both traditional and alternative methods) recommend. It's best to work with a doctor who can help you determine which supplements are right for you.

The Membrane Stabilizer

Many alternative practitioners routinely recommend a compound called phosphatidylserine to patients concerned about memory loss. This fat-soluble phospholipid that's abundant in the human brain is important in neuronal membrane functions. It both strengthens brain cell membranes and makes them more fluid, which allows the cells to function better. "It also blocks the effects of cortisol on the brain cells," Dr. Khalsa says. All of this helps to create a thicker, younger-acting brain. Clinical studies show that phosphatidylserine improves attention, arousal, verbal fluency, and memory in aging people with cognitive deterioration. Depending on your symptoms, you should take 100 to 300 milligrams a day of phosphatidylserine, Dr. Khalsa says.

Fishy Finds

Like phosphatidylserine, fish oil also helps to improve cell membrane function, but in addition it helps your thinking power by acting as a potent anti-inflammatory. Inflammation is now recognized as a component of Alzheimer's disease and age-related cognitive decline.

DHA, one of the components of fish oil, makes up as much as 40 percent of the fats in your brain. Like phosphatidylserine, it affects cell membrane stability and fluidity, allowing cell membranes to function properly, says Karin Yurko-Mauro, PhD, associate clinical director of Martek Biosciences of Columbia, Maryland.

DHA has been shown to improve blood flow in the brain and enhance learning and memory tasks. In animal models, it has also been found to reduce beta amyloid plaque and tau protein, which are known markers for Alzheimer's disease. Dr. Yurko-Mauro's research found that taking 900 milligrams a day of DHA for 6 months improved memory in healthy people over age 55 who had some memory impairment, but not those with an Alzheimer's diagnosis. "DHA appears to have a significant impact on early episodic memory changes, and its benefits are roughly equivalent to having the learning and memory skills of someone 3 years younger," she says.

As both a preventive measure and for treatment purposes, most doctors suggest that everyone take two fish oil capsules a day, which would provide about 1,000 mg of EPA and DHA combined. (Check your dosage on the label. Depending on the product you choose, you may have to take more or fewer capsules.)

The Brain Saver

The herb ginkgo has long been used to improve mental function. Ginkgo acts as a potent antioxidant, protecting your brain from oxidative damage due to aging, heart disease, or toxins, says Jay Lombard, MD, assistant clinical professor of neurology at Weill Medical College of Cornell University in New York City and coauthor of *The Brain Wellness Plan.*

It also inhibits the breakdown of some of the neurotransmitters involved in mood and memory, and it enhances the release of different kinds of these important brain chemicals.

In Europe, an extract of this herb is an approved treatment for dementia, including Alzheimer's disease. The first clinical study done in the United States found that 120 milligrams daily of ginkgo extract stabilized Alzheimer's disease and also led to significant improvements in mental function in patients. The concentration used was standardized to 24 percent ginkgoflavonglycosides and 6 percent terpene lactones, which are believed to be the active agents. Even better news: There were no reported side effects.

Further US research on ginkgo has been mixed. But, says Dr. Khalsa, "the people who prescribe it, and who do brain scans, will tell you that ginkgo is a phenomenal herb to help people improve their brain function. I've had one researcher tell me that the most beautiful brains he's seen on a brain scan are in people who are taking ginkgo."

If you do decide to use ginkgo, take 80 to 300 milligrams a day of a standardized extract (24 percent ginkgoflavonglycosides and 6 percent terpene lactones). Because ginkgo can thin blood, don't take it without your doctor's approval if you already take blood thinners.

A Triple Threat

Acetyl-L-carnitine, alpha lipoic acid, and CoQ_{10} are all natural substances that can help keep your brain healthy and active. They aid energy metabolism, so they can help all cells in the body—including the brain—make the energy they need to function properly. Alpha lipoic acid and CoQ_{10} are also powerful, fat-soluble antioxidants that help protect brain cells from damage caused by free radicals.

Acetyl-L-carnitine is structurally similar to the memory neurotransmitter acetylcholine and displays similar actions in the brain, Dr. Lombard says. Research shows that acetyl-L-carnitine might slow the rate of brain disease progression, improve memory, and improve some measures of cognitive function and behavioral performance in some patients with Alzheimer's disease.

Dr. Khalsa prefers that people combine these three nutrients, taking 100 milligrams of acetyl-L-carnitine, 100 milligrams of alpha lipoic acid, and 100 milligrams of CoQ_{10} every day.

What about Other Antioxidants?

Researchers know that inflammation is present in the brains of people with Alzheimer's disease. But just how much of a role antioxidants can play in reducing damage from inflammation is uncertain. There's evidence that people with Alzheimer's disease have significantly more free radicals in their brain tissue than normal people do, and we know that antioxidants such as vitamins C and E can reduce levels of inflammation-generating free radicals. The one long-term study that looked at disease progression in people who took high-dose vitamin E (2,000 IU a day) found that the people who took the vitamin survived 230 days longer than the people who didn't. That said, the vitamin E did not significantly slow the progression of the disease.

Both Dr. Lombard and Dr. Khalsa still recommend taking antioxidant nutrients, including vitamin E. But they favor a mixture of antioxidants and less vitamin E than was used in the study. "If you are on an antioxidant program, you just don't need that much vitamin E," Dr. Khalsa says. He recommends 400 to 800 IU of vitamin E, 3,000 milligrams of vitamin C in divided doses, and 50 to 100 micrograms of selenium (a trace mineral involved in the body's production of an important antioxidant, glutathione).

There's also good evidence that eating a diet high in fruits and vegetables can protect you from Alzheimer's and vascular dementia. Some of the best brain-boosting foods are blueberries, black raspberries, cranberries, and other berries; citrus; dark leafy greens; and nuts, such as walnuts and almonds.

Boost Your Brain with B Vitamins

Most of the B vitamins, especially B_{12} and folate, help the breakdown of blood sugar, or glucose, which is important to your gray matter because the brain relies on a perpetual supply of glucose for energy, Dr. Khalsa says. And B_{12} is needed to maintain the fatty myelin sheath that wraps around and protects nerves, including those in the brain.

One study found that older people with lower-than-average B_{12} levels were six times more likely to show signs of brain shrinkage, an early sign of impaired cognitive function and Alzheimer's disease. That's why, if you complain of initial memory problems, your doctor should start by testing your B vitamin levels, Dr. Khalsa says. The doctor might also check for high blood levels of homocysteine, a toxic by-product of protein metabolism that has been associated with atherosclerosis, which can also contribute to age-related cognitive decline. And again, the B vitamin folate has been shown to keep homocysteine in check.

To keep up on your Bs, your best tactic is to take a high-potency B-complex or multivitamin formula that includes 1,000 micrograms of vitamin B_{12} and 400 micrograms of folic acid, along with the other Bs, Dr. Khalsa says.

Turmeric Spices Up Your Memory

Growing evidence suggests that curcumin, a compound in the curry staple turmeric, is a potent Alzheimer's foe. In a study of mice genetically altered to develop Alzheimer's, curcumin inhibited the accumulation of destructive beta-amyloid protein in the brain—the "tangles" that are the hallmark of the disease.

The spice also broke up existing plaques by boosting immune cells called macrophages to clear out the plaque. Curcumin may protect against Alzheimer's disease by turning on a gene that triggers the production of antioxidant proteins, especially one called heme oxygenase-1, that help protect the brain against oxidative damage.

Population studies show that people in India, who get a ton of curcumin from foods, have the lowest incidence of Alzheimer's disease in the world. If the idea of eating that much curry makes you leery, take 100 to 200 milligrams a day of concentrated curcumin in capsules, Dr. Khalsa suggests. Some brands are formulated to be more absorbable and are worth the cost if you are serious about using curcumin to reduce inflammation.

Chinese Moss May Restore Memory

Huperzine A, a natural substance extracted from a rare moss found in the cold climates of China, is being sold in the United States as a nutritional supplement that may alleviate symptoms of Alzheimer's disease.

In several small studies, Huperzine A has improved memory, cognitive function, and behavioral function in patients with Alzheimer's and senile dementia, says Alan Kozikowski, PhD, director of the drug discovery program at Georgetown Institute of Cognitive and Computational Sciences at Georgetown University Medical Center in Washington, DC.

Huperzine A is thought to be beneficial due to its effects on acetylcholine levels. It can keep this important neurotransmitter from breaking for up to 3 hours, which means that it may have a longer duration of action than similar drugs marketed for Alzheimer's disease, such as tacrine (Cognex) or donepezil (Aricept). Huperzine A also seems to protect brain cells from some neurotoxins and helps prevent seizures.

Dr. Khalsa uses 50 micrograms of Huperzine A along with 2.5 to 5 milligrams of another plant-derived compound, vinpocetine, from the periwinkle plant, for a synergistic effect. "These are small amounts and they improve cognitive function without overstimulating or causing side effects," he says. Both of these compounds enhance the brain's blood flow and ability to produce energy, he says.

anemia

If your blood doesn't contain enough red blood cells, you have anemia. You can also have anemia if you have enough red blood cells, but they just aren't doing their jobs. If they aren't carrying sufficient hemoglobin—the iron-rich red protein that transports oxygen—you'll have anemia just as surely as if you had a red blood cell shortage.

The symptoms are noticeable, although at first you might not give them much thought. You'll probably look pale and feel pretty tired, but it's easy to write off these signs as the results of stress or not getting enough sleep.

But maybe there's another reason for feeling drained: Perhaps your blood isn't delivering the oxygen needed to create energy. If you feel weak and short of breath, if your heart beats faster and you find it hard to concentrate, it's time to ask your doctor to take a blood sample. It may take no more than a few minutes to find out whether your blood's falling down on the job.

The first thing your doctor needs to do is figure out why you are anemic. Anemia is often related to blood loss, says Michael DiPalma, ND, a naturopathic doctor and director of natural medicine at the Village of Newtown Medical Center in Pennsylvania. For menstruating women, it may mean that they are losing more blood each month than their bodies are able to resupply.

Anemia could indicate blood loss from the intestinal tract, a bleeding ulcer, hemorrhoids, or even cancer. That's why it's important to get a proper diagnosis from your doctor. He will want to order a full laboratory evaluation appropriate for your specific symptoms. If internal bleeding is suspected, for example, he may check a stool sample for blood in addition to taking a blood sample for a complete blood count.

It's also possible that a nutritional deficiency is interfering with your body's ability to make new red blood cells, Dr. DiPalma says. "Iron deficiency is the most common, and it's possible to become iron-deficient if you're regularly losing blood or if you aren't getting much iron in your

Add to Your Iron with Yellow Dock

One problem with iron supplements is their tendency to cause constipation. That's why one popular herbal tonic for iron-deficiency anemia, Floradix, includes an herb called yellow dock. While the herb is a source of iron, it also produces a gentle laxative effect. Thus, while it's contributing to your body's stores of iron, it can also help counter supplemental iron's constipating tendencies, says Dr. DiPalma.

"Yellow dock wouldn't be used alone to treat anemia, but it can be a helpful addition," says Dr. DiPalma. You shouldn't self-treat anemia without your doctor's approval, however.

diet." Other nutrients may play additional roles. Here are the things that you need to know.

Iron Out Anemia

Hemoglobin is so dependent on iron that your blood cells will look pale under a microscope if iron is lacking. And you must have healthy hemoglobin. It's the Federal Express of your blood cells, constantly picking up oxygen in the lungs and delivering it rapidly to be released in tissues where oxygen is low.

Your doctor can easily check your iron levels with blood tests, including a serum ferritin test, which can detect depleted iron stores before you actually become anemic, Dr. DiPalma says. Iron deficiency may be caused by increased iron requirements during pregnancy, an adolescent growth spurt, or heavy menstrual bleeding. It could also be a sign that you've severely decreased your dietary intake of iron—if you've gone on a diet, for instance, or switched to vegetarian meals without paying attention to the foods that provide iron.

Less commonly, the deficiency may be the result of absorption problems. You may even be donating blood more often than your body can handle. Often, the reason turns out to be a combination of factors, Dr. DiPalma says.

If your doctor determines that you are short on iron, you will need to take supplements until your anemia resolves, and then some. That is, you not only need to restore normal levels of iron, you also need to build up some excess in your system for future demands.

The amounts of iron used to correct anemia can vary widely. Some doctors initially prescribe large amounts—200 to 325 milligrams a day, usually in the form of ferrous sulfate, which is not easily absorbed and may lead to constipation. Others, such as Dr. DiPalma, use smaller amounts of a more absorbable form.

Dr. DiPalma often recommends that his patients take 30 milligrams of iron succinate or iron fumarate twice a day between meals. Or, if these supplements cause stomach upset, he may advise taking them with meals. He may also recommend an aqueous (liquid) liver extract because it provides heme iron, a natural food form that's also easily absorbed.

You should avoid using enteric-coated iron tablets or capsules containing slow-release granules, experts say. Both can interfere with the body's ability to absorb iron. Also, make sure that you continue your treatment for a sufficient period of time, under your doctor's supervision. Although your anemia will be corrected in 3 to 4 months, it takes an additional 6 to 12 months of therapy for iron stores (also called ferritin levels) to be replenished.

The B$_{12}$ Connection

A shortage of vitamin B$_{12}$ causes its own form of anemia, called pernicious anemia. Until 1934, this form was invariably fatal. That year, two Boston doctors demonstrated that a diet rich in barely cooked liver, which is rich in B$_{12}$, could ward off the deadly deficiency.

Since the symptoms of this type of anemia resemble those of other types, your doctor will need to do a blood test to figure out what's really going on, Dr. DiPalma says. If you do have a B$_{12}$ deficiency, your red blood cells suffer from what is called maturation arrest. They grow large, but they never mature into properly working cells. In fact, they may never make it out of the bone marrow, where red blood cells are normally created and released into your blood.

Doctors no longer recommend liver to correct a B$_{12}$ deficiency. Because liver is high in cholesterol, it can cause other health problems. Instead, you'll need supplemental B$_{12}$ to correct a deficiency. This deficiency is not as common as iron deficiency, but it's worth checking. It's most common in older people with reduced stomach acid or those who have had stomach surgery. People who have Crohn's disease or other stomach or intestinal problems may also be susceptible, Dr. DiPalma says. Strict vegetarians (vegans) are also at risk. Usually, B_{12} blood levels are brought up to an acceptable level (400 pg/mL or higher) with injections. Once there, people may be able to maintain their levels by taking B_{12} under the tongue, usually 1,000 to 2,000 micrograms a day. Some, however, will continue to require injections. B_{12} deficiency is best handled with medical care.

The Folic Acid Factor

If you don't get enough folic acid, another B vitamin, your blood cells don't reach maturity. Instead, they become large, immature, egg-shaped cells that can't do their jobs well.

Folate (the naturally occurring form of folic acid) is found mostly in fruits and vegetables. However, folic acid is now added to a variety of foods, such as cereals, rice, and breads. So these days, you are unlikely to experience folate-deficiency anemia, unless perhaps you have a serious malabsorption problem such as celiac or Crohn's disease. (Alcoholics may also have folate deficiency.) Besides anemia, other symptoms may include diarrhea; inflamed gums; depression; a swollen, red tongue; and elevated levels of homocysteine, an amino acid by-product that increases your risk for cardiovascular disease.

It takes only a blood test to determine if you are short on folic acid. "You may need large amounts of supplemental folic acid until blood levels are restored," Dr. DiPalma says. He recommends that his patients take 800 to 1,200 micrograms a day. High amounts of folic acid can affect the laboratory diagnosis of pernicious anemia, however, which means that some B_{12}-deficiency nerve damage could worsen even though the deficiency goes undetected. You should check with your doctor if you think you are deficient and want to take a supplement.

Add a Multi

In addition to iron, B_{12}, and folic acid, it's best to take a good multivitamin/mineral supplement when you're working to restore blood supplies, Dr. DiPalma says. For example, your body needs copper along with iron to make hemoglobin, and vitamin C helps many parts of the body function at their best, so look for a supplement that has these two nutrients. "People tend to get better faster when they are on a comprehensive program," Dr. DiPalma says.

angina

When you have angina, the pressure in your chest is a warning signal that something isn't right in the spaghetti-size arteries that deliver blood to your heart muscle.

That firm, relentless squeeze often means that the arteries have been narrowed by cholesterol-laden plaque. As plaque starts to clog those all-important pipelines, blood flow is reduced. When the arteries are starved of red blood, with its supply of oxygen and nutrients, they are more likely to go into spasm, which reduces blood flow even more.

Often, the attack hits when some other part of your body needs increased blood flow to feed your muscles or warm up your limbs. Maybe you've been exercising or are under a lot of stress. It can also occur in cold weather or after a big meal.

People with angina need to be on the same low-fat, high-fiber diet that lowers cholesterol, says Decker Weiss, NMD, director of the Weiss Center for Naturopathic Excellence in Scottsdale, Arizona, and author of *The Weiss Method: A Natural Program for Reversing Heart Disease and Preventing Heart Attacks*. He also recommends that his patients take a variety of supplements that may reduce the risk of heart disease.

Traditionally, physicians treat angina with medications such as nitroglycerin, which improves blood flow to the heart. If the blockage is bad enough, a doctor might recommend an artery-opening procedure such as angioplasty or bypass surgery.

Certain nutrients and herbs, however, can also improve blood flow to the heart and enhance energy production in the muscle cells. With the aid of these nutrients, the heart muscle can work better even though blood supply is reduced, Dr. Weiss says.

If you have a history of angina, your doctor will want you to keep a medication such as nitroglycerin on hand, and, of course, you need to check with your doctor before taking supplements. But many people are drawn to alternative treatments by the prospect of avoiding procedures such as angioplasty and bypass surgery. By taking helpful nutrients and pursuing other measures to ensure good heart health, you may be able to clear up the symptoms of angina and its causes as well, says Dr. Weiss.

Ease the Squeeze with Magnesium

At the top of Dr. Weiss's prescription list for angina is magnesium, a mineral that helps relax the muscles that wrap around blood vessels.

In several studies, intravenous magnesium was effective at stopping a type of angina characterized by spasms in the coronary arteries. In a British study that addressed another type of angina, intravenous magnesium again showed its power. People who received the magnesium had fewer angina episodes than those who didn't receive it.

"Magnesium dilates the coronary arteries, improving oxygen delivery to the heart," Dr. Weiss says. It also plays an important role in energy production in all cells, so magnesium is especially important to the high-energy-requiring heart muscle cells, he says.

Magnesium deficiency can be induced by drugs meant to help heart problems, including diuretics, which help your body excrete excess fluid. You also have to watch out for deficiency caused by the commonly prescribed digitalis heart medications digitoxin (Crystodigin) and digoxin (Lanoxin). Signs of magnesium deficiency include muscle weakness, nausea, and irritability.

If you have angina, you probably have heart disease, so it's important to consult a doctor who's knowledgeable in nutrition before taking supplemental magnesium. Dr. Weiss recommends two forms—magnesium orotate and magnesium glycinate—but check with your doctor before you settle on a dosage of either.

Get Some CoQ$_{10}$ and Omega-3s

Coenzyme Q$_{10}$ is a vitamin-like substance that plays an essential role in producing energy. CoQ$_{10}$, as it's commonly called, actually increases oxygen delivery to heart muscle cells. For anyone with angina, it's a supplement to consider.

In one study, 12 people with one type of angina who took 150 milligrams of CoQ$_{10}$ daily for 4 weeks cut the frequency of angina attacks in half compared with a group taking placebos.

If you're buying CoQ$_{10}$ for the first time, you might wonder which kind to use—gel capsules or tablets. Since CoQ$_{10}$ is fat-soluble, the gel capsules are more potent and more readily absorbed than the tablet form. Doctors also recommend two kinds of fatty acids—omega-3s, found in fish oil, for people who have angina. About 1,000 to 3,000 milligrams a day is the standard dose.

Experts also advise people with angina to cut back on saturated fats (those that are solid at room temperature), hydrogenated fats (margarine and shortening), and polyunsaturated fats (corn oil).

Get Help from Ginkgo and Amino Acids

"I absolutely recommend ginkgo for angina," says Dr. Weiss, noting that the herbal supplement can help stimulate blood flow around the damaged area of the heart.

Ginkgo also helps prevent platelets from sticking together, says Dr. Weiss. Platelets are components in blood that promote clotting, and they can also pile up at a site where an artery has been clogged by cholesterol. Dr. Weiss recommends 60 milligrams of ginkgo biloba extract (standardized to 24 percent ginkgoflavonglycosides) up to three times a day.

Another possible alternative for people who have angina is amino acids. These include acetyl-L-carnitine, taurine, and arginine, Dr. Weiss says.

"Carnitine is vital, and I recommend it because many people with heart disease need extra carnitine to utilize the essential fatty acids that their hearts need," Dr. Weiss says. This amino acid helps transport fatty acids into the mitochondria, the tiny areas within cells where energy is produced. Supplemental carnitine may help the heart muscle better utilize its limited supply of oxygen, studies show.

The daily therapeutic dose for carnitine is 1,500 to 3,000 milligrams for an average person. Take three divided doses a day, advises Dr. Weiss.

Taurine is also important for the normal function of the heart and vascular system, says Dr. Weiss. It's the most abundant amino acid found in the heart. In Japan, taurine is widely used to treat various types of heart disease.

Arginine is involved in the production of nitric oxide, a compound formed by the cells that line the arteries. With increased nitric oxide, the arteries can relax and dilate, which helps augment blood flow to crucial heart muscle.

Your best bet for using these amino acids? Ask your doctor to recommend a formula that contains a balanced mixture. Recommended doses will vary depending on your current and past history of heart disease.

Take Hawthorn for Your Heart

Hawthorn is an herb with a long history of use for heart problems, and with good reason. It improves the blood supply to the heart by dilating coronary arteries and aids the transformation of food into energy in your heart muscle cells. The herb can also help eliminate some types of arrhythmia (irregular heartbeat), says Dr. Weiss.

"It is a wonderful herb for atherosclerosis," he says. Since atherosclerosis (hardening of the arteries) is a buildup of artery-blocking plaque, it leads to angina. "Taking hawthorn can lower the frequency, duration, and severity of angina."

Hawthorn takes 2 weeks to a month to work. It is available in several different forms, Dr. Weiss says. A typical tonic dose is ¼ teaspoon of liquid extract taken two or three times a day. Many people stir this syrupy extract of hawthorn berries into a glass of hot water. If you prefer a tincture, take 30 to 60 drops daily. For capsules, take 160 milligrams three times a day. If you have a heart condition, however, check with your doctor before taking hawthorn.

Nutrients That Ease Angina

Certain vital nutrients help prevent cholesterol buildup in arteries and protect the cells lining blood vessels from damage that makes blockages more likely. These protective nutrients include vitamins C and E and the trace mineral selenium. "I routinely suggest these nutrients to people with angina," Dr. Weiss says.

In a study, supplements of vitamin E, along with vitamin C, vitamin A, and beta-carotene, reduced the incidence of angina. Vitamin E affects both cholesterol and platelets in a way that reduces the risk of heart disease, Dr. Weiss explains. He recommends 400 to 800 international units (IU) a day.

Vitamin C helps keep blood vessels open because it prevents the breakdown of nitric oxide, which helps promote blood flow, says Dr. Weiss.

Selenium, when teamed with vitamin E, can also offer some protection from angina. One study found that people with heart disease who took 200 IU of vitamin E and 1,000 micrograms (a very large dose) of selenium had a significant reduction in angina pain compared with people taking placebos. Doses of selenium over 200 micrograms must be taken with a doctor's supervision.

Doctors who recommend selenium supplements to their heart patients generally stick with no more than 50 to 200 micrograms a day. You'll also want to make sure that you're getting about 400 micrograms of folic acid, along with 1,000 micrograms of vitamin B_{12} and 50 to 100 milligrams of vitamin B_6, says Dr. Weiss. These B vitamins help your body process homocysteine, an amino acid by-product that can damage arteries by creating rough spots on artery walls that can pick up fatty deposits.

Bromelain and Curcumin: The Antiangina Duo

Dr. Weiss may also use a mixture of bromelain, a protein-dissolving enzyme found in pineapple, and curcumin, the yellow pigment found in turmeric, for people with angina. Bromelain helps reduce the formation of fibrous tissue and clots in damaged arteries, and curcumin acts somewhat like aspirin, he says. It helps to reduce the tendency for blood to clot and also reduces inflammation.

For the best therapeutic effect, Dr. Weiss recommends divided doses. A standard dose of bromelain is 125 to 450 milligrams three times a day on an empty stomach, he says. Do not take bromelain with food, though, or it will simply act as a digestive enzyme.

Usual doses of curcumin are 400 to 600 milligrams a day, Dr. Weiss says. Ask your doctor what dosage is best for you.

asthma

Asthmatic lungs are oversensitive to triggers such as airborne allergens, exercise, cold air, emotional stress, and even certain foods. When an asthma attack hits, breathing passageways are narrowed, making precious oxygen scarce. Spasms in the bronchial tubes cause tightness in the chest and fits of coughing. And when inflammation lingers in the lungs, you'll start wheezing.

Chronic asthma is often treated with medications that are inhaled directly, so the medicine reaches the lungs' deep inner passageways. If you have asthma, these drugs may help you breathe better, but they also offer their share of side effects.

If you use medication to control your asthma, supplements may help you gradually reduce the amount of medication you're taking. Giving these supplements a try may restore healthy breathing in a safe and natural way, but get your doctor's approval before taking supplements for asthma.

Try Magnesium for Relief

Quite a bit of research has linked magnesium with the improvement of asthma symptoms. In fact, magnesium is used intravenously for treating acute asthma attacks. Taking magnesium by mouth isn't recommended to stop an attack, but taking it regularly, over time, can improve symptoms, according to new research from the National Center for Complementary and Alternative Medicine.

Researchers from Bastyr University in Kenmore, Washington, and the University of California, Davis, enrolled 52 men and women ages 21 to 55 with mild-to-moderate asthma. The participants consumed either 340 milligrams of magnesium citrate or a placebo daily for $6\frac{1}{2}$ months. The researchers found that those who took magnesium experienced significant improvement in lung activity and the ability to move air in and out of their lungs. Those taking magnesium also reported other improvements in asthma control and quality of life compared with people who received the placebo.

"Magnesium definitely has an antispasmodic effect on the smooth muscle of the upper respiratory tract," says Claudia Cooke, MD, a holistic doctor in New York City. Since asthma is aggravated or worsened by spasms in the smooth muscles, which are involuntary muscles, magnesium's antispasmodic effects can be beneficial.

For an asthma attack, Dr. Cooke recommends taking 600 milligrams of magnesium along with any medications that have been prescribed by your doctor. If you get relief, she suggests, continue with a daily supplement of 600 milligrams, but don't take this much if you have any kidney problems or low blood pressure.

Keep Exercising—And Breathing— With Vitamin C

Asthma that's brought on by bouts of exercise can be particularly troubling for folks who are trying to stay fit. According to a study at Tel Aviv University in Israel, vitamin C may be able to prevent attacks among people who have exercise-induced asthma.

In the study, some people were given 2,000 milligrams of vitamin C 1 hour before they stepped on a treadmill for a workout. When researchers compared those who got the vitamin C to those who didn't, they discovered that those receiving the supplements showed less hyperreactivity in their airways. The results were probably due to vitamin C's ability to squelch certain inflammatory substances that are produced by overreactive lung cells.

Getting your vitamin C from fruits such as oranges, grapefruit, and kiwi may be even better because these fruits also contain bioflavonoids, compounds that also reduce inflammation. Research shows that eating citrus fruits once or twice a week is associated with improved lung function.

People with asthma who get the lowest amounts of vitamin C in their diets have significantly more bronchial activity in general, Dr. Cooke says. If you're not eating citrus fruits and other C-rich sources, take at least 2,000 milligrams a day in divided doses, she suggests. If you start to get diarrhea from a dose this high, you should gradually reduce the dose until this side effect goes away.

Tame Inflammation with Fish Oil

One of the newest pharmaceutical weapons against asthma is a class of drugs called leukotriene inhibitors. They work by halting the actions of compounds produced in the body that cause bronchial constriction and other allergic reactions.

In an emergency situation, drugs like these are probably the quickest route to relief, but supplements of omega-3 fatty acids—specifically fish oil—work by a similar anti-inflammatory mechanism. They reduce the body's synthesis of pro-inflammatory leukotrienes, says Joseph E. Pizzorno Jr., ND, president emeritus of Bastyr University in Kenmore, Washington. Moreover, they can be nearly as effective for long-term asthma control, especially in children, who may not be getting enough omega-3s in their diets. One study showed that children taking a fish-oil supplement had improved peak airflow and reduced their medication use.

Omega-3 fatty acids are found in the oils of certain fish, particularly cold-water fish such as tuna, mackerel, and salmon, and in the oils of some plants, including flax. Our bodies don't produce omega-3s, and our diets tend to be lacking in these important fats, Dr. Pizzorno says. "Most of us eat way too many saturated fats and not enough of the omega-3 type. You do need both kinds, ultimately, but you need them in balance with each other."

You can get more omega-3s—and cut back on saturated fats—by eating one to two servings of fatty fish a week in place of other meats. If you can't or won't eat fish, take a fish-oil supplement that is verified by the United States Pharmacopeia (USP). These products are high quality and verified to be free of contaminants such as pesticides and mercury. Doctors recommend a dose of 1,000 to 3,000 milligrams of fish oil a day. You'll need to give it some time to start working. Expect to feel some improvement by 3 months, and symptoms may continue to improve for up to 1 year.

Breathe Easier with Bioflavonoids

The best things you can eat to help with asthma? More fruits and vegetables, says Dr. Pizzorno. That's because of the special "ingredients" found only in those types of foods: All of them contain bioflavonoids.

There are almost as many different kinds of bioflavonoids as there are colors in nature. "Basically, they're the bright pigments that you see in produce," says Dr. Pizzorno. But they're more than pretty colors.

Bioflavonoids are growth regulators in plants. When you eat bioflavonoids in foods, you get the benefit of their potent anti-inflammatory and antiallergic properties.

Some of the bioflavonoids available as supplements include quercetin, pine bark extract (Pycnogenol), grapeseed extract, and ginkgo extract.

Clinical research on children ages 6 to 18 showed that taking 1 milligram of Pycnogenol per pound of body weight daily in addition to conventional asthma treatment seems to increase peak expiratory flow, decrease asthma symptoms, and decrease the need for rescue medications.

You can take any of these bioflavonoids singly or as a blended combination: Many mixtures and concentrations are available in drugstores and health food stores. For dosages, just check the label and follow the instructions on the particular bottle you choose, says Dr. Pizzorno.

binge-eating disorder

It's a vicious cycle.

First, an irresistible urge compels you to eat large amounts of food in one sitting. Days later, you're at it again, wolfing down bagfuls of potato chips, cookies, or whatever else you can get your hands on. Extreme feelings of guilt and distress follow each episode, but even that doesn't stop you from repeating this uncontrollable eating pattern over and over again. More than likely, you hide your behavior from everyone, choosing to suffer in silence.

If this pattern sounds familiar, you might be among the 1 to 2 million Americans who have binge-eating disorder. The hardest part may be looking for help.

When you are used to hiding a problem like this, it's extremely difficult to tell anyone about it—even your own doctor. Nevertheless, the first thing you should do is see your physician. You need to be diagnosed—and to find out what your treatment options are—before taking any nutritional supplement, says Nancy Dunne Boggs, ND, a naturopathic doctor in Missoula, Montana.

Most of those who have binge-eating disorder are obese, and the condition is slightly more common in women, affecting three women for every two men. Research shows that mild to moderate depression is the most common cause, says Dr. Boggs, so it's important to treat the depression with medication and counseling. Practitioners of alternative medicine say that one of the best ways to treat the depression associated with binge eating is to take a variety of nutritional supplements. Some vitamins, minerals, herbs, and other natural compounds can increase the levels of certain brain chemicals, or neurotransmitters, that lift your mood, suppress your appetite, and eliminate cravings.

Bring in the Bs

Because binge eaters tend to consume large quantities of high-fat, refined carbohydrate foods that have little or no nutritional value, many are deficient in important B-complex vitamins and the minerals chromium, magnesium, and zinc, says Susan Kowalsky, ND, a naturopathic doctor in Norwich, Vermont.

The B vitamins are needed to manufacture important brain chemicals, such as serotonin, that are responsible for regulating your moods, emotions, sleep patterns, and appetite. Vitamin B_6, in particular, helps convert tryptophan (an amino acid found in many foods) to serotonin in your brain, says Dr. Kowalsky. Serotonin is one of the chemical messengers that has been closely associated with many emotional states, including depression.

Vitamin B_{12} also facilitates brain cell communication so that other neurotransmitters can work together to help relieve depression. In addition, this vitamin helps your body make use of other mood-elevating brain chemicals such as dopamine and norepinephrine.

Dr. Kowalsky suggests taking a high-quality B-complex multivitamin daily. These are often labeled as B-50 because they contain 50 milligrams of some of the Bs and 500 to 1,000 micrograms of B_{12}. Good multivitamins often have high-dose Bs, as well, so check your labels.

Mind the Minerals

Chromium and magnesium can help eliminate cravings and stabilize levels of blood sugar, which fluctuate wildly when a person binges on large amounts of food, says Dr. Kowalsky.

Take 200 to 400 micrograms of chromium and 500 to 700 milligrams of magnesium daily, says Dr. Kowalsky, but be sure to check with your doctor first if you have heart or kidney problems.

Another mineral, zinc, is also a player. Supplementing with zinc can help derail your appetite by activating a brain signal that tells you when you're hungry and when you're full. Dr. Kowalsky recommends taking 15 milligrams of zinc daily. If you take a multivitamin, you're probably getting all you need, since that's the amount found in most multis.

Boost Serotonin with 5-HTP

Binge eaters commonly produce low levels of serotonin, the chemical messenger that plays an important role in depression. As a result, their appetites become ravenous. They tend to crave high-fat carbohydrates and are less likely to receive a signal telling them that they're full.

That's where 5-hydroxytryptophan (5-HTP) can help. Shortly after you take 5-HTP in supplement form, the compound travels to your brain, where it is converted to serotonin. The boost in serotonin will suppress your appetite and activate the brain signal that tells you that you've eaten enough. You'll be in better spirits, your binge eating will be under control, and you'll eventually lose weight, says Dr. Boggs.

She suggests taking 50 milligrams of 5-HTP three times a day as a starting point. If you don't notice any decrease in your cravings and binge-eating episodes after 6 weeks, take 100 milligrams three times a day. If there is still no improvement after 6 additional weeks, increase to 200 milligrams three times a day, but don't exceed 900 milligrams daily. (If it doesn't work after that, talk with your doctor to see if you should continue.) You can find this supplement in health food stores. But be sure you don't take it with other medications, especially antidepressants, unless you talk to your doctor.

birth defect prevention

Most people think that conception is the simple, no-planning-necessary part of having a baby. That's not quite right. Doctors say that if you want to ensure a healthy baby, you should start planning months before conception by eating a diet jam-packed with fruits and vegetables.

That little fertilized egg has a long way to go in 9 months. It has to grow and divide. Its cells specialize to become bones, nerves, and other essential tissues. What helps make all of this happen without a hitch? Nutrients.

Sure, you can take other actions to protect a developing fetus. Avoid x-rays and environmental toxins, try to stay free of infections—especially German measles—and check with your doctor before taking any medication, over the counter or prescriptive. Apart from that, however, nutrients are your best insurance. They're the stuff that cells use to build your baby.

Both the contributors and the detractors deserve special attention in this baby-building process. On the plus side, you need folic acid. On the minus side, make sure that you don't get too much of potentially harmful nutrients, such as vitamin A.

Plan Ahead

Around 1965, researchers began to suspect that a deficiency of folic acid, a B vitamin, during pregnancy could lead to central nervous system disorders called neural tube defects in the developing fetus. It seems that a high percentage of women who were taking anticonvulsant drugs (which interfere with the way your body incorporates folic acid) were giving birth to babies with these serious defects.

In a fetus, the neural tube is just a fold of tissue. When the baby is fully developed, that tissue becomes the spinal cord and brain. A baby whose neural tube doesn't close at the top is born with little or no brain and rarely lives more than a few days. A baby whose tube doesn't close at the bottom is born with spina bifida, a condition that can cause paralysis

Protecting the Unborn from Overdose

Making sure that you get the right amounts of nutrients is only half the battle when it comes to producing a healthy baby. The other 50 percent is avoiding the things that cause birth defects. One precaution you should take is to watch your daily consumption of vitamin A. Don't take daily doses of supplemental vitamin A that exceed 5,000 IU. These levels, which are almost impossible to get from food alone, have been shown to cause various types of birth defects, says Aubrey Milunsky, MD, professor of human genetics, pediatrics, and pathology and director of the Center for Human Genetics at Boston University School of Medicine. (On supplement bottles, look for the words "retinol" and "palmitate.") Also avoid putting retinols (a form of vitamin A used to treat acne and other skin conditions) on your skin.

"I tell my pregnant patients not to take anything that they don't absolutely have to, including herbs," says Priscilla Evans, ND, a naturopathic doctor at the Community Wholistic Health Center in Chapel Hill, North Carolina. Herbs that are safe to take during the second trimester, for instance, might not be safe during the first, when all of the baby's organs are being formed. "You should consult a qualified practitioner of herbal medicine before using herbs during pregnancy," she says.

of the lower body because the vertebrae don't join properly to protect the spinal cord.

Research now confirms that getting enough folate at the time of conception and for about 6 weeks afterwards can help prevent spina bifida. In 1996, the United States began folic acid–fortification of some of the most commonly eaten foods: flour, rice, cornmeal, cereals, and enriched breads. As a result, folic acid intake has just about doubled. Without even trying, you'll most likely be getting enough folic acid from foods to protect your baby during those crucial first weeks of development. If you're trying or know you'll be trying to get pregnant soon, you can also take a multi with 400 micrograms of folic acid, or talk with your doctor about taking prenatal vitamins before conceiving. (See Make Multivitamins a Must on page 338.)

Getting adequate amounts of omega-3 fatty acids, especially DHA, while you are pregnant and breastfeeding promotes brain development in infants. Research has shown that skimping on seafood during pregnancy may contribute to poor verbal skills, behavioral problems, and other early developmental issues.

But some types of seafood—particularly large, predatory fish such as shark, swordfish, king mackerel, and tilefish—may contain high levels of mercury, which is toxic and can damage your baby's brain and nervous system. And some fish, such as farmed salmon, can contain dioxins and other harmful chemicals. That's why the Food and Drug Administration (FDA) and the Environmental Protection Agency (EPA) have issued a joint advisory for fish consumption for pregnant women: www.epa.gov/waterscience/fishadvice/factsheet.html.

If you don't want to eat fish, you may want to take fish-oil supplements instead. The usual recommendation for pregnant and lactating women is 1,200 milligrams a day of fish oil. (That's the equivalent of more than a daily serving of salmon.) Look for a brand that is molecularly distilled to remove toxins.

Make Multivitamins a Must

"A good multivitamin is essential for pregnant women," says Willow Moore, DC, ND, a chiropractor and naturopathic doctor in Owings Mills, Maryland. "Probably, though, taking the full dose once a day isn't the best approach. I recommend that pregnant women take prenatal multivitamins that come in divided doses to be taken throughout the day." Your body is better able to absorb the nutrients if you take them in several smaller doses.

Researchers can't yet say exactly which vitamins within a multivitamin do the beneficial work. Apart from the effect of folic acid, there's evidence to suggest that other B vitamins, such as B_6, play vital roles. But we lack specific evidence. That's understandable, notes Dr. Moore, since researchers would never deprive pregnant women of nutrients that might prevent birth defects in order to study the effects of deficiency.

Some supplements might even make your pregnancy safer and more comfortable for *you*. Taking 500 to 700 milligrams of magnesium a day (more than is found in most multis) can significantly reduce leg cramping during pregnancy. And taking 1 to 2 grams of elemental calcium daily reduces the risk of pregnancy-related high blood pressure and preeclampsia by about 50 percent (when compared to a placebo). Don't forget vitamin D, too. Getting adequate amounts—about 4,000 IU a day—reduces rates of complications, including gestational diabetes.

bladder infections

Having a frequent "urge to go," a burning sensation when you do, and achy lower abdominal pain are symptoms that many women recognize—and dread. They are symptoms of urinary tract infections (UTIs), which account for 8 million doctor visits a year. Moreover, if a woman gets one UTI, there's a good chance that she'll have a flare-up later on.

Recommendations for preventing bladder infections include drinking plenty of water—2 quarts or more a day—and urinating often, especially after intercourse. The idea is to make sure that urine doesn't stay in the bladder very long. All those fluids passing through help to wash away the bacteria that can flourish and fester there.

Bladder infections that are already raging are a little trickier. Doctors usually recommend antibiotics. Unfortunately, frequent antibiotic use may make the troublesome bacteria immune to the medication, leading to recurrent infections.

To combat a bladder infection, you need to take measures to improve your overall immunity, says Mark McClure, MD, a urologist in Raleigh, North Carolina. You also need to target those bacteria and see if you can get rid of them as soon as they come back again. Supplements can help with both of these infection-prevention initiatives.

Add Some C to a Multi

Women with bladder infections would do well to address the cause of their problem, not just the symptoms, says Dr. McClure. "Overall wellness issues and immunity should be the foundation from which you work to get well."

Stress, in particular, can predispose you to chronic or recurrent UTIs, he says, because it depletes the immune system and weakens your defenses against bacteria. "It affects the body in many negative ways, so I recommend yoga, breathing exercises, and meditation," he says.

Stress is caused by more than a hectic schedule or overly tense muscles, however. Poor nutrition is a form of stress that can affect immune performance, too, notes Dr. McClure. If you're not getting enough dietary fiber, you're loading up on sugar, and you have a lot of caffeine in your system, you reduce your body's defenses against infection, he explains. Eating better all the time should be your ultimate goal in order to prevent future infections.

Taking a good-quality, high-potency daily multivitamin is a step in the right direction, says Dr. McClure. If you're already doing that, add some extra vitamin C, he suggests. Taking 500 milligrams every 2 hours can help improve immune function by boosting white blood cell counts—a sign of better defenses. While this much C probably isn't needed on a daily basis, the body seems to require additional amounts of this nutrient in times of infection.

Prevention with Cranberry Extract

Long discussed and debated, the tart, red cranberry's bladder-friendly effects have finally been demonstrated. Cranberry really does help prevent the occurrence of UTIs.

A study conducted by cranberry researcher Edward Walker, PhD, professor of chemistry and director of the center for chemical technology at Weber State University in Ogden, Utah, showed that cranberry can help women with recurring UTIs.

In the study, 10 women were given capsules of solid cranberry concentrate for a period of 3 months. Then researchers switched them to a concentrate that looked like the same substance but didn't have any cranberry ingredients in it (a placebo). The results showed that when the women were taking real cranberry, they had half as many infections as when they were taking the placebos.

Cranberry has long been thought to work against UTIs by acidifying urine, making it into a less hospitable environment for bacteria. It's actually bacteria's ability to stick to the bladder or urinary tract walls, however, that causes infection to set in. Urine acidity doesn't seem to have much to do with it, researchers say. Besides, for cranberry to have an acidifying effect, you'd have to eat a veritable bushel of berries, according to Dr. Walker.

His research has found the active ingredient that gives cranberry its potent antiadhesion properties, counteracting the sticky attack and making infection much less likely. When cranberry is present, the bacteria in the bladder or urinary tract can't hold on. Without firm footing, they are essentially rendered harmless.

"The bacteria will die on their own without a place to live," says Dr. Walker. Then the natural flow of urine gives the bad guys an easy ride out of town. "It's a lot gentler to just send them out of the body like this rather than use antibiotics," he says.

According to Dr. Walker's results, cranberry's strong suit is preventing—not curing—UTIs. "Our hypothesis was that cranberry would reduce the number of recurrent infections," he says—and that's exactly what happened. Other dark berries, such as blueberries, have similar antiadhesion components.

For women plagued by regular infections, this news is as good as it gets. It means that you can use a cranberry supplement as a preventive measure. Take 400 milligrams of standardized cranberry extract twice a day, suggests Dr. Walker. The extract is available in health food stores. Sugar-sweetened cranberry juice is not recommended.

An Herb to Squelch Infection

Uva-ursi, a strangely named shrub that grows in North America, can be a suitable stand-in for antibiotic infection fighters, says naturopathic doctor Tori Hudson, ND, professor at the National College of Naturopathic Medicine in Portland, Oregon, and author of *Women's Encyclopedia of Natural Medicine*. "It's really the most important, most useful herb for treating bladder infections," she says.

While you can take uva-ursi as a tea, the dosage is more precise if you take supplements. If you find capsules that contain only powdered uva-ursi leaves, you'll need to take 500 to 1,000 milligrams three times a day, according to Dr. Hudson. A higher concentration is found in an extract of uva-ursi standardized to contain 20 percent arbutin, one of the active ingredients. If you take that concentration, you'll need only 125 to 250 milligrams three times daily, she says.

Stop taking uva-ursi when you feel well again. It could cause problems if taken over the long term. Also, it may be preferable to avoid taking

Uva-Ursi Knocks Out Bad Bacteria

For more than 1,000 years, people around the world have treated urinary troubles with the leaves of uva-ursi. Tannin and arbutin, the active ingredients, have important qualities that give this herb its impressive powers. Tannin is an astringent, which means that it causes tissue to contract in a way that can make an inhospitable environment for bacteria. In the urinary tract, arbutin becomes an antiseptic, which means that it directly battles the growth of bacteria and other organisms.

"Other plants do contain arbutin, but the highest amounts are found in uva-ursi," says naturopathic doctor Tori Hudson, ND, professor at the National College of Naturopathic Medicine and director of A Woman's Time health clinic, both in Portland, Oregon.

While you can make a compress of uva-ursi and apply it directly to cuts and scrapes to help prevent infection, the herb is more often used to treat urinary problems than for minor first aid. In addition to being sold in supplement form, uva-ursi is available in some specially blended teas.

cranberry extract at the same time, Dr. Hudson cautions, since arbutin works best in a nonacidic environment. You can take cranberry afterward to prevent recurring infections, she says. Pregnant women should avoid uva-ursi completely because it may bring on uterine contractions.

Battle Bacteria with Goldenseal

Urinary tract infections are usually caused by one type of bacteria in particular—the awful organism known as *Escherichia coli*. Luckily, there's a natural weapon that has a special hatred for *E. coli*—its nemesis is the herb called goldenseal.

Goldenseal's antimicrobial and immune-stimulating properties make it a popular choice for treating infections in general, says Dr. Hudson. Berberine, the active ingredient, is what makes it specifically useful for UTIs, she says. Take 500 to 1,000 milligrams of goldenseal root extract daily, but don't take it for more than 1 week. Do not take this herb if you are pregnant, however.

cancer

There aren't many things worse than sitting in the chair across from your doctor and being told that you have cancer. Behind that dreadful scenario, however, there's a statistic that allows for more hope than ever before. Today, many experts think that at least 65 percent of all cancers can be prevented with simple lifestyle changes, such as eating right, exercising regularly, keeping excess weight off, and avoiding toxic materials. By taking the right steps, you could help reduce your risk of developing this feared disease.

There are lots of different kinds of cancer and many different causes, but ultimately, cancer comes down to changes in a cell's genetic information—its DNA. A number of things—toxins, viruses, radiation, or inherited weaknesses—can trigger that cell change. Whether or not a precancerous cell progresses to cancer depends on your body's ability to repair the DNA damage, or if it can identify and destroy the unhealthy cell.

While lifestyle plays a major role in cancer protection, certain nutritional supplements may help you avoid cancer, slow its growth, and support your body while it fights cancer and if you have to go through the stressful treatments of radiation and chemotherapy. Most of these supplements are based on nutrients naturally found in foods, says naturopathic doctor Tori Hudson, ND, professor at the National College of Naturopathic Medicine in Portland, Oregon, and author of *Women's Encyclopedia of Natural Medicine*. For example, green tea extract contains concentrated epigallocatechin-3 gallate (EGCG), a cancer-fighting ingredient in the tea; curcumin extract is concentrated (and sometimes made into a more absorbable form) from the yellow Indian spice turmeric; and resveratrol, derived from red wine, has antiaging and anticancer properties.

These food-based compounds help disarm or detoxify toxins, shield cells from cancer-causing damage, help preserve normal cell function, and help keep a cell's DNA intact. Here's a rundown of the most popular.

343

Get an Edge with Antioxidants

Antioxidants are the most familiar of the cancer-fighting biochemicals. They neutralize tiny particles called free radicals, which are formed by exposure to various environmental factors, including tobacco smoke and radiation. Free radicals are molecules missing one or more electrons, so they "grab" electrons from other molecules, which causes cellular damage. Over time, such damage may become irreversible and lead to cancer.

Antioxidants help to "mop up" free radicals, meaning they neutralize the electrical charge and prevent the free radical from taking electrons from other molecules. Therefore, they help stop the process that could lead to cancer.

You probably know about the antioxidant vitamins C and E and beta-carotene. But there are many others, such as lycopene and lutein, pigments found in foods. Still other nutrients and plant compounds are needed for the body to make its own powerful antioxidants and other toxin-neutralizing biochemicals, and those include superoxide dismutase, glutathione peroxidase, alpha lipoic acid, catalase, and coenzyme Q_{10}. Even though we make these in our bodies, we need lots of other nutrients, including selenium, magnesium, and sulfur, as well as the amino acids glutamine and cysteine, to help us do so.

The best advice? Don't drive yourself crazy trying to zero in on a few select cancer-fighting foods. Instead, eat a variety of fruits and vegetables (the main sources of antioxidants), such as: dark leafy greens (spinach, kale); orange produce like winter squash, mangoes, and carrots; red, purple, and blue berries and fruits like blueberries, pomegranate, watermelon, and plums; and whole grains, avocadoes, olives, and nuts (especially walnuts and Brazil nuts) for trace minerals like selenium and vitamin E. Include vitamin C–rich sources like citrus, red peppers, tomatoes, and kiwifruit, and use unrefined oils like extra virgin olive oil. Include spices like turmeric, ginger, cayenne, and curry, and herbs like rosemary, parsley, and thyme.

If you take an antioxidant supplement or a multivitamin/mineral supplement marketed as an "antioxidant," look for these things:

• *About 300 milligrams of vitamin C.* In one review of studies that examined vitamin C intake in different populations, researchers concluded that women who get about 300 milligrams of vitamin C a day are 30 percent less likely to get breast cancer. If you want or need to take more, take a separate vitamin C supplement.

If You're Being Treated for Cancer . . .

Some cancer drugs actually work by causing oxidative damage to cancer cells. You certainly don't want to interfere with that. And that's why some oncologists ask that you do not take large doses of antioxidant vitamins during treatment.

On the other hand, there is some research that says antioxidants may still help you during treatment. A systematic review of 19 studies found that taking supplemental antioxidants during cancer chemotherapy did not seem to interfere with treatment and may, in fact, have helped increase survival rates, tumor response, and the person's ability to tolerate chemotherapy.

All of the studies were randomized trials with a control group and included reporting of treatment response (tumor shrinkage) and survival data. Most people included in the studies had advanced or relapsed cancer. All of the studies that included survival statistics showed similar or better survival rates for the antioxidant group than the control group. None of the studies supported the theory that antioxidant supplements make chemotherapy less effective.

What to do? Get your doctor's input on this one. And once you are done with treatment, discuss again with your doctor or a nutritionist what diet and nutrients are best for you.

• *About 200 micrograms of selenium, from selenomethionine,* a highly bioavailable organic source. A study by the University of Arizona showed that taking 200 micrograms of selenium (as selenomethionine) daily for 5 years reduced overall cancer rates by 42 percent and cancer deaths by 52 percent. Selenium was particularly potent against colorectal cancer, reducing risk by 64 percent, and prostate cancer, reducing risk by 69 percent.

• *About 400 IU of vitamin E as mixed tocopherols,* and, ideally, mixed tocotrienols. Avoid dl-alpha-tocopherol, a synthetic form of the vitamin, which doesn't seem to be as helpful as getting a variety of the forms of vitamin E. (Walnuts are a great source.)

• *About 25,000 IU of mixed carotenoids.* This is preferable to beta-carotene, and taking preformed vitamin A (retinol) is not necessary. Your body can convert what it needs from carotenoids.

Puffers Beware

If you are a smoker (or a recent ex-smoker), don't take supplemental beta-carotene. Two studies showed that smokers who got high doses in supplement form were actually more likely to develop lung cancer than smokers who took no beta-carotene. Getting beta-carotene from foods, though, is fine.

The Goodness of Green Tea

Some people think that green tea—a favorite of the Japanese—is an acquired taste. If so, there's a good reason to acquire it.

The traditional pale-green brew that accompanies Japanese food appears to have potent anticancer properties, according to Jerzy Jankun, MD, a cancer researcher and associate professor in the department of urology at the Medical College of Ohio in Toledo.

Green tea contains a substance called epigallocathechin-3 gallate (EGCG). Dr. Jankun's research shows that EGCG inhibits urokinase, an enzyme that allows tumors to grow and spread. "By inhibiting urokinase, those processes could be stopped," says Dr. Jankun.

Research has also shown that EGCG can slow blood vessel formation in tumors, reducing the rate at which they can grow and spread. It can also regulate cell division and growth and cause programmed cell death in DNA-damaged cells. The cancers that green tea can possibly slow down include prostate, esophageal, bladder, cervical, pancreatic, ovarian, lymphoma, and leukemia. Green tea is also active against human papillomavirus (HPV), a sexually transmitted virus associated with cervical and anal cancer and warts.

EGCG is structurally similar to methotrexate, a drug used to treat cancer. Asian women who have had stage I or II breast cancer who drink 3 to 5 or even more cups of green tea daily seem to have a reduced risk of breast cancer recurrence. Men with high-grade prostatic intraepithelial neoplasia (a precancerous condition) who took 200 milligrams of EGCG three times daily for a year had a reduced risk of progression to prostate cancer.

How much green tea should you sip? The commonly prescribed dose of green tea is based on the amount typically consumed in Asian countries, which is about 3 cups per day, providing 240 to 320 milligrams of polyphenols.

You can get decaffeinated green tea or, if you prefer, decaffeinated green tea extract. Since potencies are different, follow the directions on the label. Aim for a dosage of 200 to 400 milligrams a day, and talk with your doctor first to make sure green tea is right for you.

Toxins and Your Body

You've probably heard about detoxing, a hot trend right now. The thinking is that toxins can build up in our bodies and cause damage. We're exposed to toxins all the time—in exhaust fumes and secondhand smoke, phthalates in plastics, pesticides and herbicides found in the foods we eat. They're in the medications we take, the junk we eat and drink—they're even formed by our bodies' normal metabolic processes. Toxins make us age faster and increase our risk for cancer and other diseases.

A safe detox program is designed to remove accumulated toxins by helping your body to break them down and excrete them. The liver is the main organ for detoxification. It produces enzymes that break down toxins so that they can be removed. But even the liver can get overwhelmed if it has too much work to do.

Instead of doing a trendy fasting detox, try these simple tips to clear your body of damaging toxins.

• *Drink plenty of clean water.* Green tea is fine, too. Get about 8 glasses a day of water that, at a minimum, has been run through an activated charcoal filter.

• *Get plenty of soluble fiber.* It binds up toxin-loaded bile so it can't be reabsorbed. Most people need to double the amount of fiber they are getting. If need be, use psyllium to add soluble fiber to your diet.

• *Take 100 milligrams of alpha lipoic acid,* a versatile, liver-friendly antioxidant, every day.

• *Eat three to five servings a week of cruciferous vegetables* such as broccoli, cabbage, cauliflower, watercress, and kale. Compounds in these plants stimulate the activity of detoxifying enzymes. If you aren't eating enough, supplement your diet with a "green foods" product.

• *Eat garlic, onions, and chives, or take garlic extract.* Compounds in these vegetables signal genes to produce two protective enzymes, glutathione-S-transferase and superoxide dismutase, both powerful antioxidants involved in the body's main detox pathways.

• *Take a high-antioxidant multivitamin/mineral supplement.* Trace minerals such as selenium, zinc, and manganese are needed to produce detoxifying liver enzymes. Antioxidants like vitamins A, C, and E protect DNA from toxin-related damage that can lead to cancer. And B vitamins like folic acid, B_{12}, and B_6 help drive metabolic pathways that reduce levels of toxic metabolic by-products like homocysteine.

• *Consider taking grape seed extract.* It's a powerful stimulant of detoxifying liver enzymes. It helps break down and clear out caffeine, nicotine, acetaminophen, and a number of other drugs.

• *Ask your doctor about milk thistle.* It supports your liver by promoting liver regeneration and the formation of new liver cells. It also helps to protect against injury to the liver by toxins. It may also help protect the kidneys and colon. Milk thistle can interact with some drugs and can decrease the effectiveness of some cancer drugs. It may also have some estrogenic effects, in which case you'd want to avoid it if you've had estrogen-positive cancer (which can include forms of breast, endometrial, uterine, and ovarian cancers).

Help Your Immunity

Supplements that strengthen your immunity are a good idea if you're trying to prevent cancer, withstand the immunity-debilitating effects of chemotherapy and radiation, and avoid a recurrence of the disease.

Probiotics can help your immune system remain vigilant and limit cancer-causing toxins in your intestines. They are especially useful if you take antibiotics, chemotherapy, or are having radiation treatment to your abdomen. Probiotics may also help prevent postradiation sepsis, a potentially fatal bodywide infection. Japanese researchers have found that use of a *Lactobacillus*-containing probiotic almost doubled the time to recurrence in people with bladder cancer. Moreover, the natural tendency of one in three new bladder cancers to have a more aggressive grade disappeared almost completely. There are many kinds of probiotics, so you'll want to pick a high-potency, proven brand. One medical-grade, prescription probiotic, VSL#3, is a high-potency probiotic safely used for inflammatory bowel disease.

Another way to boost immunity is to eat mushrooms or take a mushroom extract. Several kinds of mushrooms, such as maitake, reishi, and shiitake, have been found to help stimulate immunity and inhibit tumor growth. People receiving chemotherapy may use a mushroom extract to maintain an adequate white blood cell count so they can continue therapy. There are a number of active ingredients in mushrooms, but the "D-fraction" of an ingredient called beta-glucan appears to be the most active and potent form.

Talk with your doctor before taking a mushroom extract to make sure it's all right for you. Be careful if you are taking immune-suppressing drugs, as mushrooms can counteract these and certain other drugs.

Garlic also has impressive immunity-stimulating activity. Both fresh garlic and aged garlic extract can stimulate T-cell proliferation; restore suppressed antibody responses; stimulate the death of tumor cells; and induce the release of several important cancer-fighting biochemicals, including interleukin-2, tumor necrosis factor-alpha, and gamma interferon. Ask your doctor to check for any possible interactions between garlic and medications you are taking before you take garlic extract.

Zinc helps by building new immune system cells and getting them ready to battle disease. Zinc is responsible for three important parts of the immunity arsenal: neutrophils, natural killer cells, and T lymphocytes. Even mild zinc deficiency might adversely affect immunity function, but too much zinc can also have an adverse effect, says Jennifer Brett, ND, a naturopathic doctor at the Wilton Naturopathic Center in Stratford, Connecticut. If you meet the Daily Value by getting 15 milligrams of zinc a day, you're probably getting enough, she says.

The Pros and Cons of Phytoestrogens for Cancer Protection

Soy foods, red clover, and flaxseed all contain high amounts of phyto- (meaning "plant") estrogens. These are weak forms of estrogen that can block the action of natural, stronger forms of estrogen that women produce. So phytoestrogens can help prevent cancer, especially in younger women, who have lots of estrogen. In older women, however, the picture is less clear. Based on animal studies, researchers have speculated that, as natural estrogen levels drop, plant estrogens have the potential to promote estrogen-positive cancers, such as breast, endometrial, uterine, and ovarian. The form of phytoestrogen found to be most stimulating of cancer growth in animals is an isoflavone called genistein. That's also the most common isoflavone found in phytoestrogen supplements made from soy or red clover, which are often sold as meno-pause or hot flash remedies.

But that theory is contradicted by several recent population studies, in both Asia and the United States, which suggest that eating minimally processed, traditional soy foods like tofu and edamame seems to offer breast cancer protection, says Mark Messina, PhD, a leading soy expert and a soy industry spokesman.

For instance, a study from the University of California at Berkeley found that soy foods are not necessarily contraindicated for breast cancer patients. That study, which included 1,954 breast cancer survivors, found that increased intake of dietary sources of isoflavones was associated with a trend toward reduced risk of cancer recurrence. This trend was true for both tamoxifen users and nonusers. (Tamoxifen selectively blocks estro-gen.) In fact, among postmenopausal women treated with tamoxifen, there was an approximate 60 percent reduction in breast cancer recurrence between the highest and the lowest insoflavone intakes.

So what's the bottom line? "The default position for oncologists has been no soy for women who've had breast cancer," Dr. Messina says. "We think the evidence now supports allowing about two servings of soy a day to breast cancer patients who want to eat it, especially vegetarians and Asian women." However, he agrees that more study is needed before soy foods can be rec-ommended as improving the prognosis for breast cancer survivors. If you have or have had breast cancer, don't take any soy products or supplements without talking it over with your doctors first.

As a general rule, 1 gram of a traditional soy food such as tofu or soy milk has about 3.5 milligrams of isoflavones. Foods made from soy protein isolates, such as some protein bars, have about 1 milligram of isoflavones per gram of protein.

As for isoflavone supplements from soy or clover, there is not much evidence to support their use for cancer prevention. However, "we do know that these supplements are processed in the body the same way as isoflavones found in foods are," Dr. Messina says.

Finds about Folate

While folate has been found to be a lifesaver in terms of preventing heart disease and birth defects, you may have to watch out for it when it comes to cancer. "Adequate levels of this B vitamin are essential for DNA synthesis and therefore promote cell growth, and drugs that mimic the structure of folate and inhibit its function are used to treat certain cancers," says Patrick Stover, PhD, professor and director of the Division of Nutritional Sciences at Cornell University. "On the other hand, folate deficiency not only impairs cell growth, but also can lead to DNA mutations that promote carcinogenesis," he adds.

The theory that taking large amounts of folic acid can increase cancer risk is "highly contentious in the scientific arena, but the literature has some seriously flawed studies and the well-done studies show high levels of folic acid intake neither prevent or accelerate cancer," Dr. Stover says. Lung cancer may be an exception, but the public health message should probably be "don't smoke."

So the advice these days is: Get enough folic acid—400 micrograms a day is plenty. You'll get that amount by taking a basic multi and by eating folic acid–fortified foods such as enriched bread and cereals, pasta, rice, and cornmeal, and by eating naturally rich foods like dark leafy greens, citrus fruits, lentils, and dried beans. No need to overdo it.

The Bone Builders to the Rescue

New research suggests that having an optimal blood level of vitamin D could cut your cancer risk by as much as 60 percent. Vitamin D can activate certain proteins that suppress tumor growth and development and help prevent as many as 16 different types of cancer, including lung, pancreas, breast, colon, and prostate. Vitamin D increases the self-destruction of mutated cells, reduces the spread and reproduction of cancer cells, and reduces the growth of new blood vessels from preexisting ones, which is an important step in the growth and spread of cancerous tumors.

Research shows that up to 70 percent of Americans have suboptimal blood levels of vitamin D. The best way to figure out how much you need is to get a blood test, both before and after you have started taking supplements. Some people need 2,000 to 5,000 IU of vitamin D_3 a day, or even more, to stay at a good blood level of 50 ng/ml or higher.

Getting enough vitamin D and calcium may help prevent the spread of breast cancer to bones because it slows bone turnover, preliminary research shows. Many cancer patients are low in vitamin D, and RDA doses (400 IU) aren't enough to reach optimal levels. (Although new recommendations are 600 IU for people 70 and under and 800 IU for those over 71.)

The best way to find out how much D you need is to get your blood levels tested and then take an amount of vitamin D that will keep you in an optimum midrange level of 50 ng/ml. But you need to work with your doctor to find the perfect dose for you.

Calcium has long been thought to reduce colon cancer risk. The theory is that calcium binds bile acids and other carcinogens in the intestine. Both dietary and supplemental calcium seem to help reduce colon cancer risk by keeping normal epithelial cells in the colon from proliferating abnormally. There is also evidence that supplementing with calcium carbonate (1,200 milligrams per day) produces a moderate reduction in the recurrence of adenomas in people who have already had a colorectal adenoma removed. If you're taking calcium for cancer protection, it's important to also take enough vitamin D. That's because people with below-average vitamin D levels don't seem to get any benefit from calcium and may even see some harm. (One study found an increase in prostate cancer among high-dose calcium users.) "It seems that greatly increased calcium intake may depress the active form of vitamin D," says Robert E. C. Wildman, PhD, assistant professor of human nutrition at the University of Delaware in Newark.

So if you're using calcium for cancer protection, get about 1,200 milligrams a day from food and supplements. Take your supplements in divided doses of 300 to 500 milligrams, separate from a multivitamin. (Calcium can interfere with the absorption of some other minerals.) Experts are recommending 1,000 to 2,000 IU of vitamin D a day, but you may need more if your blood levels are low.

Heat Up Cancer Protection

Curcumin, a component of the yellow spice turmeric, has emerged as a leading cancer fighter. It can disrupt cancer cells in several stages of development. It, too, causes programmed cell death and inhibits the development of new blood vessels to feed tumors It seems to work best against colon cancer, and in some animal studies, it was as good as certain chemotherapy drugs at inhibiting the growth of cancer cells. Dosages of up to 8,000 milligrams a day for 3 months have been used with no toxicity. Lower dosages are fine if you go with a form that is more easily absorbed.

canker sores

Canker sores may be out of sight, but they're not out of mind. They lie on the inner lining of your lips and cheeks or on the base of your tongue, the floor of your mouth, or your soft palate. Eat anything hot or spicy, and they'll burn like fire.

These painful critters, also called recurrent aphthous ulcers, are yellowish gray or white with red borders. They're tiny, round, and appear individually or in bunches.

Fortunately, they're not contagious and they normally heal within 7 to 14 days. But that's faint praise. When they do make their cameo appearances, they can turn the simple pleasures of eating, talking, and even brushing your teeth into harrowing experiences.

It's a good thing that help is just around the corner. There are some dietary and other natural measures that you can take to keep these little buggers out of your mouth.

Start by eliminating the top canker sore triggers from your diet, such as chocolate, nuts, tomatoes, green peppers, strawberries, and oranges and other citrus fruits. Try to avoid eating sharp-edged corn chips and pretzels, because they can irritate and injure the lining of your mouth and produce an ulcer.

After you've eliminated the troublemakers, you can reintroduce each of these foods into your diet one at a time every two to three days to determine which is the source of the trouble.

Canker sores can also be caused by food sensitivities to wheat products. See your doctor to determine whether food allergies are causing your problem.

Once you've taken these steps, if you still suffer from an occasional canker sore or two, a certain type of licorice supplement will relieve the pain and shorten the duration of the ulcer (see page 354). You can also take a high-quality multivitamin/mineral supplement daily to prevent them altogether.

Zap Canker Sores with Licorice

The kind of licorice that stops canker sores is a far cry from the black, stringy stuff that kids love to gnaw on. What you want is deglycyrrhizinated licorice, or DGL.

"DGL has anti-inflammatory properties. It speeds the healing process and soothes the discomfort of canker sores," says Michael Traub, ND, a naturopathic doctor and director of the integrated residency program at North Hawaii Community Hospital in Kamuela.

In one study, 20 people with recurrent canker sores used a DGL mouthwash. Fifteen people experienced at least a 50 percent improvement within 1 day and were completely healed by the third day.

Among those who recovered was one patient who had had recurrent canker sores for over 10 years. He had several sores on his tongue and lips, inside his cheek, on his soft palate, and in the back of his throat. By the seventh day after he started using the DGL solution, he was completely free of sores.

To begin the healing process, take two 200-milligram tablets 20 minutes before meals, says Dr. Traub, or chew one or two tablets two or three times a day. While chewing, use your tongue to position the tablet residue on the sore to promote even speedier healing. You should use DGL, which is available at health food stores, until the sore heals, he adds.

In addition, you can empty the powder from a capsule into ½ cup of lukewarm water, dissolve the DGL, and swish the solution around in your mouth, says Dr. Traub. Repeat this at least two or three times a day until the sore has healed.

A High-Potency Multivitamin to Cover Your Bases

Deficiencies of B vitamins, including B_{12} and folic acid; zinc; and iron appear to be prevalent among people with canker sores. When the deficiencies are corrected, the sores often show improvement or complete remission. "Evidence of a vitamin deficiency often shows up inside your mouth and throat because of the rapid cell turnover rate that's characteristic of the mucous membranes," says Jennifer Brett, ND, a naturopathic doctor at the Wilton Naturopathic Center in Stratford, Connecticut.

"Low levels of some B vitamins can cause swelling of the tongue and canker sores. If you're not getting enough zinc, you won't heal as quickly from small injuries like biting the inside of your mouth. And without enough folic acid and iron, you won't maintain the necessary rapid cell division that you need to keep the lining of your mouth healthy," says Dr. Brett.

A high-potency multivitamin purchased at a health food store should give you the nutrients that are necessary to prevent recurrent canker sores, says Dr. Brett. Take 500 to 1,000 micrograms of vitamin B_{12}, 10 milligrams of iron (if you're a man or a postmenopausal woman, consult a doctor first), 800 micrograms of folic acid, and 15 to 20 milligrams of zinc, she says. If your multivitamin doesn't include all you need, simply add separate supplements to make up the difference.

C and Thiamin: More Sore Solutions

If your canker sores are a result of food allergies, take 1,000 to 1,200 milligrams of buffered vitamin C daily to help reduce the level of histamines in your body, says Dr. Brett. Histamines are the immune system chemicals that are released by white blood cells and cause inflammation and irritation. To enhance the effectiveness of the vitamin C, take 1,000 milligrams of quercetin or 100 milligrams of grape seed extract daily as a preventive, she says. These are both bioflavonoids—compounds that inhibit histamine release, reduce inflammation, and speed healing.

Other research shows that a thiamin deficiency can lead to recurrent mouth ulcers. In a study, researchers determined levels of a thiamin-dependent enzyme in 120 people. Forty-nine of the 70 participants with recurrent canker sores had low levels of the enzyme, compared to only 2 among the 50 in the group without ulcers. Dr. Brett recommends taking 100 milligrams of thiamin daily as a preventive.

carpal tunnel syndrome

What makes your foot go numb when you sit too long with your legs crossed? Bad circulation, right? That's why it helps to stand up and stomp the pins and needles out. It gets the blood moving again.

What's really going on doesn't have anything to do with blood flow, though. The numbness occurs when a nerve, not a blood vessel, is compressed. That's the same thing that happens—in a different part of the body, of course—when someone has carpal tunnel syndrome (CTS).

Instead of being compressed by a weight, the median nerve that runs to your thumb and first two fingers is constricted when your body's tendons and tissues swell and press against it. The nerve and the nine tendons that move your fingers are encased in a sheath called the synovium, making a sausagelike bundle that passes through the bony, hourglass-shaped passageway on the underside of the wrist that's known as the carpal tunnel.

When you're doing things like typing or bowling, the repetitive motions of your hand and wrist can cause the tendons and synovium to become inflamed and swollen. Even slight swelling in the wrist area can press the nerve enough to short-circuit the signal.

Women, especially pregnant women, are more prone to CTS than men. Regardless of your sex, however, you're at greater risk for CTS if you're overweight and if you don't exercise very much. Women's risk is also increased by taking oral contraceptives and during menopause.

The first symptoms of CTS aren't that far removed from the sensation you get in your foot when it "falls asleep." You may experience tingling, numbness, or pain in the hand and fingers, especially in the thumb and first two fingers. The more you use your hand, the more it will hurt. As the condition progresses, your hand can become so weak that you can't even grip a glass. For severe cases like this, a doctor may recommend surgery to relieve pressure on the entrapped nerve.

Naturopathic doctors recommend that you first take steps to avoid surgery by working on the mechanical problem of CTS as well as taking supplements. You may be able to get relief and reduce inflammation right away with simple measures like splinting your wrist in a neutral position and altering your activity. You can also use heat and cold to help relieve your symptoms.

In addition, you'll probably want to try some of the supplements that can help. Here are some vitamins and herbs to soothe and heal the irritated nerve.

Vitamin B$_6$ Gets a Boost

B$_6$ has often been recommended for CTS, and while there are some older studies showing that it works, newer studies show that it seems to work more on the symptoms of peripheral neuropathy—nerve damage in the hands or feet, often caused by diabetes—than CTS. Still, it's worth a try, says Thomas Kruzel, ND, a naturopathic doctor in Scottsdale, Arizona. To end the tingling, take 50 milligrams of B$_6$ each day, he suggests, and give it at least 12 weeks before you expect to feel a difference.

You can boost the healing power of B$_6$ by taking at least 10 milligrams of riboflavin along with it, says Dr. Kruzel. The riboflavin converts the B$_6$ to a more active form that is essential to more than 60 chemical reactions in your body.

Some Wrist Action for Pineapple

When it comes to inflammation, sometimes your body just doesn't know when to stop. With CTS, you need to reduce the inflammation in the swollen tendons and synovium in order to relieve the pain. Pharmaceutical anti-inflammatories like aspirin or ibuprofen might be all you need, but some people find that they experience side effects from these drugs, particularly upset stomach and ringing in the ears.

For relief with fewer side effects, you have the option of trying some supplements that can be very effective. One of these is bromelain, an enzyme found in pineapple; it's one of nature's own anti-inflammatory medicines. This hungry enzyme can take a bite out of pain and swelling and help you heal faster, says Dr. Kruzel. Just be sure you don't blunt its effect by taking it with meals. If you do, all of its enzymatic energy is just digested. If you take it between meals, however, it goes to work digesting the products of inflammation.

When the tingling pain of CTS strikes, take two 500-milligram tablets or capsules of bromelain between meals two or three times a day, says Dr. Kruzel. Bromelain is measured in milk-clotting units (mcu) or gelatin-dissolving units (gdu). The higher the number, the greater its potency. Look for a supplement with between 1,800 and 2,400 mcu or 1,080 and 1,440 gdu in each capsule.

Pouring On the Flaxseed Oil

You can also soothe the inflamed nerve and tissues with flaxseed oil, a supplement rich in omega-3 essential fatty acids, says Ellen Potthoff, DC, ND, a chiropractor and naturopathic doctor in Pleasant Hill, California. Any type of inflammation responds well to essential fatty acids because no matter where it hurts, they interrupt the process of inflammation early.

You should feel better in 2 to 4 weeks if you start taking 1 tablespoon of flaxseed oil every day, says Dr. Potthoff. Taste is one way to tell if you're getting good-quality flaxseed oil. "It should have a really nice, nutty flavor and a dark amber color," she says.

The Power of Turmeric

Turmeric is an herb that contains a powerful anti-inflammatory chemical called curcumin. The herb has traditionally been used in India's Ayurvedic medicine to treat pain and inflammation.

The effect of turmeric has been compared to that of cortisone, the pharmaceutical sometimes used to treat CTS symptoms. Although turmeric's pain-fighting power is not as strong as cortisone's, the herb is a lot easier on your system, says Dr. Kruzel.

Turmeric's action is similar to that of bromelain. For some relief, opt for capsules of the standardized extract. Unlike the turmeric on your spice shelf, the capsules contain 95 percent pure curcumin.

Dr. Kruzel gives people with CTS 250 to 500 milligrams of curcumin a day. Keep taking this dose until the inflammation has been reduced, he advises, then take half that dose for 1 to 2 weeks until your symptoms are gone.

If the symptoms return, repeat the high dose and return to the lower dose again after they improve. Do not use turmeric supplements without talking to your doctor, especially if you are pregnant.

You might also consider adding bioflavonoids to your supplement arsenal, suggests Dr. Potthoff. Rich in powerful antioxidants, bioflavonoids are used to treat injuries because they relieve pain and promote healing, she says. She recommends taking 1,000 milligrams of a broad-range bio-flavonoid supplement that contains citrus bioflavonoids and quercetin three times a day.

cataracts

If your doctor tells you that you're developing a cataract, it means that the lens in one of your eyes is becoming less transparent. As this normally crystal-clear disk begins to cloud over, you might have trouble seeing into the distance, words on a page may appear blurry, or you could find yourself wishing that your eyeglasses were stronger.

Cataracts ultimately interfere with clear vision, but if they are treated properly, they generally aren't blinding or life-threatening. "Ninety-nine percent of the time, cataracts are not an emergency," says Robert Abel Jr., MD, clinical professor of ophthalmology at Thomas Jefferson University in Philadelphia and author of *The Eye Care Revolution*. You should go to an eye doctor for a thorough examination at least once every 2 years. Your doctor will be able to tell you if you have cataracts, and if so, what stage they've reached.

The progression of cataracts can be slowed or even reversed with the right vitamins, says Dr. Abel, but he advises that you check with your doctor before taking supplements. "The perfect people to try supplements as treatment are those with early or intermediate cataracts—the kind they may not even be aware of yet," he says. By taking some supplements for as little as 6 months, some people can get out of what Dr. Abel calls the "cataract surgery zone."

Antioxidants Keep Things Clear

Most of the evidence for supplements' effect on cataracts points to vitamins C and E and selenium.

The lens of the eye has the second highest concentration of vitamin C of any organ in the body, says Mark Lamden, ND, a naturopathic doctor and adjunct faculty member at Bastyr University in Kenmore, Washington. Any vitamin C that you get—from food or supplements— can help your lenses in a big way.

There's another reason to take vitamin C, however. It's an antioxidant, and you need its power because the eyes are prime sites of what are called oxidative processes. Any time we burn energy, it's a metabolic process that involves oxygen molecules. The eyes, says Dr. Abel, are the most metabolically active parts of the body. "For the eyes, it's constant oxidation," he says, "and even though oxidation is a normal life process, it exerts a lot of wear and tear."

Research suggests that when it comes to vitamin C and cataract prevention, commitment is the key. A study of 247 nurses at Tufts University in Boston showed that women who took vitamin C supplements for 10 years or more were much less likely to have signs of cataracts than those who never took the vitamin.

If you have cataracts, you should take 3,000 to 5,000 milligrams of vitamin C in divided doses throughout the day, recommends Dr. Lamden.

Scavengers for Better Vision

Vitamin E and selenium are other antioxidants that have been associated with reduced risk of cataracts. Like vitamin C, they scavenge free radicals, the free-roaming, unstable molecules that wreak a lot of damage on cells. Because of their free radical–scavenging abilities, vitamin E and selenium help prevent or clear up cloudiness in the lens. Research has shown that people with cataracts often have low levels of selenium in their blood and in the aqueous humor—the fluid within the eyeball—compared to people without cataracts.

Although vitamin E and selenium are present in some foods, such as whole grains and vegetable oils, you would have a hard time getting significant amounts of either nutrient from food. "There's no way you could eat enough of the right foods to get the high doses necessary for real nutrition therapy," says Dr. Lamden. Fortunately, that's where supplements come into the picture.

For people already diagnosed with cataracts, Dr. Lamden recommends 800 to 1,200 international units (IU) of natural vitamin E and 400 micrograms of selenium a day. To help keep cataracts from forming in the first place, a lower daily dose of 400 to 800 IU of vitamin E is ample. Since these are high doses of both supplements, however, you should talk to your doctor first.

The mineral zinc is another nutrient that can help halt hazy sight, says Dr. Lamden. In studies, it has been noted that the lenses of people with cataracts tend to be lacking in zinc. If you have cataracts, Dr. Lamden recommends 30 to 60 milligrams of zinc every day. These high doses also require medical supervision.

A good dose of riboflavin—which boosts glutathione levels in the body—may also help prevent cataracts. A study at the State University of New York at Stony Brook found that people who received the most riboflavin were much less likely to have cataracts than those who received smaller amounts. The connection, once again, appears to be antioxidants. The body uses riboflavin to manufacture glutathione, a powerful compound that battles free radicals. When you don't get enough riboflavin, glutathione levels fall, and that gives free radicals more time to damage the eyes.

celiac disease

Some folks who have celiac disease find themselves in an ironic situation. They eat a balanced diet of meat, dairy, fruits, vegetables, and whole-grain foods, yet their guts growl constantly with gas, diarrhea, and stomach cramps, alternating with constipation. It's as if their insides were rebelling against what, for most people, would be a healthy and nutritious diet.

If you have celiac disease, you're intolerant of gluten, the protein in wheat, rye, and barley that makes dough sticky and gooey. Unless the condition is treated, your system can't absorb enough nutrients from food to carry on body functions, a condition known as malabsorption. If you lose weight, become listless, and appear malnourished, you may have celiac disease.

"If left untreated, it can become life-threatening. People can waste away," says Kristin Stiles, ND, a naturopathic doctor at the Complementary Medicine and Healing Arts Center in Vestal, New York. That's why it's important to get a proper diagnosis from your doctor if you experience these symptoms.

Get the Gluten Out

Fortunately, the treatment is fairly simple once you know the cause. The disease, which often runs in families, was initially identified in the first century AD. It wasn't until World War II, however, that a Dutch pediatrician discovered that his patients improved because there was no bread available. It seems that some people lack an enzyme that breaks down and helps digest gluten. When this enzyme is absent, a toxic substance builds up and damages the mucous membrane lining the small intestine. Frequently, the damaged area becomes inflamed.

When injured, the intestinal lining has difficulty soaking up the nutrients in food. That's why people with celiac disease may also develop anemia. Anemia often results from a lack of iron in the blood, and that's one of the nutrients that is blocked when the intestinal lining can't do its job. Other deficiencies may show up, too, such as shortages of folic acid and other B vitamins, as well as vitamins A, D, E, K, and beta-carotene.

The first and most effective treatment is to eliminate gluten from your diet. This isn't quite as easy as it sounds because so many processed foods use wheat, which contains gluten, for filler and flavoring. If you're aware of risky food products and avoid them, a gluten-free diet can restore small intestine function within a few days to a few months. Once the mucous membrane is no longer inflamed, the absorption problem usually disappears.

Replace Lost Nutrients

In the meantime, until the healing process does its work, it's a good idea to take vitamin and mineral supplements to prevent deficiencies and malnutrition, says Pamela Taylor, ND, a naturopathic doctor in Moline, Illinois.

At the very least, you'll want to take a multivitamin/mineral supplement that includes calcium and magnesium, says Dr. Taylor. Magnesium deficiency often occurs in malabsorption syndromes and may contribute to osteoporosis, the rapid bone loss that can lead to hip fractures and other skeletal problems. This mineral is also important for proper tissue healing, so you need to get enough to help your body heal itself. To make sure that you get magnesium, be sure that your diet consists of moderate amounts of protein and plenty of steamed leafy green vegetables like kale, collard greens, and mustard greens. These greens are also good sources of calcium, she adds.

In addition to a multivitamin each day, Dr. Stiles tells her patients to take a high-potency B-complex supplement. This type of supplement contains 50 milligrams or the equivalent of B vitamins like niacin, thiamin, and riboflavin, as well as 400 to 800 micrograms of folic acid. Typically, one or two tablets daily with food are sufficient, she says. Your doctor can determine through blood tests how much you should take, she adds. If you take more than 35 milligrams of niacin, though, be sure to let your doctor know.

"You definitely want to supplement B vitamins, because those are not well absorbed when the intestines are aggravated," says Dr. Stiles. "Also, always take the supplement with food. If you take it on an empty stomach, you won't absorb it."

Even after your intestinal inflammation has subsided and you're absorbing nutrients the way you should, you probably should continue taking a multivitamin, says Dr. Taylor. "A good multivitamin/mineral tablet can catch and fill in the deficiencies and make sure you're getting what you need each day."

Speed the Healing

The inflammation in the intestine won't go away until you eliminate gluten, but you may be able to speed healing by taking an herbal combination of echinacea and goldenseal, says Dr. Stiles. These two immune system boosters are often packaged together in capsule form. Take one capsule three or four times a day, she suggests. If you use a tincture, take 10 to 15 drops of each herb in water or juice three or four times a day, with or without food.

You may also find echinacea and goldenseal in combination with slippery elm, marshmallow, geranium, and other herbs. If you can't find this combination at a drugstore, check at a health food store. This supplement goes by the generic name of Robert's Formula, which is made by a number of different supplement makers. It is a naturopathic mixture that treats the digestive tract by creating a slimy goo that is healing to gut tissues.

Echinacea and goldenseal are important healers because they have anti-inflammatory and antibacterial properties. One cautionary note, however: Don't take these herbs continuously. Dr. Stiles recommends 2 weeks on and 2 weeks off for a period of 1 to 2 months. "You quickly build up a tolerance to echinacea, and it's no longer effective," she says.

Vitamins can also speed healing. Dr. Taylor often recommends that her patients take a combination supplement of vitamins A, E, and C, along with a chelated form of zinc supplement. She suggests that you follow the dosage directions on the bottle. A typical dose, for example, is 5,000 international units (IU) of vitamin A, 200 to 500 milligrams of vitamin C, 100 to 400 IU of vitamin E, and 15 to 30 milligrams of chelated zinc. You'll need to check with your doctor before taking more than 20 milligrams of zinc, however.

Dr. Taylor recommends taking the supplements with food. You may need to continue supplementation for 2 to 4 months, she says.

chronic fatigue syndrome

Sure, we're all tired, at least some of the time. But people with chronic fatigue syndrome (CFS) have more than that occasional pooped-out feeling.

CFS, in fact, has an official definition that's used for diagnosis in the medical community. It's defined as debilitating fatigue that lasts for at least 6 months, accompanied by a number of other symptoms such as sleep disturbances, tender lymph nodes, sore throat, trouble with short-term memory, and various aches and pains.

Needless to say, if you have such continuous fatigue, the first thing you need to do is see if you and your doctor can find a cause, since many health problems can cause a similar range of problems. (Some possible explanations: Lyme disease, autoimmune disease, hepatitis, depression, and hypothyroidism.)

CFS is actually called a diagnosis of exclusion. You're often diagnosed with it when doctors have ruled out all other causes. Unfortunately, there is no test to confirm that diagnosis, and although there are ways to treat some symptoms, there are no medical treatments that provide a cure.

There are many theories about what causes it. Researchers speculate that it may be an autonomic nervous system disorder, where the body's "master gland," the hypothalamus, fails to regulate properly, or that it may be a psychiatric or metabolic disorder that impairs the ability to produce energy. Some think it signals nutritional deficiencies; others link it to oxidative damage. In fact, CFS may have multiple causes.

The theory that an infectious agent may be involved got a boost recently when researchers discovered that a retrovirus is found in many people with CFS. However, it's not known if the virus causes the symptoms or if compromised immunity in people with CFS (yet another theory) gives the virus an opportunity to thrive.

People with CFS often have other health problems, as well, which can muddy the picture (and treatment) even further. They may need treatment for depression, sleep disorders, fibromyalgia, low blood pressure, gastrointestinal problems, food or chemical sensitivities, or any other number of issues.

Jacob Teitelbaum, MD, author of *From Fatigued to Fantastic* and director of the Fibromyalgia and Fatigue Centers, a national group of clinics, sees it in a more encompassing way. "Chronic fatigue syndrome represents an energy crisis in the body. You are expending more energy than you are able to make, just as you would blow a fuse in your house if you plugged in too many electrical appliances."

There are hundreds of ways this can happen in your body, Dr. Teitelbaum says. Chronic infections, nutritional deficiencies, hormonal imbalances, sleep disorders, chronic situational stress, and toxin exposure all deplete energy resources in the body, he says, creating the backdrop for this disease.

But there is another important component, Dr. Teitelbaum explains. Once your energy levels drop, your hypothalamus—the organ that, ounce for ounce, uses the most energy—starts to malfunction. Since your hypothalamus controls everything from your sleep to blood pressure, from your body temperature to bowels, you can easily see why so many symptoms can appear when your hypothalamus gets out of whack.

But the main symptom, besides fatigue, is insomnia, Dr. Teitelbaum says. "It is the combination of severe insomnia in the face of exhaustion that tells you that the hypothalamus is malfunctioning," he says. "People with chronic fatigue syndrome are lucky if they can sleep 4 or 5 hours a night. And even then, they don't get the deep sleep they need."

Sleep Ease

Getting adequate sleep needs to be addressed first, otherwise fatigue continues, he says. He suggests sleep-aid supplements such as melatonin, a hormone used for jet lag and insomnia. "You need only a small dose, 0.3 to 0.5 milligram a day, to normalize melatonin levels," he says. Take it half an hour to an hour before bedtime, or even at bedtime. He also recommends 200 to 400 milligrams of magnesium glycinate. "Magnesium is important because it is involved in many aspects of energy production, many people don't get enough, and, when taken at bedtime, it can help you sleep."

He also likes an herbal product called Revitalizing Sleep Formula by Enzymatic Therapy (available at health foods stores.) It contains valerian, passionflower, wild lettuce, Jamaican dogwood, and peony. "I also suggest people get some lavender oil and spray a little on their pillows," he says. Lavender has proven relaxing effects. "It's a simple thing that works," he says.

Rebalance Your Hormones

At the same time, Dr. Teitelbaum checks people's thyroid glands. Lots of people have low-normal thyroid levels and have been told that their thyroid is normal, but they still have symptoms of low thyroid function, such as low body temperature and cold intolerance. He gives them small amounts of T3, a form of thyroid hormone that can be prescribed but is also found in some over-the-counter products, to relieve fatigue and depression. He adds iodine, another essential for thyroid production, if it seems that the person is not getting enough through foods or iodized salt. Iodine is essential for thyroid hormone production.

People with CFS often have low adrenal gland function, as well, Dr. Teitelbaum says. "The way you tell is if you have 'Feed me now or I will kill you' syndrome—or irritability when you are hungry," he says. That's because your adrenal gland isn't doing its job of signaling the body to release stored energy when blood sugar drops. He recommends a product called Adrenal Stress End by Enzymatic Therapy. It contains licorice, vitamin C, 500 milligrams of pantothenic acid, and small amounts of natural adrenal glandulars. "Just 1 or 2 in the morning can help a lot," he says. "These are small doses and I have never seen it cause problems."

The most likely sex hormone imbalance is estrogen, Dr. Teitelbaum says. For that, he recommends a handful a day of edamame, a good source of phytoestrogens. For postmenopausal women, they provide a weak estrogen. For premenopausal women, they counteract too much strong estrogen. (If you've had an estrogen-positive cancer, talk with your doctor before using soy.)

Fighting Infections

People with CFS often have impaired immunity and opportunistic infections. Chronic yeast overgrowth, *candida,* is the most common and the most likely to be widespread in the body, Dr. Teitelbaum says. There's a whole protocol to treat candida (see Yeast Infections, page 621), but "the most important thing is to stop feeding the little buggers," he says. That means cut way back on sugars, refined carbohydrates, alcohol, and even fruit. You may be able to reintroduce some fruit as your symptoms clear.

Shore Up Nutritional Support

When people ask Dr. Teitelbaum what nutrients to take, he answers: "All of them." It's true that any one nutritional deficiency will affect your body's ability to function properly, but the ones most often focused on for CFS and energy production include magnesium, most of the B vitamins, vitamin D, fish oil, antioxidants (such as vitamins E and C and the trace mineral selenium), iron, iodine, and sometimes even salt. "This is one condition where I tell people to have as much salt as their body seems to require," he says.

He also may use nutrients that enhance energy production in the body, such as ribose (5 grams three times a day for 3 weeks, then twice a day), coenzyme Q_{10} (200 milligrams a day), and acetyl-L-carnitine (1,000 to 1,500 milligrams a day). Once people have their energy back, they may be able to stop taking all of these except the ribose.

Although it's possible that you may be able to initiate some of these therapies yourself, Dr. Teitelbaum suggests finding a doctor who specializes in CFS. You can do that at www.fibroandfatigue.com or holisticboard.org (the American Board of Integrative Holistic Medicine).

colds and flu

With more than 200 cold viruses floating around and a new strain of flu just waiting to claim its next victim each year, it seems almost impossible not to get sick.

When a cold or flu hits, you may want to go stock up on drugstore and over-the-counter remedies. Before you buy those cough suppressants, decongestants, and antihistamines, though, you should consider nutritional supplements to speed your recovery.

You can try a combination of nature's most powerful herbs, such as echinacea, goldenseal, and astragalus, to shift your immune system into overdrive so that your body can fight off the infection naturally. To back up this herbal defense team, you can use an array of infection-fighting vitamins and a mineral that can shorten the duration of your cold or flu, lessen the severity of your symptoms, or continue to build your immunity until you start feeling like yourself again.

If these and other remedies don't have an effect, however, you may have to be on guard for other kinds of infections. Be sure to see your doctor if your cold does not improve within 14 days or if you have green or yellow phlegm. And check with your doctor if you have trouble breathing or if your temperature tops 102°F.

Powerful Herbs to the Rescue

Echinacea and goldenseal, taken in combination, are top cold and flu fighters among medicinal herbal supplements, says Kristy Fassler, ND, a naturopathic doctor in Portsmouth, New Hampshire.

Echinacea, also known as purple coneflower, is a potent herb that forcefully stimulates the production of natural killer cells. The aptly named killer cell is a type of white blood cell that fights off viral infections.

While boosting the population of killer cells, echinacea also increases levels of immune system chemicals, such as interferon and properdin, that kill bacteria and viruses. It speeds up destruction of bacteria and viruses by enhancing the activity of cells called phagocytes.

Similar to echinacea, goldenseal stimulates white blood cell activity and contains antiviral and antibacterial compounds, chiefly berberine. It works well with echinacea because it has properties that enable it to reduce inflammation and mucus production. When you take goldenseal, it helps break up nasal and chest congestion and also reduces the swelling of mucous membranes, says Dr. Fassler.

When symptoms strike, take 300 milligrams of each of these herbs every 2 to 4 hours for the first 2 to 3 days, says Dr. Fassler. Continue with the same dosage of each three times a day until symptoms disappear.

A Root from the Orient

For thousands of years, astragalus root has been used to enhance immunity. This potent Chinese herb is considered by herbal practitioners to be a tonic that strengthens the body's resistance to disease. Astragalus can stimulate practically all of the processes of your immune system. It increases the number of stem cells in bone marrow and speeds their growth into active immune cells.

Astragalus also may help boost levels of interferon, one of your body's potent fighters against viruses, says Chris Meletis, ND, professor of natural pharmacology at the National College of Naturopathic Medicine in Portland, Oregon. A heightened level of interferon can help prevent or shorten the duration of colds and flu. Astragalus even boosts production of white blood cells called macrophages, whose mission is to destroy invading viruses and bacteria.

To stamp out a cold or flu in its earliest stages, take one 500-milligram capsule of astragalus four times a day until symptoms disappear, says Dr. Meletis. Then take one capsule twice a day for 7 days to prevent a relapse.

Tap into a Trio of Infection Fighters

It's a good idea to stock your medicine cabinet with vitamin C, vitamin A, and beta-carotene supplements, say Dr. Fassler and Dr. Meletis. These nutrients help you fight back fast, before the virus takes up residence and multiplies in your body.

Studies show that vitamin C can shorten the duration of common colds and flus. Taken in large enough doses, vitamin C can rev up your immune system by pumping enough fuel into white blood cells to destroy invading viruses and bacteria, says Dr. Meletis.

Vitamin C increases interferon levels and has interferon-like properties itself. It acts as a natural antihistamine that helps dry up watery eyes and reduce nasal and chest congestion, according to Dr. Meletis. It is also a powerful antioxidant that can help prevent the damage that your body endures when viruses or bacteria attack your immune system, he says.

At the first sign of cold or flu symptoms, take 500 milligrams of vitamin C with bioflavonoids or rose hips four to six times a day, says Dr. Meletis. "The bioflavonoids and rose hips strengthen the vitamin C's infection-fighting power by 35 percent," he says.

Vitamin A is known as the anti-infection vitamin. It battles viruses and bacteria in two ways: First, it keeps the cells healthy all along your respiratory tract, providing a barrier that resists microorganisms. If some invading microorganisms manage to breach the barrier, you want to have antibodies and lymphocytes ready to destroy them, and the second way vitamin A helps your body is by providing those reinforcements.

Get your vitamin A from its precursor, beta-carotene, which is brimming with antioxidant power and antiviral properties. It bolsters immunity and protects the thymus gland, the main headquarters where a certain type of white blood cell matures and learns to recognize foreign invaders, says Dr. Meletis.

"Beta-carotene also protects you from viruses by enhancing mucous membrane secretions. By producing the secretions, the beta-carotene prevents the virus from setting up housekeeping in your body," says Thomas Kruzel, ND, a naturopathic doctor in Scottsdale, Arizona.

If you feel a cold or flu coming on, take 100,000 IU of beta-carotene for 10 to 14 days, says Dr. Kruzel, then cut the dosage to 30,000 IU a day to prevent future respiratory infections.

A Zinc Prescription

Of all the trace minerals found in multivitamins, zinc is probably the most important for keeping your immunity strong. It stimulates the immune system by generating new white blood cells and whipping them into shape to battle viruses. If you have too little zinc, your production of white blood cells may drop, and that can increase your risk of catching a cold, flu, or other upper respiratory infection.

In one study, children who got 10 milligrams of zinc daily for 60 days were much less likely to get respiratory infections than children getting less. In fact, the children who got enough zinc were 70 percent less likely to have fevers, 48 percent less likely to have coughs, and 28 percent less likely to have mucus buildup.

While it's best to get zinc from foods, you can get what you need from supplements. Be careful not to take too much, though—more is not necessarily better. In fact, doctors recommend taking no more than 15 milligrams a day. If you check with your physician, you can take 30 milligrams a day with food for 7 to 10 days, but don't take more than that unless you have your doctor's consent.

Also, beware of zinc nasal sprays. There have been reports of an impaired sense of smell as a result of using them, whereas zinc lozenges seem to be safe.

cold sores

A tingling sensation outside your mouth or above your lips is usually the telltale sign. Within 2 to 3 days, a painful, fluid-filled blister appears. It swells, ruptures, and oozes fluid that forms a yellow crust. Eventually, it peels off and reveals new skin underneath. The blister usually lasts 7 to 10 days, but while it's in full view, you may be tempted to go into hiding or cover your mouth with your hands until the unsightly sore disappears.

What causes cold sores, commonly called fever blisters, is herpes simplex virus type 1 (HSV-1). About 90 percent of all people are infected with this virus, and if you get a sore once, you can be pretty sure that you'll get one again. If you change your diet and take some other natural measures against these sores, however, you might be able to shorten the time that they stay on your mouth and lips.

To prevent cold sores, some naturopathic doctors advise that you eat more foods that are high in the amino acid lysine, such as yogurt, chicken, fish, and vegetables. At the same time, they say, you should cut back on foods that are high in arginine, another amino acid. The foods to avoid include chocolate, nuts, seeds, and gelatin.

As for supplements, lysine is near the top of the list. Also, certain vitamins and minerals stimulate your immune system so that your body can fight off the virus more effectively. They can shorten the time it takes for cold sores to heal, inhibit the growth and spread of the virus, and reduce pain and swelling. You should also know about some herbal supplements that are chock-full of antiviral compounds that can destroy the virus. They, too, can help build up your immune system.

Heal Them with Lysine

Lysine is an amino acid that inhibits the replication of herpes simplex. Research suggests that a diet high in lysine and low in arginine can prevent the virus from multiplying. Although it relies on arginine to thrive, the virus can't distinguish between lysine and arginine, so it's easily tricked into attaching itself to the lysine. But unlike arginine, lysine blocks the steps the virus must take to replicate.

To keep lysine levels high, take 500 to 1,500 milligrams daily at the first sign of symptoms, says Jennifer Brett, ND, a naturopathic doctor at the Wilton Naturopathic Center in Stratford, Connecticut. Continue with that dosage until symptoms disappear.

If you're having an outbreak, take 3,000 milligrams of lysine daily until the lesions go away. Applying a lysine ointment to the sore also works and may be easier for you to do. One lysine product called Super Lysine Plus has been scientifically proven to work: It has been found to decrease symptoms and duration of herpes lesions when applied every 2 hours.

Zap 'Em with Vitamin C and Bioflavonoids

Vitamin C with bioflavonoids should be your next line of defense. These supplements will boost your immune system by stimulating production of white blood cells, the infection fighters in your body. The blisters will heal faster as a result, says Dr. Brett.

Bioflavonoids, chemical compounds related to vitamin C, can help reduce the inflammation and pain that's associated with cold sores, says Dr. Brett. You can buy a formula that includes both bioflavonoids and C or take each as a separate supplement.

In one study, 20 people with cold sores took 600 milligrams of vitamin C and 600 milligrams of bioflavonoids three times a day for 3 days. Another 20 took 1,000 milligrams of C and 1,000 milligrams of bioflavonoids five times a day for the same amount of time. Ten participants received look-alike pills that didn't contain either of the active ingredients.

At the end of the study, researchers found that the vitamin C and bioflavonoids stopped the cold sores from blossoming into unsightly blisters. They also concluded that the therapy achieved the best results when people took the supplements at the first sign of symptoms.

This research also showed that taking the two together inhibits the progression of the virus. Those who were treated with 1,000-milligram doses had cold sores for a little more than 4 days. Those treated with placebos had sores for more than twice as long—at least 10 days.

To prevent cold sores, take 1,000 milligrams of vitamin C with bioflavonoids daily, Dr. Brett advises. To speed the healing of existing sores, she recommends taking 3,000 milligrams of vitamin C daily in divided doses and 1,000 milligrams daily of quercetin, a commonly used bioflavonoid.

Zinc 'Em, Too

Upping your intake of zinc can also reduce the frequency, duration, and severity of cold sore outbreaks. This mineral has been shown in test tube studies to block the reproduction of the virus. It produces T lymphocyte cells, which are important body defenses against viral infections.

During a cold sore outbreak, take no more than 40 milligrams a day of zinc in divided doses with food, says Michael Traub, ND, a naturopathic doctor and director of the integrated residency program at North Hawaii Community Hospital in Kamuela. As a preventive, take 20 milligrams a day. Also, since zinc supplementation can lead to copper deficiency, you should take 1 to 2 milligrams of copper for every 20 milligrams of zinc you take, says Dr. Traub. Don't exceed 2 milligrams of copper daily, however.

Applying a cream of zinc sulfate directly to the cold sore also helps, reducing further blistering, soreness, itching, and tingling.

An Antiviral Herb

Medicinal herbs such as echinacea can also speed healing, lessen the severity, and shorten the duration of cold sores, says Dr. Traub.

Echinacea strengthens the immune system. It also increases the levels of a chemical called properdin, which activates the part of the immune system responsible for shoring up defense mechanisms against viruses and bacteria.

Dr. Traub recommends taking one 300-milligram capsule of echinacea four times a day during a cold sore outbreak. For prevention, take one 300-milligram capsule daily during times of stress or as soon as you feel a cold sore coming on, he says.

constipation

Constipation is defined as difficult or infrequent bowel movements.

Difficult? We know what that is. But what does infrequent mean? Surely, each person's routine is different.

Even if the definition isn't crystal clear, most of us know when we're constipated. We might not know what's causing the problem, however.

"A lot of constipation just comes down to diet, water, and exercise," says Melissa Metcalfe, ND, a naturopathic doctor in Los Angeles. See a doctor, though, if you are constipated frequently and every attempt at a bowel movement involves a lot of pain. There may be a blockage, and you may need a doctor's immediate attention to have it removed.

If that's not the problem, and you just have occasional, ordinary, run-of-the-mill constipation, it might be a long-term and fairly constant struggle. There are many possible causes. You may be suffering from stress, dehydration, hemorrhoids, or anal fissures. A colon with weak muscle tone can also cause constipation.

"If there aren't serious underlying causes, the cure is pretty simple," says Dr. Metcalfe. That's where some diet and lifestyle changes, and possibly supplements, can help set things in motion and spare you the strain.

Drink Up

Your first self-treatment is an all-natural combination of two hydrogen molecules and one oxygen molecule joined together in a glass.

That's right—H_2O. Water adds soft bulk to stools. It's also required by the cells of the colon to lubricate the stool's passage, says Dr. Metcalfe.

At the very least, you should drink eight full 8-ounce glasses of water a day, says Dr. Metcalfe. If you're physically active or drink coffee and other caffeinated beverages that make you urinate often, you should drink 12 glasses a day, she says.

"You need to compensate for that dehydration," says Dr. Metcalfe. "I tell patients to put 2 liters of water in the fridge and make sure they're both gone at the end of the day."

She believes that most people probably don't drink enough water because they don't like the taste of water that comes from the tap. In that case, buy bottled water or some type of filtering system, she suggests. "If dehydration is your only problem, you can be having a normal bowel movement in less than 24 hours," Dr. Metcalfe says.

Fill Up with Fiber

Dietary fiber absorbs water and makes stools fuller and easier to pass. The result is faster transit time through the intestines.

Both soluble and insoluble fiber absorb water. Soluble fiber essentially turns into a kind of gel in your intestine. Good food sources include prunes, apples, kidney beans and other legumes, barley, and oats.

For insoluble fiber—the kind that doesn't turn jellylike but helps to "sweep" your system clean—you'll need to turn to different sources. You can get it from bran, wheat, and vegetables like celery, carrots, and spinach. Fiber is so important to digestion and regularity that experts hold to the recommendation that you should get 25 grams a day.

"Fiber works wonders pretty quickly. Within a few days of getting your daily fiber, you'll notice a difference," says Dr. Metcalfe.

Although it's best to get your fiber from food sources, you can also take a supplement when your meals aren't supplying enough. Dr. Metcalfe recommends taking 2 tablespoons daily of a fiber/nutritional supplement that contains psyllium. You can also add 2 tablespoons of ground flaxseed to yogurt or make a "smoothie" with blended yogurt, fruit, and ground flaxseed. "At the same time, though, you should be working to get more fiber in your diet," she says.

Move to Have Movement

If you think sitting on your bottom all day can give you constipation, you're not wrong. To get things moving down below, you have to get off your duff, says Pamela Taylor, ND, a naturopathic doctor in Moline, Illinois.

Two layers of muscles around the small intestine work together in a process called peristalsis, the wavelike contraction that moves digested food and waste products through the gastrointestinal system. People who are sedentary, particularly if they're older, often lack muscle tone in the abdominal area.

"Exercise can tone abdominal muscles, massage the abdominal organs, and increase blood flow to the area. All of that can help restore good bowel function," says Dr. Taylor. Even just sitting in a rocking chair and rocking can help, if that's all you can do.

depression

The ups and downs of everyday life can often leave you feeling blue. When your low spirits turn into a never-ending state of sadness, however, you may have depression. While you may not be able to tell the difference between feeling blue and being depressed, a doctor usually can.

In fact, a diagnosis of depression needs to be made by a doctor. There are many possible signs, ranging from sleeplessness and irritability to feelings of guilt or thoughts of suicide. Whether or not you have these symptoms, though, you should seek professional help if you have a blue mood that lasts more than 2 weeks.

Many doctors prescribe medication for depression, and if you're already taking medication, you shouldn't take supplements without talking to your doctor. Often, dietary and lifestyle changes can help lift your mood, says C. Norman Shealy, MD, PhD, founder of the American Holistic Medical Association and director of the Shealy Institute, a holistic and alternative medicine clinic in Springfield, Missouri. In fact, just 20 minutes of aerobic exercise 5 days a week can put the pep back in your step, says Dr. Shealy.

Studies show that any kind of exercise prompts the release of mood-enhancing brain chemicals called endorphins, which help restore your sense of well-being. Also, if you avoid caffeine, alcohol, sugar, and refined carbohydrates (found in cakes and white bread, for instance), you'll prevent brain chemical imbalances that are known to cause depression.

Some natural antidepressant supplements might also be helpful. Certain vitamins can cheer you up by helping to create and stabilize a variety of brain chemicals responsible for mental and emotional health.

Feel Better with Fish Oil

Getting enough omega-3 fish oil from fatty fish like salmon, mackerel, and sardines, or from supplements, can help lift depression and actually help you to calm down in the face of stress. People with high blood levels of omega-3s are less likely to report feeling depressed than people with low levels, they're less likely to try to commit suicide, and they respond better to antidepressant therapy. The latest research suggests that fish oil promotes structural improvement in areas of the brain related to emotional arousal and regulation. It may stabilize and improve the function of brain cell membranes and improve neurotransmission—signaling between nerve cells. Its anti-inflammatory action may also improve neurotransmitter action.

"You won't see as immediate a result as you will with some other supplements," says Kevin Passero, ND, a naturopathic doctor with a private practice in Annapolis, Maryland. "It can take 8 to 12 months to be really effective. But that doesn't discount how valuable it really is."

Take a supplement that has a good amount of DHA in it compared to other fish oils. (A 2:1 ratio of EPA to DHA is acceptable.) Take 2,000 to 5,000 milligrams a day of combined EPA and DHA for a few months, then try cutting back to about 3,000 milligrams a day. It's safe to take fish oil along with antidepressants. In fact, they can help antidepressants to work better.

Save Yourself with SAMe

SAMe (pronounced *Sammy,* short for S-Adenosylmethionine) is a naturally occurring substance composed of amino acids and found in every cell in your body. It drives a chemical process called methylation, which is vital to the production of serotonin, dopamine, and norepinephrine, all of which are important for regulating mood, sleep, and appetite. SAMe also seems to improve cell membrane fluidity, helping brain cells signal better to one another. Brain imaging studies indicate that SAMe affects the brain similarly to the way conventional antidepressants do. Low levels of SAMe are linked with higher rates of depression. There's a good deal of evidence linking SAMe with better depression results.

It also helps osteoarthritis, fibromyalgia, and chronic back pain, so it's a good choice for people with depression and chronic pain. Dosages range from 400 to 1,600 milligrams a day. It's best to take SAMe as a butanedisulfonate salt in individually blister-wrapped tablets. This is the most bioavailable and stable form.

For SAMe to work, you also need at least 500 micrograms of B_{12} and 400 micrograms of folate. Give it about 2 weeks of use to see a peak effect.

SAMe can be used in conjunction with fish oil and exercise, but it should not be used along with prescription antidepressants unless you have close medical supervision.

Pump Up Some Essential Vitamins

Supplemental vitamin D has been shown to improve mood in people who aren't getting enough in their diets or from sunshine. And, as it turns out, that's a lot of people: More than 50 percent of women and 40 percent of men over age 60 are low in vitamin D.

While sunlight can help, you may need more than the sun can provide. Take at least 800 IU a day in vitamin D supplements. Plus, get your blood level of vitamin D checked. Most practitioners who are knowledgeable about vitamin D like to see levels at or above 50 ng/ml.

People who have depression are often found to be deficient in B-complex vitamins and vitamin C, says Dr. Shealy. The B vitamins help energize brain cells and manufacture important chemicals to keep your moods soaring. Vitamin B_6, for example, plays a starring role in the making of serotonin, a brain chemical that has a direct impact on your emotions, appetite, and sleep patterns. Too little serotonin, and you're feeling down in the dumps.

What's more, B-complex vitamins enhance communication between brain cells so that other important brain chemicals can work together to keep things running smoothly, says Ray Sahelian, MD, a physician in Marina del Rey, California, and author of *The New Memory Boosters: Natural Supplements That Enhance Your Mind, Memory, and Mood.*

Another B vitamin that has been linked to depression is folate, the naturally occurring form of folic acid. In fact, depression is considered the most common symptom of a folate deficiency.

Harvard Medical School researchers reviewed the literature on depression and found that as many as 38 percent of adults diagnosed with depression had low levels of folate in their blood. Other research shows that low vitamin B_{12} levels are common in elderly people with depression and that folic acid and B_{12} work together to boost low spirits, says Dr. Shealy. Vitamin B_{12} also helps metabolize other mood-elevating brain chemicals and keep nerve tissue healthy.

Another vitamin that's just as important in maintaining high spirits is vitamin C. Low levels can leave you feeling gloomy, says Dr. Sahelian. Vitamin C helps manufacture serotonin and two other essential brain-related chemicals, dopamine and norepinephrine, which lift your mood, keep you alert, and sustain your sex drive.

For mild to moderate depression, you may want to take a high-potency multivitamin/mineral supplement daily after talking to your doctor, says Dr. Shealy. He also suggests 100 milligrams each of thiamin, riboflavin, niacin, and B$_6$, along with 400 micrograms of folic acid, 100 micrograms of B$_{12}$, and 2,000 milligrams of vitamin C in divided doses daily.

Help from St. John

St. John's wort does help mild to moderate depression. In fact, it is one of the most researched natural antidepressants around. The herb's active ingredients include hypericin, flavonoids, and other compounds that work in unison to raise serotonin levels in the brain, says Jennifer Brett, ND, a naturopathic doctor at the Wilton Naturopathic Center in Stratford, Connecticut.

While it's not understood exactly how the herb increases serotonin levels, researchers speculate that the underlying mechanism is probably similar to that of prescription antidepressants, says Dr. Brett. St. John's wort may inhibit an enzyme that breaks down serotonin molecules and other brain chemicals, or it may increase the action of serotonin at the nerve endings in the brain. The serotonin is available so that your brain can further utilize it to regulate your moods and emotions more effectively, she says.

Unfortunately, St. John's wort does have some side effects. It can cause photosensitivity, which means you may sunburn easily. It also interacts with quite a number of drugs, so before you take it, you should check with your doctor to see how it might affect any drugs you are taking. Don't take it if you're pregnant, and don't take it if you are already taking antidepressant medication.

If your doctor approves of you taking St. John's wort, Dr. Shealy suggests taking one 300-milligram tablet or capsule three times a day with meals if you have mild to moderate depression. For maximum effectiveness, buy a standardized extract containing 0.3 percent hypericin, he says. If you don't feel better after 4 to 6 weeks, it's unlikely to help, he adds.

Some Good from Ginkgo

Ginkgo helps improve blood flow to the brain, and therefore improves mental alertness and memory, and—as a by-product—relieves depression, says Dr. Sahelian. "Poor blood circulation to the brain can cause the brain to malfunction, which can lead to imbalances in serotonin levels and other neurotransmitters that regulate moods and emotional stability." It can be especially helpful for older people who have a combination of depression and cognitive decline.

If you're over age 50 and have mild to moderate depression, take one 40-milligram capsule of ginkgo three times a day, says Dr. Shealy. Choose capsules or tablets that contain 24 percent ginkgoflavonglycosides for maximum strength.

Brain Chemicals in a Pill

Another natural supplement that might have the edge over antidepressant prescription drugs is 5-HTP. This is a natural compound produced by the body from tryptophan, an amino acid found in many foods. It's also a precursor of serotonin, which means that more serotonin is produced when 5-HTP is present.

When you take 5-HTP in supplement form, it's absorbed in your gastrointestinal tract and then journeys to your brain, where it's converted into serotonin, says Dr. Sahelian.

If you've been diagnosed with depression and you have a doctor's approval, you can take 50 milligrams of 5-HTP late in the evening, says Dr. Sahelian. But he doesn't advise taking larger amounts. Any dosage over 50 milligrams can cause vivid dreams, nightmares, and nausea.

dermatitis

Dermatitis is a general term for an inflammation of the skin. The symptoms are usually itching, crustiness, blistering, and a watery discharge from pustules. In other words, just about any annoyance on the surface of your skin—ranging from the mildly itchy to the downright distressing—is dermatitis. One of the most common forms is eczema, an itchy kind of skin rash.

As for the causes, they're numerous. In some people, stress alone can lead to dermatitis. Others have allergic reactions to any number of things, from poison ivy and poison oak to certain metals. In other cases, a general infection or even a food allergy displays itself through dermatitis as well as other symptoms.

If you get standard medical treatment, your doctor might prescribe creams, lotions, or ointments that contain cortisone, or you might buy an over-the-counter hydrocortisone cream that helps soothe itching or quell the inflammation. There are natural alternatives, however.

Get Enough Vitamin D

People with atopic dermatitis, the most common form of eczema, sometimes have a defect of the immune system that interferes with the skin's ability to produce a biochemical called cathelicidin, which helps protect against microbial invasion. Researchers from the University of California, San Diego, found that giving people with moderate to severe atopic dermatitis 4,000 IU a day of vitamin D_3 boosted cathelicidin levels. Other studies have found that it can reduce symptoms of dermatitis and provide some relief for people with psoriasis. "We test just about everyone for nutritional deficiencies, and vitamin D is one of the most common," says Michael Gazsi, ND, a naturopathic doctor in private practice in Danbury, Connecticut. Ideally, you want to take a dose that maintains your blood level of vitamin D at 50 ng/ml or higher, he says. You can start at 1,000 to 2,000 IU a day and then adjust as needed.

Probiotics to the Rescue

If your symptoms seem to be associated with food allergies or irritable bowel syndrome, try taking a probiotic—friendly bacteria found in yogurt and supplements, Dr. Gazsi says. Probiotics such as *Lactobacillus* and *Bifidobacterium* seem to decrease markers of hypersensitivity reactions, including those on your skin, he says.

Combination products that contain three or more types of probiotics, those found in the refrigerated section of a health food store, and those guaranteeing 8 to 10 billion CFU (colony-forming units) are your best bets. Two good brands are Culturelle, which is available over the counter, and VSL#3, which is available by prescription.

Interrupt Inflammation

New research shows that getting plenty of DHA, a component of fish oil, can reduce the symptoms of eczema. The study used 5.4 grams a day—an amount you could only get by taking supplements. It reduced symptoms of itching and blistering by about 25 percent after 8 weeks of use.

Fish oil helps by reducing the body's production of pro-inflammatory biochemicals, Dr. Gazsi says. Flaxseed oil can also be helpful. "I tell people to try taking 1 to 3 grams of fish oil and 1 to 2 tablespoons of ground flaxseed oil every day," he says. It can take a few months, but your skin should look and feel healthier.

Combine Vitamin A and Zinc

People who have chronic skin problems may be deficient in vitamin A or zinc, says Dr. Gazsi, and some people lack both. These deficiencies show up in people with liver disease, vegetarians who don't eat healthy meat substitutes like beans or wheat germ, and people who are eating nutritionally poor diets or following faddish weight-loss diets. Alcoholism can also cause these deficiencies.

You need vitamin A for your body to properly regenerate outer layers of skin. If this critical vitamin is absent, your skin may develop a sandpaperlike texture. Zinc, too, is necessary for the skin to produce new cells and maintain new layers of skin.

"Vitamin A and zinc really work together, which is why I usually recommend them in combination," says Dr. Gazsi.

You can begin by taking a multivitamin/mineral supplement that contains the recommended daily amounts of vitamin A and zinc. Frequently, though, those amounts aren't enough if there are some problems with a person's vitamin absorption or diet, says Dr. Gazsi. Your doctor can perform a test to determine whether you have absorption problems.

"If you're looking to clear up dermatitis, I'd recommend 10 to 12 milligrams of zinc and 5,000 IU of vitamin A," he says.

Attack the Rash Topically

Since dermatitis involves the skin, topical treatments are helpful in combating itching and any resulting rash, says Kathy Foulser, ND, a naturopathic doctor at the Ridgefield Center for Integrative Medicine in Connecticut.

If your dermatitis is caused by an allergic reaction—to a poison plant, for example—you can get some relief by taking an oatmeal bath. Simply pour a cup of regular or colloidal oatmeal (such as Aveeno) into lukewarm water and soak for 15 minutes, recommends Dr. Foulser.

Aloe is another topical standby. Studies show that aloe extract cream can improve symptoms of psoriasis, decreasing skin flaking, redness, and spread of the condition. At most health food stores, you can buy aloe in gel, cream, and liquid forms. Just rub the aloe onto the itchy, damaged skin, says Dr. Foulser.

"Aloe makes a really nice, gooey mix that sits on the skin," she says. "It's really soothing for most skin problems."

diabetes

If there's one good thing that can be said about type 2 (non-insulin-dependent) diabetes, it's that this disorder usually responds very nicely to diet and lifestyle changes. And while many people with diabetes or who are at risk for diabetes (more on that in a minute) are turning to some form of alternative medicine, there's no substitute for the fundamental lifestyle changes you need to make to help control this condition.

That said, surveys show that about 60 percent of people with diabetes use some form of nontraditional medicine. There are more than 170 different natural medicines that can be used to treat diabetes, and hundreds more dietary supplement products marketed to people with diabetes. No matter what you use, you should not stop using your conventional treatment, and you should never add any natural supplement without checking with your doctor. Otherwise, it could lead to problems such as low blood sugar, says Marianna Abrams, MD, ND, medical director of Water's Edge Natural Health Center in Seattle, Washington.

Dr. Abrams specializes in diabetes (about 80 percent of her patients have either diabetes or prediabetes) and has found some common alternative treatments that work for everyone who wants to control or avoid this disease, she says. Here is what she recommends.

Focus on Fiber

Dr. Abrams has her patients slowly but surely increase their fiber intake, mostly by eating fiber-containing foods, such as root vegetables and beans, but also by taking 2 tablespoons of ground flaxseed a day, one in the morning and one later in the day. You can add flaxseed to yogurt, smoothies, cereal, and salads. "Increased fiber intake is an important way to help regulate blood sugar levels," she says. "It can also help people feel fuller so they eat less." You should aim for a total of at least 25 grams a day.

Get More Fish Oil

Fish oil is also at the top of the must-take list. The fatty acids in fish oil may help to improve insulin sensitivity over time. Plus, Dr. Abrams says, "background inflammation is what is damaging to the body in diabetes. Fish oil, having anti-inflammatory properties, is very helpful." Add fatty fish like salmon, sardines, and mackerel to your diet, or take fish oil supplements. A standard dose is 1 to 3 grams a day.

Chromium Helps Insulin Work Better

Chromium deficiency is associated with impaired glucose tolerance, high blood sugar, sugar in your urine, a decrease in the number of insulin receptors, poor insulin binding, and neuropathies. Studies of people with diabetes have shown that supplementing the diet with chromium can lower fasting blood sugar levels, improve glucose tolerance, and reduce insulin levels. It helps insulin bind to glucose so that glucose can enter a cell. For people with high sugar and high insulin levels, it's worth trying. "Chromium is our big helper. We use it a lot to help our patients," Dr. Abrams says.

How much each person needs varies. Some research suggests taking up to 1,000 micrograms a day in divided doses. Less than 200 micrograms a day doesn't seem to be enough; however, taking more than 400 micrograms a day should only be done with close medical supervision, experts say. That's because a dosage that high could cause low blood sugar or interact with other medications you are taking. If you supplement, keep it between 200 and 400 micrograms a day and make sure your supplement contains chromium picolinate. (And again, work with your doctor.) You should see an improvement in blood sugar levels after about 3 months, if not sooner.

Mind Your Magnesium

Magnesium is another nutrient deficiency linked to symptoms of diabetes. It's involved in several important aspects of carbohydrate metabolism and plays a central role in energy production. People with diabetes tend to have low levels of magnesium, and there's some evidence that getting enough may help prevent complications such as eye, heart, and kidney damage.

In addition to eating more magnesium-rich foods such as beans, whole grains, leafy greens, tofu, nuts, and seeds, shoot to get 300 to 500 milligrams a day of supplemental magnesium glycinate.

Why You Need the Bs

The B vitamins are essential for your body to convert sugar and starches to energy, a chemical process called carbohydrate metabolism. A shortage of any one of them can cause problems such as glucose intolerance—a high rise in blood sugar after eating. Shortages can also lead to nerve damage, including diabetic neuropathy and memory loss. And guess what? People with diabetes tend to come up short in these vital nutrients. If you think you need more Bs, take them as a B-complex supplement. Look for one that includes 50 milligrams of most of the B vitamins and 500 to 1,000 micrograms of B_{12}. You may also want to ask your doctor to check your B_{12} levels, since neuropathy can also signal B_{12} deficiency.

Do the "D"

One study found that more than 91 percent of people with diabetes were low in vitamin D. This vitamin has long been suspected of being a factor in glucose intolerance. Research shows that getting adequate amounts of vitamin D seems to help prevent diabetes complications. So if you think you're running a bit low on this vital nutrient, ask your doctor to test your vitamin D levels, then work with him or her to set a dosage of vitamin D that maintains your blood level at about 50 ng/ml. In general, you should be getting at least 800 IU of vitamin D a day from food or a multivitamin.

Antioxidants Provide All-Around Aid

Antioxidants don't prevent or cure diabetes, but they can help protect you from some of the debilitating side effects, such as blindness, kidney disease, and nerve damage due to high sugar levels.

Both vitamins C and E, for instance, help prevent a process called glycosylation, a reaction between sugar and protein that alters the protein's structure so it can't be used, says John Cunningham, PhD, professor of nutrition at the University of Massachusetts in Amherst. Glycosylated proteins are thought to contribute to many of the long-term complications of diabetes.

Vitamin E improves insulin action, as well. "Because vitamin E helps to protect cell membranes, some speculate that it might help insulin receptor sites on the surfaces of cells to remain functional," Dr. Cunningham says. Vitamin C protects cells by preventing sugar from being converted to sorbitol, an alcohol that cells can neither expel nor burn for energy. "Sorbitol buildup has been implicated in diabetes-related eye, nerve, and kidney damage," Dr. Cunningham says.

Studies have shown benefits from 100 to 1,000 IU a day of vitamin E and 100 to 1,000 milligrams a day of vitamin C, Dr. Cunningham says.

In addition to these, Dr. Abrams uses some less common antioxidants that zero in on diabetes problems. "We use acetyl-L-carnitine and N-acetylcysteine a lot because they both are helpful in improving energy metabolism." Both work inside the cell's tiny energy plants, called mitochondria. And she also uses alpha lipoic acid to treat diabetic neuropathy. She usually recommends 600 to 1,200 milligrams of alpha lipoic acid a day in divided doses; 600 to 1,200 milligrams of n-acetylcysteine a day in divided doses; and 1,000 to 1,500 milligrams of acetyl-L-carnitine a day in divided doses.

Head-to-Toe Help from Ginkgo

Another botanical Dr. Abrams frequently uses is ginkgo. It's especially helpful for treating the poor circulation people with diabetes experience, which, if left unchecked, can lead to amputation. Ginkgo also acts as a powerful antioxidant and enhances use of oxygen and blood sugar. Look for a standardized extract that contains 24 percent ginkgoflavonglycosides. She recommends taking 40 milligrams three times a day.

diarrhea

For most people, diarrhea is not a serious problem but rather an awkward issue for a day or two. Usually, it goes away on its own, unless it is a symptom of a more serious problem such as food poisoning, Crohn's disease, ulcerative colitis, or an adverse drug reaction.

If you try some remedies and use the supplements that doctors recommend, they should start to work in 24 to 48 hours. However, if your diarrhea lasts for more than 3 to 4 days, if there is blood in your stool, or if you feel dehydrated and very weak, see a doctor.

One thing you have to be concerned about is the loss of fluids. You may not feel like drinking when your stomach is doing somersaults, but it's necessary. You should always try to sip water to avoid dehydration, says Kristin Stiles, ND, a naturopathic doctor at the Complementary Medicine and Healing Arts Center in Vestal, New York.

Whenever you lose fluids and don't replace them, you also lose calcium and electrolytes, including sodium, magnesium, and potassium. These minerals regulate many of the body's essential processes, such as blood pressure, heart rate, and muscle movements.

If an infant or elderly adult has diarrhea that lasts for more than 12 to 24 hours, the nutrient loss can be severe, so they should get medical attention as soon as possible. In an otherwise healthy adult, the most important task is to make up for lost fluids and electrolytes.

Sports drinks may be intended for athletes, but they're perfect for anyone with diarrhea, too. These drinks contain a hearty dose of electrolytes—sodium and potassium along with simple sugar. Sip at least 4 ounces every hour for as long as the diarrhea lasts, says Dr. Stiles.

Help Out with Herbals

If your diarrhea is due to bacteria or some type of food poisoning, goldenseal and garlic can help your body do away with the bad bugs. Both have antibacterial properties. Take 100 to 250 milligrams of goldenseal or 200 to 400 milligrams of garlic three times a day until your diarrhea subsides, recommends Dr. Stiles.

When your digestive system is trying to get rid of the contents of your stomach and intestines, there's a lot of inner activity called peristaltic movement, which sometimes causes cramping. Plus, you may get gas because the material in your intestines is starting to ferment, says Pam Taylor, ND, a naturopathic doctor in Moline, Illinois. To help alleviate spasms in the gastrointestinal tract, Dr. Taylor recommends taking a capsule or two of ginger, or a dosage of 200 to 400 milligrams.

Ginger helps prevent stomach spasms and stimulates the release of gastric juices, pancreatic juices, and the enzymes that enhance digestion. "Ginger normalizes peristaltic movements and has pain-relieving properties, and it's a good tonic for the stomach," Dr. Taylor says.

Another herb that's good for relieving intestinal spasms is valerian. "Most people think of valerian only as a sleep tonic, but it also relieves stomach cramping and reduces the formation of gas," says Dr. Stiles. She recommends taking a 100- to 300-milligram capsule of valerian twice a day.

Glutamine for GI Health

With severe diarrhea or a bout that lasts a few days, the intestines may remain inflamed, says Dr. Stiles.

Try glutamine, an amino acid supplement frequently used by naturopathic doctors for gastrointestinal diseases, she says. Glutamine encourages the quick turnover or production of cells along the walls of the stomach and the small intestine, she says. It makes the body heal a bit faster.

"While you're healing, I would recommend 500 milligrams of glutamine three times a day," suggests Dr. Stiles. Continue this dosage for about 2 weeks or until you have no more discomfort, she adds.

With these remedies, you can expect diarrhea to clear up within 24 to 72 hours.

diverticulitis

It's a series of intestinal developments just waiting for trouble to happen.

Maybe you've been straining a lot during bowel movements, or maybe the walls of your colon have weakened a bit. Either way, little pouches and sacs called diverticula have formed in the lining of your colon.

In these little dead-end streets, bits of bacteria-laden waste may become trapped. When those troublemakers are not completely cleared out, they ferment, decay, and inflame tissues—and you have diverticulitis, inflamed pockets in your lower colon.

People who develop diverticulitis often have had previous symptoms of constipation and difficult bowel movements with hard stools, according to Kristin Stiles, ND, a naturopathic doctor at the Complementary Medicine and Healing Arts Center in Vestal, New York.

The problem announces itself with a wide range of symptoms. Among the signs are alternating diarrhea and constipation, gas, bloating, and chronic cramping and pain in the intestines. Since these mimic many of the symptoms of irritable bowel syndrome (IBS), it takes some medical sleuthing to determine what you have. Your doctor will make the initial diagnosis through information that you give her and through a colon examination. Left untreated, diverticulitis can lead to perforation of the bowel, or even deadly peritonitis—infection of the abdominal cavity.

Once you know you have diverticulitis, your doctor can talk to you about changes to your diet that can help prevent future attacks. Here's what experts recommend.

Prevent It with Fiber

"When I see this problem, it's usually because the person is eating a high-fat, high-sugar, low-fiber diet—basically a junk diet," says Dr. Stiles. "I immediately get him onto a high-fiber diet."

You should consume between 25 and 30 grams of soluble and insoluble fiber each day, advises Dr. Stiles, and she advocates getting most of that through diet. Fiber is found in fruits and vegetables, legumes, and grains like whole wheat, oats, and rye. If you're not getting the recommended amount of fiber from food, Dr. Stiles recommends taking 2 tablespoons daily of a fiber supplement that contains psyllium.

The standard advice used to be to avoid nuts and seeds, as well as foods containing them (like strawberries, cucumbers, and tomatoes) because it was thought that the seeds could get stuck in your colon. But there is no scientific evidence to support that advice, says Michael Picco, MD, a gastroenterologist at the Mayo Clinic in Rochester, Minnesota. Current advice is to avoid these foods only if you find that they aggravate your condition.

Since fiber absorbs large amounts of water, make sure that you drink plenty, whether you're increasing your food fiber or taking supplemental fiber. Dr. Stiles suggests that you drink eight to 10 glasses (8 ounces each) of water daily. The water adds bulk to the stool and helps soften it for easier transit through the colon.

Healing Your Irritation

When you're in the throes of diverticulitis, your immediate problems are inflammation, infection, and irritation of the colon. Several herbs, called demulcents, have the ability to soothe and coat mucous membranes. By direct contact, they help heal irritated and inflamed tissues, says Pamela Taylor, ND, a naturopathic doctor in Moline, Illinois. These herbs form a coating that bathes the walls of the large intestine and helps heal the lining.

Some health food stores carry a naturopathic herbal combination known as Robert's Formula that is very good for gastrointestinal irritation, she says. The combination includes herbs such as slippery elm, marshmallow root, and geranium. It may also contain echinacea and goldenseal, two botanical ingredients that help boost your immune system.

Robert's Formula is produced by a number of different companies with varying combinations of ingredients. It is generally available in capsules or as a tincture. If you choose to try it, simply follow the directions on the label, recommends Dr. Taylor. A usual dose is two "00" capsules three times a day. Capsules are best taken with food so the herbs will be carried to the large intestine.

A Soothing Spice for a Grumpy Gut

If you need an excuse to go out and eat some hot Indian food tonight, here's one: It's good for you.

Turmeric, the main ingredient in curry powder, is a powerful anti-inflammatory that can help reduce the puffiness and soreness of irritated tissue. It's also an antioxidant, so it helps defuse the free-roaming, unstable molecules called free radicals that can seriously damage your cells. Plus, it's a digestive aid. For all of these reasons, naturopathic doctors sometimes recommend it as a way to help prevent a flare-up of diverticulitis.

Turmeric was used as a healing herb in China. In the tradition of Ayurvedic medicine practiced by doctors in India, it has been used as a medicine for thousands of years. Today, Indian doctors use it for many inflammatory conditions, from rheumatoid arthritis to sprains. They sometimes even make poultices of turmeric that are applied directly to sore muscles and painful joints.

Ayurvedic practitioners believe that the herb has a number of benefits for the gastrointestinal system. In animal studies, it has been shown to reduce the amount of gas that's produced in the intestine and increase the secretion of gastric juices. It protects the stomach, possibly helping to prevent ulcers. Given in combination with other herbs, it has also been used to help treat liver disorders.

Although turmeric has several active ingredients, curcumin seems to be the most important for medicinal purposes. In fact, because it comes in a highly concentrated form, curcumin alone can be more effective than turmeric. It is available in capsules at health food stores. Follow the directions on the label.

You can also take some of the herbs separately. Slippery elm alone is a powerful demulcent. It's usually available in 100-milligram capsules. Take three a day, recommends Melissa Metcalfe, ND, a naturopathic doctor in Los Angeles.

Turmeric also works well as an anti-inflammatory, she says; try taking a 200- to 400-milligram capsule twice a day.

You can continue to take any of these supplements for as long as you have problems with diverticulitis, Dr. Metcalfe says.

Preventing Infection

Infection is always a concern with diverticulitis. If it is not controlled, doctors sometimes recommend surgery to remove affected portions of the intestine. If you suspect an infection—symptoms include abdominal tenderness, pain, and fever—see your doctor as soon as possible. Drugs can help knock it out fast. Then, to help prevent a recurrence of infection, you can try natural medicines.

You can help your body stave off any infection in the colon by taking a combination of echinacea and goldenseal, says Dr. Stiles. Both herbs have anti-inflammatory and antibacterial properties. Goldenseal is also astringent to the mucous membranes in the intestine, says Dr. Stiles, which means it helps to tighten the tissues, which can help provide some relief.

"You don't want to take either of these herbs for too long, however. I'd recommend 2 weeks on and 2 weeks off," says Dr. Stiles. "You can quickly build up a tolerance to echinacea, so it becomes less effective."

A typical dose is one 200- to 250-milligram capsule of echinacea and one 50- to 60-milligram capsule of goldenseal three or four times a day, she suggests. Health food stores and some drugstores also carry combination capsules. Alternatively, you can take 10 to 15 drops of an extract of each herb in water or juice three or four times a day, with or without food.

Vitamins for Healing

To heal the damaged mucous membranes, Dr. Taylor sometimes recommends that her patients take vitamins A, E, and C, and a chelated form of zinc. Many companies market these nutrients in a single supplement, says Dr. Taylor. She uses the following daily amounts, based on a body weight of 150 pounds: 5,000 to 10,000 international units (IU) of vitamin A, 200 to 500 milligrams of vitamin C, 100 to 400 IU of vitamin E, and 15 to 30 milligrams of chelated zinc. You'll need to check with a naturopathic doctor to determine the dosages appropriate for your weight and follow his advice on when to take the supplements.

As you recover from diverticulitis, the inflammation will heal, but you still need to pay attention to the factors that may have contributed to the problem in the first place. Be sure to maintain a high-fiber diet, exercise regularly, and drink adequate amounts of water, says Dr. Stiles.

"If you keep things moving and improve the muscle tone of the bowel, the pouches won't be such a problem," she says.

emphysema

Somewhere in your grade-school education, you probably yawned your way through a science class in which your teacher compared your lungs to inflatable party balloons. Like balloons, our lungs hold air and are very elastic, expanding and contracting easily. But what would happen if you let the air out of a balloon and it didn't deflate? As weird as it sounds, that's basically what happens when you have emphysema or, as it's also called, chronic obstructive pulmonary disease (COPD.)

This smoking-related disease causes your lungs to lose the resilience they need to fully collapse every time you exhale. Since you're not pushing out all of the "waste" of breathing—the carbon dioxide—that toxic gas begins to build up in your semideflated lungs. Breathing becomes difficult and not very efficient. You may have a constant sensation of breathlessness. Often, you have a cough along with the other symptoms.

If you're a smoker with emphysema, the doctor will certainly tell you to stop smoking. She'll also urge you to stay away from environmental air pollution.

Currently, there's no cure for emphysema, but people in advanced stages of the disease who need to use supplemental oxygen may find that nutritional supplements will protect their lungs from further damage.

Emphysema can be prevented, however. The most obvious step, if you're still smoking, is to quit. There is no substitute for that good bit of advice. And if you stop, good nutrition can help your body recover more fully.

Use Antioxidant Synergy

For severe emphysema, some people take supplemental oxygen to help them breathe more easily. There's something you should know about O_2, however: While it's true that humans can't live without it, oxygen in its purest form isn't purely beneficial.

"Oxygen itself is what we call an oxidizing agent," explains James Scala, PhD, a nutritionist in Lafayette, California, and author of *Prescription for Longevity*. Oxidation is what happens to bananas when they brown, iron fences when they rust, and people when they age. The process involves unstable molecules called free radicals that circulate in the body. In order to regain its electrical balance, a free radical must swipe an electron from another molecule, and this starts a chain reaction of cellular damage.

Some free radicals are produced in our bodies when we're breathing in normal amounts of oxygen, but many more of these troublesome molecules are generated by outside forces like the sun's rays, alcohol, cigarette smoke, and other forms of air pollution. Supplemental oxygen also generates an oversupply, according to Dr. Scala.

Antioxidant supplements can help prevent emphysema from worsening. Plus, says Dr. Scala, if your lungs are already in the pink, antioxidants can help keep them that way.

Recent research shows that people with emphysema tend to eat a diet that's low in several vital nutrients, including antioxidant vitamins C, E, A, and D, as well as selenium. Another study found that getting adequate vitamin D doesn't prevent COPD, but it does appear to help people with lung disease to breathe easier and more deeply. The study showed that people who had never smoked but who were getting little vitamin D had 35 percent worse lung function than did former smokers who were getting adequate amounts of the vitamin. That makes a big difference when it comes to daily activities like walking up stairs, carrying groceries, or even carrying on a conversation.

Vitamins C and E have long been considered important for lung health, but these other nutrients are vital as well, says Dr. Scala. Getting your five-a-day-plus of fruits and vegetables is the place to start, but if you're like many people with COPD, even eating and chewing can take your breath away. For that reason, he also recommends supplements. A good multivitamin/mineral supplement plus extra vitamin D may be all you need. Look for one that contains 200 to 800 IU of vitamin E, ideally as mixed tocopherols; 500 milligrams of vitamin C; 200 to 400 micrograms of selenium, ideally as selenomethionine, an organic, bioavailable form; up to 3,000 IU of preformed vitamin A (retinyl palmitate or acetate); and 1,000 to 2,000 IU of vitamin D. Ask your doctor to check your blood levels of vitamin D, and then adjust your intake to an amount that maintains your blood levels in the range of 35 to 50 ng/mL.

One antioxidant you won't want to take if you continue smoking—or even if you are a former smoker—is supplemental beta-carotene. Research suggests that it can increase the risk of lung cancer and death in smokers and ex-smokers. It's fine, though, to get beta-carotene from foods such as carrots, mangoes, peaches, sweet potatoes, orange winter squash, and dark leafy greens.

endometriosis

For some reason, in women with endometriosis, the tissue that normally lines a woman's uterus begins to migrate and grow in other areas within the abdomen while still behaving like uterine tissue. That means that other internal organs may have an island of tissue that swells and sheds blood every month. Since that foreign tissue is not supposed to be there and your organs don't know how to handle its strange behavior, you may begin to feel a lot of pain.

This is what doctors call endometriosis. It affects an estimated 10 to 15 percent of all premenopausal women.

Hormone therapies and surgery are the favored treatments in conventional medicine. If you have endometriosis, you should work with a doctor to help manage the condition. There aren't any known cures. There are, however, a number of ways to help relieve the pain and influence the hormonal balance that plays an important part in the condition, according to naturopathic doctors.

Getting your diet in order can be a big step. First, cut down on foods that might be increasing your estrogen levels, says Barbara Silbert, DC, ND, a chiropractor and naturopathic doctor in Newburyport, Massachusetts, and president of the Massachusetts Society of Naturopathic Physicians. Commercially raised animals are often given hormones for more robust growth and milk production, so if you eat meat or dairy products, you might be absorbing extra estrogen. Another possible concern with meat is that foods that are high in saturated fat have a tendency to make estrogen more available to the body.

Phase out meat and dairy products in favor of soy foods (tofu, tempeh, miso, and soy milk) and fiber-rich foods, says Dr. Silbert. Soy contains phytoestrogens, compounds that help regulate estrogen levels. Fiber makes stools firm and easy to pass, which is especially important if endometrial tissue is encroaching on the bowel area.

She also recommends regular exercise—at least 30 minutes three times a week—to help relieve the pain and cramping associated with endometriosis. With exercise, you step up production of endorphins, your body's natural pain blockers. Losing excess weight also helps, since the more fat you have on your body, the more estrogen you produce.

Then there are supplements. "Because endometriosis is a complex thing to deal with," says Dr. Silbert, "I always use a combination of herbs, vitamins, and minerals." It may take a few months for supplements to work, but there are many to try. She cautions, however, that you need to get a proper diagnosis and then work with your doctor to see if supplements are right for you.

Some supplements can lower estrogen levels by helping you excrete it. Others can help your liver and kidneys flush out as much as possible, which may help you control endometriosis. Still others can help relieve the pain. Here's what experts recommend.

Three Estrogen Reducers

"In order to get endometriosis under control, you have to reduce the amount of estrogen in your body," says Jennifer Brett, ND, a naturopathic doctor at the Wilton Naturopathic Center in Stratford, Connecticut. The herbs red clover and black cohosh, as well as genistein, a supplement derived from soybeans, can help your body excrete estrogen.

These three supplements are phytoestrogens, or plant forms of estrogen. They bind with estrogen receptor sites, which are like dedicated landing sites on your cells. These sites would normally be occupied by your body's much stronger estrogen, but when plant estrogens start to hog the sites, your estrogen has no place to go and ends up being excreted, says Dr. Brett. "That's exactly what you want to happen with endometriosis."

If you reduce the amount of estrogen circulating in your body, you'll probably also reduce the pain of endometriosis, says Dr. Brett.

When taking red clover or black cohosh, follow the directions on the package. A typical black cohosh dose is one 540-milligram capsule three times a day. Black cohosh is particularly effective at relieving cramps, notes Dr. Brett.

You can get genistein by taking a supplement of mixed soy isoflavones according to the directions on the label. A typical dose is one 540-milligram capsule a day.

Use the Cabbage Cure

Eating more of the cruciferous vegetables—like cabbage, cauliflower, brussels sprouts, watercress, mustard, and kale, among others—can help reduce estrogen levels in your body. That's because these vegetables contain a compound, indole-3-carbinol (I3C), that changes a stronger estrogen in your body (estradiol) into a weaker one (estrone). A "dose" of I3C is 200 to 300 milligrams a day, but many experts recommend that you simply add these foods to your diet and enjoy all of their benefits: fiber, folate, vitamin C, *and* I3C. Aim for at least one serving a day.

Feel Better with Fish Oil and Flaxseed

Several studies have found that fish oil can be beneficial for women with endometriosis. Because it has anti-inflammatory properties, it can relieve pain by reducing levels of an inflammatory biochemical, prostaglandin E2. Other research suggests that it can even slow the growth of endometrial tissue. A usual dose is 1 to 3 grams of fish oil a day, or two to three servings a week of fatty fish such as salmon, mackerel, or sardines.

Flaxseed contains alpha-linolenic acid, an omega-3 fatty acid that can also help reduce inflammation. It's not as strong as fish oil, but flaxseed has another good thing going for it when it comes to endometriosis: lignans. These are phytoestrogens that, like soy and clover, can block stronger forms of estrogen in your body and reduce endometrial growth. Use 1 or 2 tablespoons a day of freshly ground flaxseed. Or, if you choose to use flaxseed oil, make sure it is "high lignan." It's fine to take a combination of fish oil and flaxseed.

Flush Out Toxins

The other strategy to take with endometriosis is to get your body working to flush out as much estrogen as it can, says Dr. Brett. In the case of endometriosis, estrogen could be considered a toxin. Your body has too much of it and it's causing harm.

Your liver and kidneys are your body's main toxin filters. Enzymes in your liver help to break down toxins, including excess estrogen. Your kidneys then excrete them.

You can help your liver do its job better with certain nutrients, Dr. Silbert says. Make sure you get enough magnesium, which is about 400 milligrams a day. One of magnesium's many jobs is to transmit fluids to and from cells, your bloodstream, your lymphatic system, and your tissues, so it helps move toxins out of your body.

Vitamin B_6 and milk thistle (silymarin) both help the liver break down and dispose of excess estrogen. Try taking 50 milligrams a day of the active form of B_6, pyridoxal-5-phosphate (P5P).

For milk thistle, follow the dosage directions on the package. Typically, that means taking one or two 150-milligram capsules three times daily. N-acetylcysteine is also good for detoxifying because it helps your liver make one of its main detoxifying enzymes, glutathione. Doses range from 400 to 1,200 milligrams a day. Look in health food stores for a product labeled "lipotropic factors" with these ingredients, Dr. Silbert recommends. See your doctor for guidance if you're unsure of what or how much to take. Some detoxifying nutrients can also reduce the effectiveness of drugs you may be taking.

Finally, to make sure that your kidneys are doing their share of the work, drink plenty of water—at least eight full 8-ounce glasses every day, advises Dr. Brett.

fibromyalgia

Fibromyalgia isn't a disease. It is considered a "syndrome," a group of symptoms that include tender muscle points on the body, widespread pain, and a variety of other problems such as "fibro fog," sleep disturbances, morning stiffness, sensitivity to light and noise, headaches, and irritable bowel problems, among others.

Fibromyalgia is similar to chronic fatigue syndrome in many ways, says Jacob Teitelbaum, MD, author of *From Fatigued to Fantastic* and director of the Fibromyalgia and Fatigue Centers, a national group of clinics. "Both represent an energy crisis in the body, where basically you have blown a fuse," he says. "You are expending more energy than you are able to make, just like in your home. If you plug in too many blow dryers or space heaters, you blow a fuse and the same thing is happening here." With chronic fatigue, the main symptom of the energy crisis is, you guessed it, fatigue. With fibromyalgia, the main symptom is tight, knotted muscles.

In fact, there is a good reason for the tight muscles, Dr. Teitelbaum says. "It actually takes more energy to relax a muscle than it does to contract it," he says. Muscles contract and stay that way, and being contracted deprives them of adequate oxygen and nutrients. The pain makes people unable to sleep and unwilling to exercise. Other things going on in the body, such as hormonal imbalances, feed the problem.

There are lots of theories as to why this energy crisis occurs, but the bottom line is that you need to address the symptoms with lifestyle changes, including diet and exercise, and with supplements that increase your energy. What works for one person may not work for someone else, but there are often some common factors, Dr. Teitelbaum says. (Also see Chronic Fatigue Syndrome, page 366.)

Although fibromyalgia is often associated with fatigue that makes exercise difficult, regular exercise has been shown to be one of the most beneficial treatments, decreasing pain and tender points and improving

405

sleep and mood. "But many patients have a hard time maintaining an exercise program, and other things often need to be addressed before exercise becomes an option," says Hope Fay, ND, a naturopathic doctor on Whidbey Island, Washington.

Improve Your Sleep

Just as with chronic fatigue, sleep is a problem with fibromyalgia. Sleep apnea, where you stop breathing briefly while you sleep, is common, and it's wise to ask your doctor to check for that. Being treated for sleep apnea seems to help relieve fibromyalgia pain. (For other sleep recommendations, please see Chronic Fatigue Syndrome, page 366.)

Get Enough Vitamin D

Researchers have known for a long time that vitamin D deficiency can cause all sorts of bone and muscle pain. But they didn't connect the dots between those symptoms and fibromyalgia until recently, as vitamin D deficiency has become more recognized as a widely prevalent problem. Doctors now recognize that even a mild deficiency may cause such problems as muscle weakness, fibromyalgia, impaired balance, and depression.

The connection is rooted in vitamin D's metabolic function. Scientists believe it may begin with lower levels of circulating calcium due to inadequate vitamin D. A cascade of biochemical reactions then occurs that hinders bone metabolism and health. Low levels of calcium elevate parathyroid hormones, and that elevation impairs proper bone mineralization. That causes a spongy matrix to form under periosteal membranes covering the skeleton. This gelatin-like matrix can absorb fluid, expand, and cause outward pressure on periosteal tissues, which generates pain because these tissues are highly innervated with sensory pain fibers, reports study author W. Michael Hooten, MD, medical director and anesthesiologist at the Mayo Clinic Comprehensive Pain Rehabilitation Center in Rochester, Minnesota.

Up to 90 percent of people may be vitamin D–deficient. To find out if you are one of them, ask your doctor to test your blood, recommends John Cannell, MD, executive director of the Vitamin D Council. He suggests that people supplement with vitamin D before getting their blood tested, then

Treat the Whole Person

As with chronic fatigue, people with fibromyalgia often have underlying problems that are contributing to their energy deficit, experts say. This can include bacterial or yeast overgrowth in the intestines, food sensitivities, chronic infections, stress, and hormonal imbalances—and the list goes on and on. See a doctor who can address these issues. For a doctor who specializes in the treatment of fibromyalgia, see www.fibroandfatigue.com or holisticboard.org.

adjust their dose so their vitamin D level is between 50 and 80 ng/ml during both the summer and the winter. Dr. Teitelbaum recommends that everyone with fibromyalgia take 2,000 IU a day of vitamin D_3, the active form.

Use Magnesium to Relax Muscles

Magnesium is needed for your body to make energy, and many people don't get enough, says Michael Gazsi, ND, a naturopathic doctor in private practice in Danbury, Connecticut. He recommends about 300 milligrams a day of magnesium glycinate, an easily absorbed form. That usually relaxes the muscles, allows blood to flow into the constricted areas, and flushes out the waste products of inflammation.

Put Fat on the Fire

Reducing any kind of inflammation usually brings about some improvement in fibromyalgia symptoms, says Dr. Gazsi. "In fibromyalgia, there is clearly inflammation in the muscles and probably in the intestinal tract, as well." One good way to do this is to reduce your consumption of pro-inflammatory fats, such as saturated fats and trans fats, by cutting back on fatty meat and processed foods and increasing your intake of anti-inflammatory fats, such as fatty fish like salmon, mackerel, and sardines. You can also take fish oil supplements. How much you take may depend on your symptoms, but aim for 1 to 2 grams a day of EPA and DHA (the fatty acids in fish oil), combined. If you are a vegetarian, you can take 1 to 2 tablespoons a day of ground flaxseed.

Get Some Rub-On Relief

Although it's not a long-term treatment, lots of people can get some pain relief using topical treatments. "I especially like using castor oil," Dr. Fay says. People also relieve aching muscles with an Epsom salts bath. "This is a magnesium salt, and people really do absorb some through their skin and relax their muscles," she says. Add 2 cups to a tub of warm water.

Some research also finds that the same capsaicin (hot red pepper) cream used for joint pain can provide some relief when rubbed into knotty muscles.

fingernail problems

Take a look at your hands—specifically, your fingernails. What do you think they say about your health?

A lot, actually. Fingernails that crack or break, or are heavily ridged, "spooned," or too soft can be a sign of a health problem, says Michael Gazsi, ND, a naturopathic doctor in private practice in Danbury, Connecticut. Dr. Gazsi always looks first for a thyroid problem. In fact, low levels of thyroid hormones can cause fingernails to start to separate from the nail bed. Ouch!

Next he looks for a nutritional deficiency. Too little protein or low intake of minerals such as calcium, zinc, or iron can impair nail strength. And some B vitamins, like biotin, play a role in nail strength, too.

Make Yours a Multi

When it comes to healthier nails, your first action should be to take a high-potency multivitamin/mineral supplement, says Dr. Gazsi. That should cover your bases for most nutrients, but you may need to take extra of some, such as calcium, vitamin D, and the Bs. You need about 1,000 to 1,200 milligrams a day of calcium and at least 1,000 to 2,000 IU a day of vitamin D.

Reach for Bs

In a few cases, fingernail problems may be related to a B-vitamin deficiency. Dr. Gazsi recommends taking a B-complex or B-50 supplement—one in the morning and one in the evening. Make sure it contains enough biotin. Supplementation with this B vitamin has been a long-standing practice for hoof problems in horses and pigs, and research shows that taking 2.5 milligrams a day for 6 months can reduce splitting and increase nail thickness by about 25 percent. Supplements sold as "hair and nail" formulas are most likely to have this amount. You can be low in biotin if you take anticonvulsants, are pregnant, have diabetes, or are on long-term antibiotic therapy.

Pack In More Protein

Nails are made of protein, so if you're not getting enough of this building block, you may see it in your nails. Most people in the United States get more than enough protein. But those who might not include vegans (strict vegetarians) and dieters who aren't paying enough attention to this important nutrient. A minimum amount of protein is 0.8 grams per kilogram of body weight. One kilogram equals 2.2 pounds, so a 130-pound woman should be getting at least 48 grams of protein a day. You can get 7 grams in just one egg; 1 ounce of fish, chicken, beef, pork, or cheese; 4 ounces of tofu; or 1 tablespoon of peanut butter. One cup of milk has 8 grams of protein. Get enough servings to get the protein you need.

Fatty Acids Are Essential

Fats and oils do the same thing for your nails that they do for your hair and skin: They help nails retain moisture so they are less brittle and resist damage from detergents.

We get most of the fats we need from a regular diet, but we often come up short on one type of essential fatty acids: omega-3s, found in fish oil and converted in small amounts from some plant oils such as alpha-linoleic acid, found in flaxseed. The best way to get these fats? Eat fatty fish such as salmon, mackerel, or sardines two or three times a week, or take 1 to 2 grams a day of fish oil. As an alternative, you can take 1 to 2 tablespoons a day of ground flaxseed, Dr. Gazsi says. "Don't expect anything to happen overnight, though," he says. "It might take several months."

gallstones

Whenever you eat a high-fat meal, your body has to secrete bile to help you digest the fat. Bile is manufactured in the liver and stored in the gallbladder. From there, it's dumped into the small intestine, where it goes to work helping to break down the fat that comes from foods like steak, ice cream, and potato chips.

As you might conclude from this scenario, if you're regularly eating high-fat items, your gallbladder is working overtime.

Just because it takes a lot of gall to break down fat doesn't necessarily mean that you're going to have a lot of gallstones. Gallstones form from excess cholesterol, the same notorious fat that has a reputation for clogging arteries, and some people are just more prone to them than others. Doctors have found that women are more likely to get gallstones than men, particularly if they're pregnant. Both sexes are at higher risk if they're overweight. So you have yet another reason to try to keep off the pounds or lose them for good.

If you've had gallstones, you're definitely at risk of getting them again, so it makes sense to take preventive steps. When gallstones are inside the gallbladder, they sometimes cause intestinal discomfort or nausea, but only a doctor, with the help of x-rays, can tell you whether those symptoms are being caused by stones.

Once the stones start to move into the bile ducts—the exit ramps from the gallbladder and the liver—pain is not far behind. This movement can be dangerous, too, because blocked ducts can cause jaundice or serious infection. If this happens, you need immediate medical help. You might need to have the gallstones dissolved or have the stones or your gallbladder surgically removed.

But if you've had mild symptoms or have already had gallstones removed, here is what you can do to keep the condition from progressing or prevent a recurrence.

Fill Up with Fiber, Not Fat

"I believe that your first defense against gallstones is to change what you're eating," says Kristin Stiles, ND, a naturopathic doctor at the Complementary Medicine and Healing Arts Center in Vestal, New York. "You have to cut back on the fat and get more fiber in your diet."

Getting more fiber into your diet is a simple way to decrease excess fat. Dietary fiber binds with bile salts (which are a primary part of bile) and cholesterol in your intestines and prevents both from being absorbed by your body. You can up your fiber intake by eating as many fruits and vegetables as possible, along with brans and whole grains like wheat, oats, and rye, says Dr. Stiles.

Fiber absorbs large amounts of water, and water-soaked fiber bulks up and softens the stool. A well-hydrated stool absorbs lots of waste and by-products of digestion, such as fat. With less fat around, the process of gallstone formation may be interrupted.

The recommended daily amount of fiber is 25 to 30 grams, says Dr. Stiles. If you find that you can't eat enough high-fiber foods to achieve that level, an alternative is to try one of the soluble fiber supplements found in drugstores and health food stores. Dr. Stiles recommends a supplement that contains psyllium. She suggests stirring 2 tablespoons of the supplement into a glass of water and drinking it at breakfast each day.

Turning to Lecithin

According to naturopathic doctors, one nutritional substance that might help prevent gallstones is lecithin. Also called phosphatidylcholine, lecithin is a major ingredient in cell membranes. It's found in animal tissues, especially the nerves, liver, and semen.

Lecithin is important because it helps water and fat mix together more easily. Usually, fat stays separate from water, but lecithin is an emulsifier, a kind of go-between that reconciles these opposites and allows the two substances to combine.

In the body, lecithin can help make cholesterol (a fat) mix with water. Because lecithin is such a good emulsifier, naturopaths believe that cholesterol is transported more easily when there's plenty of lecithin around.

Indeed, some naturopathic doctors say that low levels of lecithin in the body have been linked to the formation of gallstones. If you supplement with lecithin, gallstones are less likely to occur. You can also get lecithin from foods such as soybeans, wheat germ, and peanuts.

Lecithin can't dissolve stones that are already in your gallbladder, says Dr. Stiles, but it might help prevent new ones. The typical dose of lecithin is 500 to 1,000 milligrams a day, she says. You should supplement for several months while simultaneously working to improve your diet.

Making Bile Flow

If you can just "keep the juices flowing," you may help prevent gallstone problems, herbalists believe. You can get some aid from herbs that have what are called choleretic properties, meaning the ability to increase the amount of bile the liver produces and also boost the flow of bile from the gallbladder. At the same time, herbalists believe that herbs with choleretic properties stimulate gallbladder contraction.

Milk thistle is one herb with these properties. "It gets things moving and helps flush out the small stones," says Dr. Stiles. It is also believed to help improve the digestion of fats, she adds.

Although some supplement formulas are made up of a number of choleretic herbs, William Warnock, ND, a naturopathic doctor in Shelburne, Vermont, favors milk thistle taken by itself. "What usually happens when you put a lot of herbs into one capsule is that you don't end up with high concentrations of any of them," he says.

For the most effective concentration, you need a standardized extract of milk thistle that contains 80 percent silymarin, the herb's primary active ingredient, says Dr. Warnock. The typical dose is 70 to 210 milligrams three times a day. A naturopathic doctor can recommend a specific amount.

"It may take 3 to 6 months before it has a beneficial effect," says Dr. Warnock. You should never take it during a gallstone attack, however. If you already have gallstones that begin to cause persistent pain or a fever, you should see a doctor immediately, not wait months to find out whether the herb is effective.

Eat to the Beet

"I've had people get really effective relief from gallbladder pain with beet greens," says Dr. Warnock. When steamed, beet greens are unusually high in minerals, vitamin A, and a substance called betaine. According to Dr. Warnock, betaine stimulates the production of bile and simultaneously thins it out. Also, betaine causes the muscles surrounding the gallbladder and bile ducts to contract and move things along.

genital herpes

Genital herpes is more common than you might think. At least 45 million Americans have it—twice as many women as men—and there has been an increase among older women who have it. (Women can get genital herpes and some other sexually transmitted infections more easily than men do.)

Most of the time this herpes simplex virus lies dormant in your body. But sometimes you get a flare-up, very often when your defenses are down—during times of stress or illness, for example.

Fortunately, you can keep this annoying virus in check by making a few significant adjustments to your lifestyle and diet. Daily exercise such as brisk walking, cycling, jogging, and stretching can melt away stress and fatigue, two of the most common triggers of recurrent outbreaks, says Susan Kowalsky, ND, a naturopathic doctor in Norwich, Vermont.

Moreover, doctors say that if you eat more foods high in the amino acid lysine, such as chicken, fish, and vegetables, you can help keep the virus at arm's length. They also say you should try to avoid fare such as chocolate, nuts, seeds, and gelatin—foods that are high in another amino acid, arginine.

In addition, a variety of nutritional supplements, topical and oral, can give you extra protection. Certain herbs, vitamins, and minerals can all reduce the number of recurrent infections, shorten the duration of the episodes, and speed the healing of lesions.

The Bee's Remedy

Honeybees produce a dark, sticky, resinous substance called propolis to seal small cracks in their hives and keep out microbes. Propolis has been analyzed and found to be a strong antibacterial, antiviral, antifungal agent. Research has found that a 3 percent propolis ointment can significantly improve healing of recurrent genital lesions caused by herpes simplex 2. In fact, it may help heal sores faster and more completely than the acyclovir ointment that's usually prescribed. Follow directions on the product. It's available as a tincture and as ointments. (Beehive Botanicals specializes in propolis products.)

Line Up Lysine

Lysine is an amino acid that, in large amounts, can inhibit herpes simplex replication. Research supports increasing lysine and reducing arginine (an amino acid needed for viral replication) as a way to fight herpes infections. Foods that are high in lysine but low in arginine are mangoes, apricots, pears, apples, figs, papayas, beets, milk and dairy products (including ice cream, cheese, and yogurt), eggs, avocadoes, and tomatoes.

But applying lysine topically is easier to do and may be just as effective. The one lysine product that's scientifically proven to work is Super Lysine Plus, a product containing lysine and zinc oxide, plus 14 other ingredients. It has been found to decrease the symptoms and duration of herpes lesions when applied every 2 hours.

Zap It with Zinc

Zinc cream—yes, the same stuff lifeguards slather all over their noses—has its own antiviral activity. It, too, has been found to reduce symptoms such as blistering, soreness, itching, and tingling. It can also reduce the duration of sores by about a day and a half if it's started as soon as you notice the symptoms of an outbreak. Zinc oxide is available over the counter as a cream.

Lay On the Lemon Balm

Applying an ointment containing 1 percent lemon balm extract has been found to shorten healing time, prevent the spread of infection, and reduce symptoms of recurring genital herpes. Lemon balm contains a number of active ingredients with antiviral and antioxidant effects. To get a good product, look for one that is verified for potency by the US Pharmacopeia (USP).

Add Echinacea

Some lemon balm ointments also contain echinacea, a potent antiviral and antibacterial herb that activates the parts of your immune system that destroy viruses and raise levels of interferon, a biochemical that blocks the replication of herpes virus proteins. You can also take 500 milligrams of a tincture of echinacea twice a day at the first sign of symptoms to help prevent an outbreak or to speed the healing of lesions if you're already having a recurrence, says Thomas Kruzel, ND, a naturopathic doctor in Scottsdale, Arizona. Echinacea is best used for 2 to 3 weeks at a time, at most. It tends to lose effectiveness if used continually.

Boost Immunity with Vitamin C

Since herpes tends to resurface whenever your immunity is low, a vitamin that supports your immune system is a real ally in your battle with herpes. Vitamin C is such a vitamin. It can recharge your immune system by strengthening white blood cells that will fight off the virus. Vitamin C can also help speed healing—and the faster you heal, the less pain and discomfort you'll experience from the lesions. According to Dr. Kowalsky, this vitamin can also prevent damage to healthy cells and boost interferon levels.

"It's known that viruses deplete vitamin C residing in white blood cells, so we know that if you want your immune system to stay strong, you need to take extra vitamin C," says Dr. Kowalsky. To prevent herpes outbreaks, she recommends taking 1,000 to 3,000 milligrams daily in divided doses.

If you're having an outbreak, Dr. Kowalsky recommends you take even more: 3,000 to 12,000 milligrams of vitamin C. Along with that, she recommends taking 1,000 to 3,000 milligrams of citrus bioflavonoids, compounds that may help fight inflammation, halt viruses, and control the oxidation process that can lead to premature aging of cells. Citrus bioflavonoids boost the absorption of vitamin C and shorten the duration of herpes outbreaks, according to Dr. Kowalsky.

A Trio of Infection-Fighting Nutrients

Vitamin A, beta-carotene, and vitamin E all qualify as strong contenders in the fight against recurrent herpes infections.

Vitamin A arms your immune system with the ammunition it needs to battle the virus. It can alleviate symptoms of an impending outbreak and reduce the number of recurrences. Since doses of vitamin A above 10,000 international units (IU) are not usually recommended, a safer alternative is to take beta-carotene, according to Dr. Kowalsky. Beta-carotene is the antioxidant that increases antibody production and white blood cell activity, and it converts to vitamin A in the body.

"Beta-carotene encourages new cell growth and strengthens your cells' outer layers so that the virus can't penetrate, duplicate itself, and spread like wildfire," says Dr. Kruzel.

When you feel the symptoms of a possible outbreak coming on, take 100,000 IU of beta-carotene daily in divided doses to jump-start your immune system, says Dr. Kowalsky. Although you should also check with your doctor before taking this high daily dose, beta-carotene doesn't pose the same risks as vitamin A.

Vitamin E also protects your white blood cells from invading viruses and strengthens other aspects of your immune system. It can help speed the healing of herpes lesions as well, says Dr. Kowalsky. She recommends taking 400 IU a day during an outbreak and continuing with it, as that's a safe daily dose.

gingivitis

Gingivitis, or gum disease, isn't just about bad breath or losing teeth, although both of those things are bad enough. As gum disease progresses, the underlying inflammation and infection can affect other organs in your body, especially your heart and pancreas. It's been linked to an increased risk of heart attack and stroke, as well as pancreatic cancer.

In the early stages, gingivitis is reversible as long as you conscientiously clean your teeth at home and visit your dentist a couple of times a year for professional cleanings. Untreated, gingivitis can lead to periodontitis, an advanced stage of gum disease that causes receding gums, pockets forming between the teeth and gums, infection, loss of bone, and, finally, tooth loss.

Your best weapons against gum disease are a soft-bristle toothbrush, fluoride toothpaste, and dental floss. To prevent plaque buildup, brush your teeth after every meal, making sure you focus on the gum line, and floss at least once a day. Combine that with regular visits to your dentist, and you should be fine, says Meena Shah, DDS, a dentist in Lake Grove, New York.

If you're already practicing good dental hygiene but your gums are still a little inflamed and bleed periodically, visit your dentist. Meanwhile, you can make some dietary choices that can reduce the progression of gingivitis.

To start with, eat lots of high-fiber foods and less sugar-laden fare, says Dr. Shah. Dietary fiber acts as a cleaning agent for your teeth. Raw veggies are especially cleansing. Sugary foods like cookies, cake, and candy, and sticky foods like raisins and other dried fruit, including fruit "roll-ups," increase plaque buildup on your teeth and breed bacteria, she says.

Supplements can help control gingivitis, too. Taking extra vitamin C, folic acid, and other nutrients can rev up your immune system to battle the infection, reduce inflammation, and stop the bleeding. Certain medicinal herbs, such as echinacea, can also boost immunity as well as heal and strengthen damaged gum tissue. Here's how the supplement lineup can help keep your gums and teeth in tip-top shape.

Combine Vitamin C with Bioflavonoids

One important nutrient that can help heal red, swollen gums is vitamin C. This antioxidant boosts your immune system, brings down inflammation, and speeds up wound healing. In fact, a deficiency of vitamin C can lead to gingivitis, which may cause teeth to become loose and even fall out.

Vitamin C has proven to be vital for the production of collagen, the basic protein building block for the fibrous framework of all tissues, including gums. The vitamin strengthens gum tissue and helps the gum lining resist bacteria.

Vitamin C can repair and rebuild connective tissue. "Moreover, it will boost your immune system so that you can fight off the infection," says Liz Collins, ND, a naturopathic doctor and co-owner of the Natural Childbirth and Family Clinic in Portland, Oregon.

Dr. Collins recommends taking 3,000 to 4,000 milligrams of vitamin C daily in divided doses. As part of your daily vitamin C regimen, Dr. Collins also recommends taking bioflavonoids. Naturopathic doctors believe that these nutrients are very effective at reducing inflammation and repairing and healing gum tissue. They're strong antioxidants that can prevent damage from free radicals, the free-roaming, unstable molecules that harm cells. Bioflavonoids are also known to boost the effectiveness of vitamin C.

"You should always take bioflavonoids with vitamin C," says Dr. Collins. You can buy a vitamin C and bioflavonoid combination formula or take the bioflavonoids separately.

Two of the most effective bioflavonoids are quercetin and grape seed extract. Take 1,000 to 2,000 milligrams of quercetin or 100 to 200 milligrams of grape seed extract daily, says Jennifer Brett, ND, a naturopathic doctor at the Wilton Naturopathic Center in Stratford, Connecticut.

Get Optimal Vitamin D

Vitamin D has been found to have anti-inflammatory effects and may reduce susceptibility to gum disease. Researchers at Boston University evaluated the association between vitamin D levels and gingivitis. They analyzed data from 77,503 teeth in 6,700 people in the third National Health and Nutrition Examination Survey and found that people with higher blood levels of vitamin D were less likely to experience bleeding gums during gingival probing.

Many people don't get enough vitamin D. Take a multi with extra vitamin D, or take a supplement with up to 800 IU. If your gum disease persists, ask your doctor to test your blood levels. Experts recommend that you take enough to keep your vitamin D blood levels in the healthy range of 50 to 80 ng/ml.

Treat With Tea Tree

Tea tree oil has proven antibiotic properties. In one study, people with severe chronic gingivitis who brushed with a tea tree oil gel had a significant reduction in inflammation and bleeding. Use only commercial tea tree toothpaste, not tea tree oil, which is too concentrated to put directly in your mouth. Brush twice daily with it until your symptoms are under control, then alternate its use with an antiplaque toothpaste.

Swish and Swallow Cranberry Juice

Research shows that cranberry juice may help gum disease by preventing bacteria from sticking to teeth. Look at your local health food store for cranberry juice with no added sugar in it. (You can add a little stevia extract for sweetness.) Simply swish 4 ounces or so around in your mouth like mouthwash, then swallow it.

Coenzyme Q_{10} for Healthy Gums

Coenzyme Q_{10}, or CoQ_{10}, is a vitamin-like compound found in human tissue that stimulates the immune system. It's chemically similar to vitamin E and is a powerful antioxidant that helps treat gingivitis and maintain healthy gums and other tissues by increasing the flow of oxygen to cells. Food sources include salmon, sardines, beef, peanuts, and spinach. In Japan, CoQ_{10} is widely used to treat gum disease.

When researchers reviewed seven studies that used CoQ_{10}, they found that 70 percent of the 332 people with periodontal disease who took supplements of the substance showed signs of improvement. In one of these studies, the group taking CoQ_{10} showed a reduction in inflammation, receding gums, and tooth mobility.

Dr. Brett recommends taking 150 to 200 milligrams daily if your gums are inflamed and bleeding. As soon as the bleeding stops and the inflammation goes down, you can stop taking it.

Herbal Remedies Fight Infection

Medicinal herbs like echinacea can help battle a gingivitis infection, says Ellen Evert Hopman, a professional member of the American Herbalists Guild, a lay homeopath in Amherst, Massachusetts, and author of *Tree Medicine, Tree Magic*. She recommends taking this herb in capsule form.

Dosages vary, so follow the directions on the label. If the echinacea supplement is 380 milligrams, a typical dose would be one to three capsules three times daily with water at mealtimes.

Echinacea stimulates the immune system by galvanizing white blood cell production, Hopman says. It increases levels of a chemical in the body called properdin, which activates the part of the immune system responsible for shoring up defense mechanisms against bacteria and viruses.

gout

If you have gout, you don't just have a red, swollen, throbbing toe or other joint. Gout means that your body has a buildup of uric acid, a toxic waste product that should be excreted by your kidneys. You may be having a kidney problem, have become dehydrated, or have a genetic tendency to develop gout, in which case you can curse your ancestors.

With gout, needle-sharp uric acid crystals form in the fluid surrounding a joint, says Luc Maes, DC, ND, a chiropractor and naturopathic doctor in Santa Barbara, California. Over time, gout can damage joints and other parts of the body. High blood levels of uric acid can lead to high blood pressure and an increased risk for heart disease. "That pain in the joint is the end result of a long breakdown process," Dr. Maes says. It means that your body is not detoxifying itself properly. Purine-rich foods just make matters worse. Purines are chemicals found in foods such as alcohol, seafood, and organ meats. Normally, they don't do any damage, but if you're prone to gout, these foods can cause crystal formation. You may love these things, but if you have gout, they've gotta go. It helps to drink as much water as possible to help your kidneys flush purines and uric acid from your system. Make a conscious effort to drink at least eight glasses of water a day, and even more if you sweat a lot. And avoid too much caffeine. Having three or more caffeinated drinks a day increases your risk for recurrent gout attacks by up to 80 percent. Another step: Reduce your intake of sugared drinks. A high intake of sugar-added foods elevates uric acid levels. Aspirin can also raise uric acid levels, so don't use it to relieve gout pain.

Along with those measures, nutritional and herbal supplements are good allies, say alternative medicine experts. Many can help improve the kidneys, the liver, and the blood, according to Dr. Maes. Others can help fight inflammation. But he emphasizes that supplements can't make amends for a gout-promoting diet. "If you eat a poor diet for a long time, your body gets too much of certain nutrients and not enough of others," he says.

Get Enough Vitamin C

Men who get more than 500 milligrams a day of vitamin C from foods and supplements have serum uric acid levels that are 0.5 to 0.6 mg/dL lower than men who consume less than 90 milligrams daily. They also have about one-third less risk of developing gout. Fill up on citrus fruits and other high-C foods, and then take a supplement containing up to 500 milligrams of vitamin C.

Fight the Flame with EPA

When you eat saturated fats—the kind that come from meat and dairy foods—you're inviting the overproduction of inflammatory chemicals. "Gout is a state of inflammation," says Dr. Maes. "Things are on fire."

Studies have shown that you can help reverse this pattern and correct the nutritional imbalance by taking fish oil or flaxseed oil. Fish-oil supplements are particularly rich in an omega-3 fatty acid called eicosapentaenoic acid (EPA), which discourages inflammation, says Priscilla Evans, ND, a naturopathic doctor in private practice in Cary, North Carolina. EPA is only available from fish.

EPA reroutes the chemicals in your body early in the inflammation process so your body produces fewer pro-inflammatory biochemicals. But supplements can't do the whole job, Dr. Evans emphasizes. "It's very important to cut back on oils and saturated fats that promote inflammation. Just adding fish oil is not enough if you're still eating a lot of red meat and fat."

Dr. Maes advises people with gout to take 1,500 milligrams of fish oil a day, but not all at once. Divide the doses and take the supplements with meals.

You should also take 400 IU of vitamin E a day with the fish oil, she says. It works along with the EPA to act as an anti-inflammatory and also serves as an antioxidant.

If you're a vegetarian or don't like fish, you may be able to get similar benefits by taking 1 to 2 tablespoons of flaxseed oil every day, says Dr. Maes. This oil contains alpha-linolenic acid, however, not the more valuable EPA, and only a portion of it is converted to EPA by the body.

The Bromelain Benefit

The enzyme bromelain, derived from a favorite tropical fruit—the pineapple—is one of nature's anti-inflammatory medicines. "Bromelain helps to break down proteins in the body that are causing inflammation," Dr. Evans says. Take 300 milligrams three times a day, between meals. Although an attack of gout can last as long as a few weeks, you should only take this high dose of bromelain for 4 or 5 days. After that, take 125 to 250 milligrams three times a day until the gout subsides, advises Dr. Evans.

Boon from Berries

Help in another form comes from bioflavonoid molecules, which are found in cherries, blueberries, and other fruits. In the 1950s, researchers discovered that cherries could decrease uric acid levels and prevent a gout attack. You'd have to eat a lot of cherries—a half-pound a day—or the equivalent amount of unsweetened juice to make a dent in gout. Blueberries work, as well.

For the same results, you can take a bioflavonoid supplement or 2,000 milligrams of berry extract a day, says Dr. Maes. The best are those that have a combination of all the bioflavonoids or the extracts of several different berries, he says.

Bioflavonoids affect other body processes as well as uric acid production. Researchers have found that they help in tissue building and can prevent the release of some compounds that promote inflammation.

hair loss

If you're looking for a cure for male pattern baldness, you won't find it here. Hair loss is a trait inherited through the maternal side of the family.

If your mom's dad or her brothers are bald, the cards are stacked against you. Unless you're willing to spend hundreds of dollars a year on hair-raising new drugs that may or may not produce results, you'll just have to resign yourself to a future of diminishing strands.

Not all hair loss is inevitable, however, nor is the decline entirely controlled by genes. Stress; hormone changes; extreme weight loss; and vitamin, mineral, or protein deficiencies can lead to fast fallout. Moreover, you're likely to lose hair faster if your hair follicles become inflamed or if you get skin disorders that affect your scalp.

Even women aren't immune to some of the fallout from these problems. "I've had women patients who have lost all their hair due to major stresses in their lives," says Hope Fay, ND, a naturopathic doctor in Seattle. "When you're under stress from illness or work, sometimes the circulation in the scalp is so constricted that the hair follicles lose blood supply, which causes them to die and fall out." Dr. Fay is quick to add, however, that if women lose their hair, it often grows right back in when they're no longer under extreme stress.

To help the hair return when the loss isn't a matter of inherited baldness, you can try a number of tactics. The solution usually lies with improving your diet and making lifestyle changes to relieve stress, says Dr. Fay. In addition, you can supplement your diet with nutrients that aid in hair growth, she says.

Take a Good Multivitamin/Mineral Supplement

When a vitamin or mineral deficiency is at the root of your hair loss, you simply need to correct the deficiency. Maybe it's the result of improper digestion, or perhaps you're not absorbing the necessary vitamins and minerals as well as you need to, notes Elizabeth Wotton, ND, a naturopathic doctor at Compass Family Health Center in Plymouth, Massachusetts.

Iron, selenium, and zinc deficiencies generally lead to hair loss, researchers have observed. These minerals aid in immune function and in the utilization of protein that your body needs to help produce hair. They are also involved in the production of thyroid hormones, and if those hormones aren't being pumped out properly, you can lose your hair. Low levels of some of the B vitamins, especially B_{12} and biotin, can also contribute to thinning hair.

A good multivitamin/mineral supplement should provide all you need of these nutrients, and more. If hair loss is accompanied by extreme fatigue, see your doctor. If you're seriously deficient in iron or B_{12} (both also vital for energy), you may need prescription-strength dosages of these nutrients to restore proper blood levels.

Regulate Your Hormones

In the first few months after their children are born, some women are distressed to find that their hair begins to fall out. The problem is usually due to hormonal changes. The body's hormone ratios are radically revised during pregnancy. After delivery, the body has to establish a new balance.

Hormone upsets aren't limited to new mothers, however. Stress, menopause, and illness can also bring on changes.

To ease hormonal transitions, Dr. Wotton suggests giving your body the nutritional building blocks it needs to manufacture and regulate hormones. You can begin by eating more foods containing phytoestrogens, plant compounds that mimic the biological activities of female hormones. These foods include soybeans, such as edamame, and soy products, such as tofu.

In addition, you might consider supplementing with essential fatty acids from flaxseed, says Dr. Fay. These kinds of fats form the biological backbone of many hormone molecules. The oils are rich sources of omega-3 and omega-6 fatty acids—good fats that are important for healthy skin and hair. To get the most phytoestrogen effect out of flaxseed, use 1 or 2 tablespoons of ground seeds or use a "high-lignan" flaxseed oil for salad dressings.

headache

If you are prone to headaches, chances are you were born with a slightly different brain chemistry than people who get don't get them. (Sorry about that.) Your brain may have a hard time regulating levels of the neurotransmitter serotonin, which is a messenger that helps regulate the diameter of blood vessels.

Medical researchers now believe that in the majority of headaches, certain factors trigger fluctuations in serotonin levels. Once the serotonin is out of balance, the blood vessels in your brain become inflamed and you end up with a head that's throbbing with pain.

More than 90 percent of all headaches are classified as tension headaches, which occur when the muscles in the back of your neck and scalp tighten. When you have a tension headache, you'll probably feel a generalized dull head pain. That's a signal that the nerves running through the muscles have become inflamed and irritated.

Migraines are another animal entirely. The pulsating throb of a migraine headache is less common but more likely to send you to the doctor in search of relief. You may also experience other symptoms such as an aura, sensitivity to light, and nausea in addition to your head feeling like it's about to explode. Migraines occur more often in women than in men and can last from a few minutes to a few days.

A third type, the cluster headache, is even more acute but also much more rare. A cluster headache is one-sided head pain that may involve tearing of the eyes and a stuffy nose. Attacks occur regularly for 1 week to 1 year, separated by long pain-free periods that last at least 1 month, possibly longer.

Whichever type of headache you're prone to, chances are that the underlying cause is your genetic makeup. "We are clearly dealing with a biological disorder, not a psychological one," says Fred Sheftell, MD, a psychiatrist, headache specialist, and cofounder of the New England Center for Headache in Stamford, Connecticut.

Pay Attention to Triggers

Just because you were born with a predisposition for headaches doesn't mean that you have to get them, according to Dr. Sheftell. If you can avoid the pain triggers, you might be able to avoid the headaches.

Heading up Dr. Sheftell's Top 10 List of triggers are sensitivities to foods such as chocolate, certain food components such as alcohol and caffeine, and the food additive MSG. Other possible triggers are hormone fluctuations during the menstrual cycle, changes in the weather or season, sleeping late or not enough, bright lights, and odors. Last but certainly not least is that old bugbear, stress.

Traditional over-the-counter medications may get rid of the pain once it hits, but they won't help you have fewer headaches. In fact, many chronic headache problems are really "rebound" headaches that happen after you go off pain medications.

But with nutritional measures, you can take a preventive approach, says Dr. Sheftell. Which supplement you try will depend on which type of headaches you get and what's causing them. Each supplement acts in a different way. You can take headache-reducing supplements in combination without any problems, but your best approach, says Dr. Sheftell, is to try one or two at a time until you find the custom formula that works for you.

Try Riboflavin for Migraines

Riboflavin is a B vitamin. In superhigh doses, it can help ward off a migraine attack by helping the brain cells utilize energy, says Dr. Sheftell.

In a Belgian study of 49 people who frequently got migraines, researchers got good results with daily doses of 400 milligrams of riboflavin. At that dose, about half of the people in the study became migraine free. Among the others, the intensity of pain was reduced by about 70 percent.

How does riboflavin work? Researchers have found that some people who get migraines may not have enough energy stored in their brain cells. Riboflavin helps the enzymes in the body tap into the energy stored in those cells.

Researchers speculate that flooding the system with riboflavin stirs up more energy in the cells. Helping to regenerate the lethargic cellular energy system defuses the migraine, says Seymour Solomon, MD, professor of

A Mineral for Facial Pain

It's not hard to recognize a headache when it's happening, but what if you're having pain in your face rather than your head?

Frequently, the source of facial pain—sometimes called trifacial neuralgia—is the trigeminal nerve. Known as the great sensory nerve of the head, it comes out of the cranium right above the jaw. The extensions of that nerve form a web across much of your face. If you have inflammation or infection or if the nerve is injured, you might feel the pain signals all around your face.

Many people have this kind of facial pain as the result of temporomandibular disorder (TMD), a problem with the temporomandibular joint in the jaw. If your jaw doesn't line up correctly, it may grind or click whenever you're chewing and talking. TMD can lead to muscle spasms, pain, and eventually inflammation, which in turn leads to more pain, says Anne McClenon, ND, a naturopathic doctor at the Compass Family Health Center in Plymouth, Massachusetts.

If you have facial pain caused by TMD, try some kind of physical bodywork, suggests Dr. McClenon. Chiropractic, craniosacral therapy, or massage therapy can relax the muscles and allow the joint to line up properly. If this doesn't help, you may need to see a dentist who specializes in TMD, she says.

For TMD, Dr. McClenon also recommends magnesium, which is an effective headache cure. Magnesium is the critical mineral in getting muscles to relax. Take 300 to 350 milligrams a day, suggests Dr. McClenon. "Usually, people take it in the evening so that muscle relaxation hits about bedtime," she says. "That way, they can get a good night's sleep."

neurology at the Albert Einstein College of Medicine of Yeshiva University in the Bronx.

Riboflavin is found in milk. Four glasses will give you the Daily Value of 1.7 milligrams. The doses needed to help prevent migraine are many times higher, however. In fact, since you would need to drink about 62 gallons of milk a day to get the 400-milligram dose that was used in the Belgian study, supplementing is essential. "Almost as a matter of routine, all of our patients are put on riboflavin. We start them on 200 milligrams for a week and then bring them up to 400 milligrams," Dr. Sheftell says.

According to Dr. Sheftell, some people experience nausea when they take as much as 400 milligrams. If that happens, you can just return to the 200-milligram dose. It may take some time to get relief, so stick with the supplements for 2 to 3 months before you decide whether they have any benefit, says Dr. Sheftell.

Add Some Magnesium

Another promising migraine fighter is magnesium. This mineral plays a key role in regulating both blood vessel size and the rate at which cells burn energy. Researchers estimate that 50 percent of migraine sufferers are magnesium deficient, says Burton M. Altura, MD, professor of physiology and medicine at the State University of New York Health Science Center in Brooklyn. At the center, studies on more than 1,000 migraine sufferers have shown that an intravenous dose of 1,000 milligrams of magnesium sulfate can relieve some acute headache attacks.

Does this mean that you can pop a few magnesium tablets to get rid of a headache? Not quite, but the supplement may be useful in preventing them.

"We believe that everyone should be taking 500 to 600 milligrams of magnesium a day in a combination of diet and supplements," says Dr. Altura. "If people would bring up their total consumption of magnesium, they could reduce the frequency of recurring migraine headaches." To avoid possible loose stools, take a form of magnesium that is easily absorbed, such as magnesium gluconate or glycinate.

Feed on Feverfew

Don't wait until you're hurting to take feverfew, says Dr. Sheftell. A cousin of dandelion and marigold, feverfew has long been used to prevent headaches of all kinds, but medical doctors took little notice of this folk remedy until 1985. That was the year that a British survey of 270 migraine sufferers found that 70 percent had fewer headaches and less pain when they ate feverfew leaves daily. Experts suggest chewing one to four fresh leaves daily.

"It's important to understand that when you use a remedy preventively, it takes a fair amount of time to evaluate its effectiveness," says Dr. Sheftell. "You need to take 125 milligrams of feverfew every day for 6 to 8 weeks." Don't use this if you have ragweed allergy.

Pain Relief from Fatty Acids

If you're not getting the relief you need from other pharmaceuticals and supplements, you might try adding omega-3 essential fatty acids to your diet. Found in high amounts in fish oil and flaxseed oil, these key fats fight inflammation and reduce pain. High doses (15 grams a day) have even been helpful for severe migraines. A usual dose of 1 to 3 grams a day may be all you need for a more common tension or PMS headache. You need to take fish oil daily, not just when you have a headache, and it may take a few months before you begin to notice benefits.

An Herbal Massage

When your head is in the viselike grip of a tension headache, take small doses of an herbal supplement that includes a mixture of valerian, passionflower, and skullcap, says Priscilla Evans, ND, a naturopathic doctor in private practice in Cary, North Carolina. This trio of herbs can help relax muscles in your shoulders, neck, and scalp. "Valerian is great for relaxing the nervous system, relieving tension, and providing general pain relief. Passionflower and skullcap help to calm stress," she says.

Stick with the manufacturer's recommendations if you choose a premixed supplement. Typical instructions are to take 225 milligrams with meals or water twice a day. If you're using a tincture that combines the three herbs, take 10 drops three or four times a day, says Dr. Evans.

Peppermint oil, a well-known muscle relaxant, is also used for tension headaches. Add about 2 drops of the oil to 20 drops of a base oil, such as almond oil, and massage it on your forehead, temples, or wherever your muscles feel tight. You should feel some relief about 15 minutes after application.

Better Than Aspirin

For pain relief from tension headaches, use a supplement of white willow bark. This is the same salicylate-containing herb that led to the development of aspirin, says Brent Mathieu, ND, in Boise, Idaho. For effective relief, take one or two 400-milligram doses of dried bark capsules every 2 to 4 hours as needed.

If willow bark and aspirin both have the same components—salicylates— why not just take an aspirin? "Willow bark is naturally buffered and acts gently, so it generally does not upset and irritate the stomach," Dr. Mathieu says.

The herb also contains small amounts of vitamin C and quercetin and other bioflavonoids, which combine with the salicylate to relieve both pain and inflammation. The trade-off is that it's hard to regulate the dosage with herbs. "There's a wide variation in the quality of the plant and how it was prepared, so you never know exactly how much of the active substance you're getting," says Dr. Mathieu.

Although its active ingredients are less concentrated than the drugstore product, you shouldn't take willow bark if you are allergic to aspirin, says Dr. Mathieu.

Chase Premenstrual Headaches with Chasteberry

Even if you don't suffer from migraines, you may still get that aggravating PMS headache once a month. These headaches may result from fluid buildup and hormonal changes. For these particular head pains, try the herb chasteberry, also called vitex. It's thought to relieve PMS symptoms by affecting brain neurotransmitters and hormones. Don't expect instant results, though, since it can take 1 to 4 weeks of daily use to see a benefit. Studies have found 20 to 40 milligrams a day to be an effective dose.

heart arrhythmia

A heartbeat is a highly coordinated event. Nerves need to fire in precisely the right sequence to stimulate muscles that contract the chambers of the heart. When a heartbeat goes perfectly, blood flows through your heart and out to your lungs and the rest of your body.

When this process goes awry, it results in heart arrhythmia. If nerves fire out of sequence, the chambers of the heart don't contract properly.

Usually, arrhythmia is the result of damage to the heart muscle. The cause could be coronary artery disease or even a viral infection, says Decker Weiss, NMD, director of the Weiss Center for Naturopathic Excellence, in Scottsdale, Arizona, and author of *The Weiss Method: A Natural Program for Reversing Heart Disease and Preventing Heart Attacks.* "Anything that affects the heart adversely can affect the nerve conduction system of the heart, which is what controls the heartbeat."

Sometimes, and often in conjunction with heart disease, mineral imbalances can interfere with the heart's normal nerve function. These imbalances may be brought on by drugs that have been prescribed to treat high blood pressure or congestive heart failure.

You need to be under a doctor's care if you have arrhythmia, but there are some mineral and herb treatments that can go hand in hand with medications to help keep the nerves firing smoothly. Just make sure your doctor works with you, and don't take any supplements without his or her knowledge.

Two minerals, potassium and magnesium, play an especially important role in helping your heart beat properly.

Potassium Powers the Pump

If you're a heart patient, your doctor will monitor your blood levels of potassium. Low potassium can cause heart arrhythmia, and certain types of diuretics, such as thiazide (Hydrodiuril), can leach this mineral from your

433

body, says Carla Sueta, MD, PhD, assistant professor of medicine and cardiology at the University of North Carolina at Chapel Hill School of Medicine. Digitalis, a common heart medication, can also lower potassium.

Potassium deficiency affects more than your heart. It can also weaken your muscles and lead to mental confusion.

The Daily Value for potassium is 3,500 milligrams, and a diet with plenty of fruits and vegetables gives most people what they need. Too much potassium is as bad as too little, so it is essential that you work with your doctor if you need supplemental potassium to control your heartbeat, Dr. Sueta says.

Magnesium Keeps the Beat

When magnesium levels in the heart are low, people can develop certain types of heart arrhythmia. Some of them are potentially dangerous, Dr. Sueta says. The effects of magnesium are so well proven that doctors sometimes give it intravenously to prevent certain kinds of arrhythmia. Studies have shown, for instance, that intravenous magnesium reduces the incidence of death from ventricular arrhythmia, which involves the lower chambers of the heart. "In fact, intravenous therapy with magnesium now is considered standard for two types of ventricular arrhythmia," Dr. Sueta says.

Just as diuretics and digitalis can cause potassium deficiency, these medications can also induce a shortage of magnesium. Moreover, magnesium is often at the bottom of what's called refractory potassium deficiency, says Michael A. Brodsky, MD, professor of medicine at the University of California, Irvine, and director of the cardiac electrophysiology/arrhythmia service at the university's medical school.

"The amount of magnesium in the body determines the amount of a particular enzyme that determines the amount of potassium," says Dr. Brodsky. "If you are magnesium deficient, you may in turn be potassium deficient, and no amount of potassium is going to correct this unless you are also getting enough magnesium."

It's best if your doctor monitors your blood levels of magnesium, because how much you need depends on the amount that's in your blood. A test that measures ionized magnesium—the active form of magnesium in the blood—can detect a deficiency before it reaches a critical level, Dr. Sueta says. Most doctors test only for serum magnesium, which detects only severe deficiency, so make sure to ask for the ionized test.

Smoother Beating with CoQ$_{10}$

Along with magnesium, Dr. Weiss may recommend coenzyme Q$_{10}$ (CoQ$_{10}$) for heart arrhythmia.

This vitamin-like substance is made in the body, particularly in the cells of the heart muscle, where it is used to produce the energy that the muscle needs. Additional CoQ$_{10}$ seems to provide more energy to the muscle cells, an action that can be of great benefit for heart disease, Dr. Weiss says.

CoQ$_{10}$ also seems to help reduce stiffening of the heart muscle. This stiffening can produce abnormalities called diastolic dysfunction, says Peter Langsjoen, MD, a cardiologist in Tyler, Texas. Dr. Langsjoen has been using CoQ$_{10}$ in his practice to treat heart disease since 1985.

The diastolic, or filling, phase of the cardiac cycle actually requires more energy than the systolic, or contraction, phase, Dr. Langsjoen says. "Relaxation of the muscle actually requires energy," he points out. "This stiffening of the heart muscle returns to normal with supplemental CoQ$_{10}$, and people have less fatigue." In his observation, CoQ$_{10}$ not only improves irregular heart rhythm but also reduces chest pain. "It's as dramatic as watering a dried-up houseplant."

The need for additional CoQ$_{10}$ depends on your symptoms. Dr. Weiss starts with a minimum dose of 120 milligrams a day divided into four 30-milligram doses. To aid absorption, he suggests taking it between meals with omega-3 and omega-6 fatty acids. If you're taking the blood thinner warfarin (Coumadin) for heart disease, though, be sure to talk to your doctor, since taking CoQ$_{10}$ can cause a slight decrease in its effectiveness.

Dr. Langsjoen starts people on twice that much, 240 milligrams a day, and may raise the level as high as 360 milligrams, divided into three daily doses, if symptoms are severe.

Some people respond quickly to CoQ$_{10}$, while others show little or no response for weeks or months, says Dr. Weiss.

This supplement is expensive, so you'll want to stay with the lowest dose that relieves your symptoms. Studies show that there are no side effects or toxicity associated with CoQ$_{10}$.

CoQ$_{10}$ is fat soluble, which means that your body will absorb more of the active ingredient if it's in a gelcap, rather than in powder or tablet form. A new form, called liposomal CoQ$_{10}$, adds an emulsifier to the enzyme, then breaks the mixture into tiny, easily absorbed spheres. This process increases absorption several hundredfold and allows you to take a lower dose.

Fats That May Help Your Heart

Dr. Weiss recommends cutting back on the fats that can harm your heart, including the saturated fats that come from animal sources and hydrogenated fats found in many high-fat food products. Instead, he urges getting more of two essential fatty acids that help to protect your heart: omega-3 fatty acids found in fish oils and omega-3s and omega-6s from flaxseed oil and borage oil, respectively (among other sources). Dr. Weiss recommends that people with heart arrhythmia get 1,000 to 3,000 milligrams a day of a mixture of these two fats. They are available as gelcaps or, in the case of flaxseed or borage oil, in liquid form. It's possible that some forms of arrhythmia can worsen with use of fish oil, so check with your doctor before you start taking it.

Strengthen with Hawthorn

When someone's heart is additionally weakened by cardiovascular disease or congestive heart failure, Dr. Weiss may add hawthorn, an herb known for its heart-strengthening effects. Hawthorn contains bioflavonoids, compounds that act as heart-protective antioxidants.

"Hawthorn's bioflavonoids are considered to be very specific for blood vessels," Dr. Weiss says. German researchers report that it gently increases the strength of the heartbeat. Typically, it also helps the heart muscle beat at a normal rhythm and simultaneously increases blood supply to the heart.

Hawthorn is used while the current problem exists, explains Dr. Weiss. If a patient's heart function is improving due to diet and lifestyle changes such as exercise and weight reduction, Dr. Weiss will wean the patient off hawthorn.

Although Dr. Weiss says that he has monitored patients on hawthorn for many years without seeing any problems with the supplement, he still advises that you get your doctor's advice before you use it, especially if you are taking other heart drugs. You may require lower doses of other medications, such as blood pressure drugs, since hawthorn has been shown to lower blood pressure.

As for dosage requirements, the amount of hawthorn you should take depends on your symptoms and the type of hawthorn you're using. A typical dose is ¼ teaspoon of standardized extract taken two or three times daily.

heartburn

Heartburn has always been misnamed—this annoying and painful condition has nothing to do with your heart.

Chronic heartburn has a more correct moniker—GERD, or gastro-esophageal reflux disease—and with that long name comes a million-dollar business in stomach acid–reducing drugs. While those remedies may work in the short term, you shouldn't rely on them since they don't address the underlying cause of that burning sensation. And some people find that if they take them for too long, they can't go off them at all because they experience a rebound effect once they stop taking the drugs.

In fact, many natural healers believe that we should try to do more than just reduce the acid. For one thing, it helps to improve your diet and digestion so the acid stays where it belongs—in your stomach. It also helps to use herbal and nutritional supplements that can heal the irritation and burning caused by any acid backup, says William Warnock, ND, a naturopathic doctor in Shelburne, Vermont.

"Normally, stomach acid is confined to the stomach by a valve between the stomach and the esophagus," says Dr. Warnock. "When that valve malfunctions and the acid is able to pass from the stomach into the esophagus, it can cause irritation there, so the first thing you want to do is prevent the irritation from continuing."

If you're plagued by the symptoms of heartburn, you may want to consider changing your eating habits. Fatty, fried, or high-protein foods; alcohol; and coffee are often the culprits behind heartburn, says Pamela Taylor, ND, a naturopathic doctor in Moline, Illinois.

People who eat quickly and gulp their food often get heartburn, says Dr. Warnock. He advises people to eat regular meals and, above all, to chew food slowly, savoring the smell and taste.

Also, pay attention to the final meal of the day, suggests Dr. Taylor. "I tell patients not to eat within 4 hours of their bedtimes and that their last meal of the day should be oriented toward foods such as steamed vegetables, baked or broiled fish, and nonwheat grains such as rice or quinoa," she says.

Coat, Soothe, and Heal

Even if you're a deliberate eater, you may have chronic heartburn. There are many possible causes, including stress, age, and poor digestion. You may even have chronic heartburn because you've been infected with *Helicobacter pylori,* the same bacteria that contribute to stomach ulcers.

People are more prone to heartburn if they take medications that affect the muscles of the esophagus. And they're more likely to get it if they have a hiatal hernia (a hernia of the diaphragm).

Whatever the source of the problem, the mucous membranes of your esophagus are probably inflamed and irritated, says Melissa Metcalfe, ND, a naturopathic doctor in Los Angeles. That's one area where supplements might be able to lend a helping hand.

An excellent herb to soothe those tissues is deglycyrrhizinated licorice, or DGL, according to Dr. Metcalfe. For one thing, DGL has antispasmodic action, which means that it helps to control various muscle actions that can affect your digestive tract. The herb also helps reduce acid reflux by calming a cramping stomach, she says.

The primary medicinal benefit of DGL, however, is its ability to increase and build up the protective substances that line the digestive tract. By stimulating the body's natural defense mechanisms, licorice helps prevent the formation of ulcers and lesions due to the irritating acid, says Dr. Metcalfe. It's also a powerful, localized anti-inflammatory.

"It's the first thing I recommend to people—it's a great initial treatment," says Dr. Metcalfe. The typical dose is two 250-milligram capsules taken 20 minutes before mealtime.

Rather than swallowing the DGL with water, Dr. Metcalfe suggests that you suck on the capsules and let them dissolve slowly in your mouth. You can also get DGL in chewable tablets that dissolve as you chew them. "You want the licorice to coat the inside of your throat and esophagus to cover those inflamed and irritated tissues," she says.

Use it for 4 weeks and then assess if it's working, she suggests. If it is, your throat should feel less irritated. If not, see your health-care practitioner.

A Cure with a Peel

No one knows exactly how it works, but a product called Orange Peel Extract helps to reduce symptoms of heartburn, says Bernie Noe, ND, a naturopathic doctor with a private practice in Montpelier, Vermont. The product is rich in a substance called D-limonene, a citrus bioflavonoid that seems to strengthen the esophageal sphincter muscle (it's that muscle that keeps stomach contents from entering the esophagus). D-limonene also floats on top of stomach acid and prevents the acid from coming into contact with the delicate tissues of the esophagus.

Clinical studies have found that people taking 1,000 milligrams of D-limonene either every day or every other day dropped 1 or 2 points on the heartburn severity index, a scale that rates pain from 1 to 10, with 10 being the most severe. Additionally, after 2 weeks on the supplement, 83 percent of the participants reported no higher than a 2 on the severity scale, and 75 percent experienced no heartburn symptoms for up to 6 months after the study.

Get at the Inflammation

Another healing substance for damaged mucous membranes is glutamine, an amino acid that's available as a nutritional supplement. Dr. Metcalfe frequently recommends it for gastrointestinal disorders whenever inflammation is a problem.

Glutamine encourages the turnover or disposal of damaged cells, and it increases the production of new cells along the gastrointestinal walls, says Dr. Metcalfe. It's also a potent antioxidant, helping to protect cells from the damage caused by free-roaming, unstable molecules called free radicals. All of these actions equate with faster healing, she says.

"I tell people to take one 500-milligram capsule four times a day until they are feeling better," says Dr. Metcalfe. "Usually, that's about a month."

Kill the Bacteria

If bad bacteria—usually *H. pylori*—are the source of your problem, you could consider taking goldenseal, says Dr. Metcalfe. First, though, get a proper diagnosis from your doctor.

For best results, Dr. Metcalfe recommends that you combine a golden-seal supplement with colloidal bismuth, which is the active ingredient in many over-the-counter stomach medications like Pepto-Bismol Maximum Strength Liquid. Besides coating the stomach, the bismuth helps the herb adhere to the mucous membranes of the stomach.

Take two or three 400-milligram capsules of goldenseal daily along with 1 tablespoon of Pepto-Bismol Maximum Strength Liquid four times daily, Dr. Metcalfe suggests. "When you take bismuth, be aware that your stools will turn black. It's nothing to worry about." Don't use goldenseal if you are pregnant, however.

Relief on the Run

You don't need to go to the health food store for relief. In fact, you don't have to look any farther than the spice rack.

"When people are traveling and have heartburn, I tell them to stop at a supermarket and buy some ginger," says Dr. Taylor. You can get either fresh ginger in the produce section or the powdered spice.

Ginger relaxes the smooth muscle along the walls of the esophagus, says Dr. Taylor. "If your digestion is working better, you're less likely to get that reflux, or backwash, of stomach acid," she says. "Ginger is an excellent tonic for the whole gastrointestinal tract."

If you're using ginger to prevent heartburn, take it 20 minutes before a meal. Take it as a capsule, a tincture, make a tea from the fresh root or the powder, or eat candied or pickled ginger as it comes from the jar.

To use it in capsule form, take one or two "00" capsules and wait for a half-hour. If your symptoms don't improve in that time, you may repeat the dose. You can also empty the contents of the capsules into hot water and drink it as a tea, Dr. Taylor says.

Candied ginger has a long history as a digestive aid. It only takes a small amount—about the size of the tip of your little finger. Chew it slowly and well, incorporating a fair amount of saliva before swallowing, Dr. Taylor says. You can repeat this dose in 10 minutes or so if your symptoms persist.

If you choose a tincture, she recommends a dose between 15 and 60 drops. "Always use the smaller amount, in a little water if possible. Repeat the 15-drop dose every 15 minutes, up to a total of 60 drops, if necessary."

Because ginger is considered a "hot bitter," people with very sensitive stomachs may find it too strong.

high blood pressure

If you have high blood pressure (consistently higher than 140/90) and see a conventional doctor, chances are pretty good that the doctor will tell you that you'll have to take drugs, probably for the rest of your life.

If you're willing to make some changes in your diet and lifestyle, though, there's a good chance that you can bring your blood pressure into the normal range—or at least reduce it somewhat. Losing just a little weight can work wonders. So can a modest cutback in salt. In one study, dropping about 8 pounds and reducing sodium intake by 25 percent allowed half of the participants to lower their blood pressures enough to stop taking medication. Eating less saturated fat and more fiber can also reduce pressure, studies have shown.

There's more. Doctors and practitioners who use alternative medicine have an arsenal of nutritional supplements—including herbs—that go hand in hand with dietary measures and weight loss. Some of these supplements help regulate blood volume and relax blood vessel muscles so that arteries can dilate, which reduces blood pressure. Others reduce your risk of developing atherosclerosis (hardening of the arteries), which eventually also causes high blood pressure. Still others, such as coenzyme Q_{10} (CoQ_{10}), help your heart pump more efficiently, which also reduces blood pressure, especially in people with damaged hearts. If you have high blood pressure, though, always check with your doctor before you take any supplements.

A Trio of Helpful Minerals

The people who are most sensitive to salt's blood pressure–elevating effects may be low in other minerals, such as potassium, magnesium, and perhaps calcium, says David McCarron, MD, professor of medicine and head of the division of nephrology, hypertension, and clinical pharmacology at Oregon Health Sciences University in Portland.

441

Potassium, magnesium, and calcium have a direct effect on blood volume or influence the ability of blood vessels to relax. Increasing blood volume is like opening up a faucet, and it increases blood pressure. If blood vessels are constricted, pressure also rises. When the vessels relax, blood pressure tends to go down.

"Each of these minerals has some effect separately, but all three interact and may have a better combined effect," Dr. McCarron says.

Potassium Power

Potassium affects blood volume because it helps you excrete sodium, says David B. Young, PhD, professor of physiology and biophysics at the University of Mississippi Medical Center in Jackson. When you excrete sodium, you also excrete water, which reduces blood volume and in turn reduces blood pressure.

How much should you get? The Daily Value (DV) is 3,500 milligrams, an amount provided by eight or nine servings of fruits and vegetables, and that much will help to reduce blood pressure. "More potassium will reduce it even more, however," says Dr. Young. "I'd like people to aim for twice that amount—7,000 milligrams or more a day."

The safest way to get potassium is from foods, he says. In supplement form, a prescription is needed for dosages higher than 99 milligrams per tablet. If you are taking a non-potassium-sparing diuretic for high blood pressure, though, you may need supplemental potassium, Dr. Young says. In this case, your doctor will give you prescription potassium and monitor your blood levels.

More Magnesium?

Magnesium helps to relax the smooth muscles in blood vessels, which allows them to dilate, says Decker Weiss, NMD, director of the Weiss Center for Naturopathic Excellence in Scottsdale, Arizona, and author of *The Weiss Method: A Natural Program for Reversing Heart Disease and Preventing Heart Attacks.* Supplemental magnesium has been effective in people who have high blood pressure due to kidney damage, pregnancy-induced high blood pressure, and the type of high blood pressure that's caused by diuretics.

If you're taking non-potassium-sparing diuretics such as thiazides to treat high blood pressure, they will begin to deplete your body of magnesium and potassium, the very minerals that you need to help regulate your pressure, notes Dr. Weiss. If your doctor has prescribed a diuretic for blood pressure control, it may stop working after 6 months or so because magnesium has been drained from your system. "Supplemental magnesium sometimes makes the diuretic more effective again," he says.

It's safe for most people to use up to 350 milligrams a day of supplemental magnesium, Dr. Weiss says. The preferred forms are magnesium orotate and magnesium glycinate.

Calcium sometimes also helps to reduce blood pressure, although it has less effect than potassium or magnesium. It seems to work best in women who develop high blood pressure during pregnancy and in children who are calcium-deficient, says Matthew Gillman, MD, assistant professor of ambulatory care and prevention at Boston University Medical School. In one study, pregnant women who took 2,000 milligrams a day of calcium reduced the incidence of high blood pressure by 54 percent.

The DV for calcium is 1,000 milligrams, an amount that many of us fail to consume in our daily diets. Even if you're not getting the DV, though, if you already have high blood pressure, you should check with your doctor before taking supplemental calcium, Dr. Weiss says. "I don't normally recommend it for high blood pressure unless I'm seeing an older woman who also has osteoporosis, because too much calcium can interfere with magnesium's muscle-relaxing ability."

Don't Forget D

Any time you are taking calcium, you should make sure you're also getting enough vitamin D. Studies show that getting enough vitamin D can lower blood pressure, because the vitamin works like an ACE inhibitor, a blood pressure–lowering drug. Vitamin D and blood pressure drugs both control a substance called angiotensin II, which does a number of things to increase your blood pressure and raise your risk of disease. First, it constricts blood vessels. Excess angiotensin II also leads to abnormal thickening of both the heart muscle and blood vessel walls. It increases output of adrenaline and similar substances, and generates another blood pressure–raising hormone called aldosterone. As if that wasn't enough, it also increases salt retention by the kidneys.

Experts now recommend 800 to 4,000 IU or more of vitamin D each day. Start taking the suggested 800 IU of vitamin D, and if you can, have your doctor monitor your blood levels and continue to take a dosage that maintains your vitamin D blood level at 50 to 80 ng/ml, recommends John Cannell, MD, executive director of the Vitamin D Council.

Fiber Fills the Bill

Dr. Weiss routinely prescribes a high-fiber diet for people concerned about heart disease, and there's some evidence that fiber can also help reduce high blood pressure. In a large study of more than 40,000 nurses whose lifestyles and diet patterns were followed for 4 years, researchers discovered that those who got the highest amounts of fiber were least likely to develop high blood pressure. In another study, with animals whose blood pressures had been elevated by a high-fat diet, switching to a low-fat diet and fiber supplements reduced pressure by 10 to 15 points.

Of the two kinds of fiber—soluble and insoluble—it's the soluble type that's more important for lowering blood pressure, Dr. Weiss says. This fiber is found in fruits, beans, and oats. If you want additional fiber, look for a supplement that contains mixed soluble fibers such as psyllium, gums, and pectin, he says.

Fish Oil and Flaxseed Oil Smooth the Way

Doctors recommend that you do some serious fat-swapping if you have high blood pressure. Cut back on saturated fats, they say, including animal fat, butter, and the kind of fat that's in many baked goods. As much as possible, avoid trans fats, the kind found in margarine and shortening, and polyunsaturated fats, such as corn oil.

Instead of these "unhealthy" fats, Dr. Weiss suggests that you get more omega-3s from fish oil and flaxseed oil. Aim for 1,000 to 3,000 milligrams a day.

"I recommend 1,000 to 3,000 milligrams a day of a mixture of these two essential fatty acids," he says. The fatty acids change your body chemistry so that you produce fewer harmful prostaglandins, hormonelike substances that can jack up blood pressure.

Vitamins to the Rescue

High blood pressure can also develop over time from atherosclerosis, as arteries clogged with fatty deposits become narrow and hardened, like pipes clogged with mineral deposits. Not everyone with high blood pressure has atherosclerosis, but if you have high cholesterol and high blood pressure, Dr. Weiss recommends adding nutrients that help prevent atherosclerosis. These include vitamins C and E, which help reduce the formation of fatty deposits and clots inside blood vessels.

Vitamin C may have additional blood pressure–lowering effects, Italian researchers report. They found that it helped blood vessels dilate normally. In some people with high blood pressure, the vitamin stopped the breakdown of nitric oxide, a blood vessel–dilating chemical that is secreted from the walls of the blood vessels.

"I routinely prescribe these to anyone who wants to prevent heart disease and related problems," Dr. Weiss says. He recommends 400 to 800 international units of vitamin E and suggests using the type labeled "mixed tocopherols." "And I recommend 1,000 to 2,000 milligrams a day of vitamin C in divided doses," he says.

You'll also want to make sure that you get about 400 micrograms of folic acid, 1,000 micrograms of vitamin B_{12}, and 100 milligrams of vitamin B_6, Dr. Weiss says. Doses of vitamin B_6 above 200 milligrams a day should only be taken under medical supervision.

These three B vitamins are important because they help your body clear out homocysteine, an amino acid by-product that can damage arteries, says Dr. Weiss. Homocysteine creates rough spots on artery walls, and those roughened areas can pick up fatty deposits that harden into artery-clogging plaque. Taking these B vitamins can help preserve smooth-walled arteries.

Coenzyme Q_{10} Helps Your Heart Help You

This substance is made naturally in the body, but production declines with age, and CoQ_{10} is depleted by cholesterol-lowering statin drugs. If high blood pressure is accompanied by heart damage or weakness, you might need CoQ_{10}, Dr. Weiss says. It improves energy supplies to the heart muscle cells, so it helps your heart to pump more efficiently, with less effort. That in turn helps to lower blood pressure.

In one study of 109 people with high blood pressure, more than half were able to stop or reduce their medication after 4 months of treatment with CoQ_{10}. Dr. Weiss recommends 30 milligrams three times a day. To improve absorption, he says, it's best to take it at the same time you take fish oil or flaxseed oil.

high cholesterol

High cholesterol isn't a disease—it's more like an alarm signal. The state of your cholesterol levels tells you something about your risk of developing the United States' number one killer, heart disease, or coronary artery disease.

The higher your blood levels of "bad" low-density lipoprotein (LDL) cholesterol, the greater your risk of developing coronary artery disease, the life-threatening condition that occurs when the arteries to your heart become clogged with cholesterol. One form of LDL cholesterol, called lipoprotein (a), or Lp(a), has been found to be even more damaging than ordinary LDL. In fact, the risk of heart disease for people with high levels of Lp(a) is 10 times higher than that of people who simply have elevated levels of LDL cholesterol. That's because Lp(a) sticks to artery walls much more easily than LDL does.

When doctors look at cholesterol levels for a profile of your risks, they also consider other kinds of fats, or lipids, that affect arterial health. Two of those factors, one bad and one good, are triglycerides and high-density lipoprotein (HDL) cholesterol. Triglycerides are simply partners in crime with LDL, and when your blood profile shows high triglycerides, there's reason for concern. HDL, on the other hand, is a fat that campaigns for free-flowing blood, and it never sticks around to cause trouble in your arteries. For this reason, it's easiest to think of HDL as the good cholesterol; the higher your HDL levels, the lower your risk of heart disease.

Eating a diet low in fat, especially saturated fat, and high in fiber is always a primary strategy for lowering the bad cholesterol and raising the good. You need to pursue that diet even if your cholesterol is so high that your doctor has prescribed cholesterol-lowering drugs, says Decker Weiss, NMD, director of the Weiss Center for Naturopathic Excellence, in Scottsdale, Arizona, and author of *The Weiss Method: A Natural Program for Reversing Heart Disease and Preventing Heart Attacks*.

If you know that your LDL cholesterol is high and you're already on cholesterol-lowering drugs, some vitamin or herbal supplements might come in handy for reducing the side effects of those drugs. Other supplements directly lower cholesterol levels or reduce your risk for atherosclerosis, the notorious hardening of the arteries that results from a buildup of blood-slowing plaque along the arterial walls. Supplements can reinforce your cholesterol-control efforts on a number of different fronts. Here's how they stack up.

Antioxidants Help Disarm Cholesterol

"Cholesterol doesn't hurt you when it's just floating around in your blood," Dr. Weiss says. As soon as the fatty substance clings to your artery walls, however, it becomes a threat, and a serious one at that.

Harmful LDL cholesterol doesn't go looking for trouble when it's traveling along in its free-floating form. Before it can stick to your artery walls, it has to be oxidized. To prevent the chain of events that leads to oxidation of cholesterol, you need a good dose of the antioxidant nutrients that can disarm free radicals, the free-roaming, unstable molecules that do the damage. Many antioxidants are found in foods. Others are most available from supplements, particularly when you want vitamin E or large amounts of vitamin C.

Dr. Weiss recommends taking 400 to 800 international units (IU) of vitamin E every day. "While it doesn't actually affect cholesterol levels, vitamin E does help to lessen the potential harmful effects of high cholesterol levels," he says.

In your body, vitamin E helps prevent LDL cholesterol from being oxidized. A study showed that at least 400 IU is needed to significantly reduce LDL oxidation.

C: What It Does

Vitamin C apparently can have a more direct effect on cholesterol levels. Dozens of studies have shown that higher blood levels of vitamin C correspond to lower total cholesterol and triglyceride levels and higher HDL levels. In a study at the Jean Mayer USDA Human Nutrition Research Center on Aging at Tufts University in Boston, researchers found that people with low blood levels of ascorbic acid (vitamin C) who took 1,000 milligrams a day for 8 months had an average 7 percent increase in HDL. Researchers say that eating five servings of fruits and vegetables a day would bring your vitamin C levels into the normal range.

Dr. Weiss recommends taking 1,000 to 3,000 milligrams of vitamin C daily in divided doses.

More on the Antioxidant Front

Additionally, Dr. Weiss recommends alpha lipoic acid, an antioxidant that plays a role in energy production. This antioxidant has a unique property: It is effective against both fat-soluble and water-soluble free radicals. It has been found to raise blood levels of vitamin C and of glutathione, another powerful antioxidant that is made in the body. You can get alpha lipoic acid in either capsules or tablets. Doses of 300 milligrams twice a day are used for artery disease.

Dr. Weiss also recommends bioflavonoids, or proanthocyanidins. These powerful antioxidant compounds are found in many plants and in red wine. The proanthocyanidins in supplements come from grape seeds and pine bark.

Laboratory studies indicate that, in theory, "proanthocyanidins can trap a variety of free radicals and inhibit the damaging effects of several enzymes, including enzymes that degrade collagen, the body's main connective tissue," says Dr. Weiss. If you're using proanthocyanidins to prevent heart disease, a daily dose of 50 milligrams is enough. If you already have heart disease, you should raise the dose to 150 to 400 milligrams a day, he says. Of course, be sure to tell your doctor which supplements you are taking.

Lipotropic Compounds Aid Your Liver

Believe it or not, most of the cholesterol floating around in your bloodstream is made in your liver. In order to make that cholesterol, the liver relies on the fats you eat for raw material. That's why it deserves attention if you have high cholesterol, Dr. Weiss says.

He recommends a combination supplement of lipotropic compounds that have multiple benefits for the liver. The mixture may include choline, betaine, methionine, vitamin B_6, folic acid, vitamin B_{12}, milk thistle, and dandelion. The combination helps to promote the flow of bile to and from the liver, in effect decongesting it. It helps to promote improved liver function and improve the way your body burns fat.

Take enough lipotropic compounds to get a daily dose of 1,000 milligrams of choline and 1,000 milligrams of either methionine and/or cysteine, recommends Michael Murray, ND, a naturopathic doctor and coauthor of *Encyclopedia of Natural Medicine.*

Double Up on Fiber

Along with a lipotropic compound, Dr. Weiss recommends a high-fiber diet. Fiber, especially the soluble kind, can bind up the bile that's secreted by your liver into the small intestine. Bile is laden with cholesterol. When fiber binds with the bile and escorts it from your body, it means that the fats won't be reabsorbed, "so the combination of fiber and a lipotropic compound is often an effective way to lower cholesterol," Dr. Weiss says.

You need to get somewhere between 15 and 30 grams of fiber a day in order to see an impact on your cholesterol levels, according to Dr. Weiss. The average intake in the United States is about 12 grams, so he says that you should aim for about twice that amount. Beans, berries, whole grains, and bran, such as oat or wheat bran, can provide good amounts of fiber.

If you need to get more, use a supplement of mixed soluble and insoluble fibers, including pectin, gums, psyllium, and oat bran, Dr. Weiss recommends.

Fatty Acids Protect the Heart

Our bodies use both blood sugar (glucose) and fat as fuel. The energy that the heart muscle relies on, however, is supplied mostly by fatty acids. Dr. Weiss recommends cutting back on the fats that can harm and going for one that can heal. The harmful kinds are saturated and hydrogenated fats, found in red meat, hydrogenated oils, and many processed foods.

The essential fatty acid that helps to protect your heart is omega-3 fatty acid, found in fish oil. Studies show that substituting it for saturated fats or other unsaturated fats can significantly reduce triglycerides.

Dr. Weiss recommends that people with high cholesterol get 1,000 to 3,000 milligrams daily of fish oil from fatty fish such as wild Alaskan salmon or from fish oil capsules.

Niacin Nixes the Bad Stuff

In large doses, niacin, a B vitamin, is sometimes used to lower LDL cholesterol. Niacin also raises HDL and lowers levels of Lp(a) and triglycerides. It also lowers fibrinogen, a blood protein that causes clot formation. Dr. Weiss cautions, however, that niacin is not universally effective, since there are some inherited forms of high cholesterol that it won't improve.

Also, niacin is not a supplement that you can automatically substitute for a cholesterol-lowering drug. Some people are better off with one of the "statin" drugs, such as simvastatin (Zocor), says Dr. Weiss. "Either niacin or a statin drug may be an appropriate choice for a particular patient, depending on the patient's lipid profile."

If triglyceride levels are high, you might get better results from niacin, or even fish oil, Dr. Weiss notes. Statin drugs, on the other hand, are more likely to be your doctor's first choice if you've just had a heart attack and have very high LDL levels that need to be reduced quickly.

Even though niacin is available at health food stores, you need to talk to a doctor before you take the high doses—1,000 to 3,000 milligrams a day—that are needed to lower cholesterol. At high doses, niacin can cause liver damage, especially timed-release niacin.

Your doctor will want to monitor your liver enzymes while you are taking niacin. If you are taking a cholesterol-lowering drug, never add large amounts of niacin without your doctor's approval. Such a combination can cause serious liver damage.

Added Protection: Coenzyme Q_{10}

If you're taking a statin drug, Dr. Weiss recommends taking coenzyme Q_{10} (CoQ_{10}), a vitamin-like compound that's made in your body. It acts as an antioxidant and is also essential for the production of energy. "Statin drugs deplete your blood of CoQ_{10}, so I have my patients use supplements while they're taking a statin drug," says Dr. Weiss.

CoQ_{10} may help your liver cells withstand the toxicity of the statin drugs and reduces side effects such as liver problems and muscle aches. As for how much to take, 100 to 300 milligrams a day has proven to be an effective dose for reducing statin-related muscle soreness, but some people may need more, depending on their age and the dosage of statin they are taking.

An Ayurvedic Approach: Gugulipid

Doctors will sometimes use a compound from an herb from India to lower cholesterol. The compound, called gugulipid, is derived from the resin or sap of the mukul myrrh tree.

"I might use gugulipid to lower cholesterol if someone has liver damage, is intolerant of niacin, or has diabetes along with high cholesterol, since niacin sometimes makes blood sugar levels harder to control," says Decker Weiss, NMD, director of the Weiss Center for Naturopathic Excellence in Scottsdale, Arizona, and author of *The Weiss Method: A Natural Program for Reversing Heart Disease and Preventing Heart Attacks.*

Gugulipid has a long history of medical use in India, especially for lipid disorders and obesity. Studies show that it can indeed lower cholesterol and triglyceride levels, raise HDL levels, and promote weight loss. Like niacin, it acts in the liver, stimulating liver cells to increase the amount of LDL cholesterol they gather from the blood. In 1986, gugulipid was approved in India for marketing as a lipid-lowering drug.

There's no standard dose, and how much you need to take depends on a number of factors, says Michael Murray, ND, a naturopathic doctor and coauthor of the *Encyclopedia of Natural Medicine.* In studies, people were able to lower their cholesterol if they took doses of 25 milligrams of guggulsterone—the active ingredient—three times a day.

To get that amount of the active ingredient in an extract that's labeled as 5 percent guggulsterone, you'd need to take a dose of 500 milligrams three times a day. Gugulipid has an excellent safety record and does not affect liver function, blood sugar control, or kidney function, according to Dr. Murray.

Garlic Gobbles Up Cholesterol

If you're a garlic fan, go ahead and eat your fill. Having plenty of fresh raw or lightly cooked garlic may be all you need to do to lower your cholesterol, Dr. Weiss says.

The benefits of whole garlic are well known, and Dr. Weiss has found that the experience of his patients supports the good press about garlic. "I had one lady whose cholesterol and blood pressure were really out of whack, and the only thing she did was to eat 10 to 15 steamed cloves of garlic a day—she loved it. Everything normalized in 3 weeks."

For many people, however, consistently eating five or more cloves a day to lower cholesterol is just a bit more than they can relish. If you're among the lukewarm fans of whole garlic, the pills are worth a try before you consider cholesterol-lowering drugs, Dr. Weiss says.

Look for dried garlic powder preparations in enteric-coated tablets or capsules. These are designed to pass through the stomach and then degrade in the alkaline environment of the intestine, where the beneficial conversion of one compound, alliin, into the active ingredient, allicin, takes place.

In studies, it's been found that people can lower total cholesterol by 10 to 12 percent and LDL and triglycerides by about 15 percent with supplements. HDL levels usually increased by about 10 percent. For these kinds of results, you'll need a preparation that provides a daily dose of at least 10 milligrams of alliin or a total allicin potential of 4,000 micrograms. You'll probably need to allow 1 to 3 months before you begin seeing a change in your cholesterol levels.

What about Red Yeast Rice?

If you've been taking a statin drug to lower cholesterol, you may be dealing with the common side effects of these drugs: muscle pain, fatigue and weakness, cognitive problems, and peripheral neuropathy, which causes tingling, pain, and numbness in the feet and hands. Statins may have some benefits, but for some people the side effects are bad enough that they'd like some other options.

And that's where red yeast rice comes in. This yeast that grows on rice contains a number of cholesterol-lowering substances, including monacolin K, which is identical to the cholesterol-lowering drug lovastatin. Red yeast rice has been used in China for centuries to treat poor circulation. It has recently gained popularity in the United States, as the side effects of statins become more widely known.

Can it deliver? A new study from China showed that red yeast rice lowered the risk for heart disease by about 30 percent after an average of 4½ years of use. It also decreased the need for bypass surgery, lowered triglycerides, and raised beneficial HDL. But here's the best part: It was safe and had few side effects.

If you're really having a problem with statins, this may be your savior. Research conducted in the United States shows that people who couldn't stand taking statins because of muscle pain were able to take red yeast rice without significant side effects. Two 1,800-milligram doses each day lowered LDL cholesterol an average of 35 mg/dl, a drop comparable to that seen when using statin drugs.

"Usually, about half the people who are intolerant of one statin drug are also intolerant when they switch to a different one," says David J. Becker, MD, the study's main investigator. "But people who switched to red yeast rice were able to tolerate it better. Only three people (about 10 percent) on red yeast rice dropped out of the study because of muscle pain."

Researchers think red yeast rice may be easier on the body than statins are because it works at a lower dosage. Another possibility is that its many cholesterol-lowering compounds work synergistically.

But because red yeast rice is so similar to statin drugs, Dr. Becker suggests several precautions if you're going to use it to lower cholesterol or if you're planning to switch from a statin drug you're currently taking.

- Don't take both red yeast rice and a statin drug without medical supervision.
- Take 100 to 200 milligrams of CoQ_{10} a day, to prevent the depletion of this important energy-producing biochemical. Both statins and red yeast rice interfere with the body's production of CoQ_{10}.
- Get your liver enzymes checked about 6 weeks after starting red yeast rice, and then every 6 months thereafter, for as long as you take it.
- Consider also taking additional phytosterols to further reduce LDL cholesterol.
- Dosages ranging from 600 to 1,800 milligrams twice a day have been shown to be effective. Don't take more than 1,800 milligrams twice a day of red yeast rice. Taking more doesn't lower cholesterol further.

HIV and AIDS

For people living with HIV/AIDS, progress literally means a new lease on life. HIV/AIDS is no longer a death sentence, as it was in the '70s and '80s. "It's now considered a manageable chronic disease," says Steve Milkis, ND, supervisor of naturopathic medicine at the Bastyr Center for Natural Health's Immune Wellness Clinic in Kenmore, Washington. Smarter use of the drugs available to treat HIV/AIDS has made treatment more tolerable, with fewer side effects. While natural treatments such as supplements can help even more, you shouldn't expect them to replace traditional HIV medications. "We can certainly help people become healthier, but there is nothing in natural medicine that reduces the viral load and increases CD4 counts as well as the antiretroviral drugs," he says. (CD4 cells are the immune cells depleted by HIV.)

With that in mind, here is what he and others recommend.

Live Healthy

Diet and lifestyle are always the starting point, from a naturopathic perspective. "We look at eliminating smoking, alcohol use, excess caffeine, and recreational drugs, as well as getting enough sleep and exercise—everything," Dr. Milkis says.

Dietwise, he says, the aim is to reduce foods that are inflammatory, such as red meat, dairy, sugar, and refined carbohydrates, and to increase anti-inflammatory foods like fresh fruits and vegetables. "I tell people to eat a rainbow of colors every day, because all those bright colors are nature's chemicals to protect the plants, and they protect us, too."

Dr. Milkis also increases his patients' protein intake beyond the normal 0.8 gm/kg of body weight, to 1.0 to 1.3 gm/kg, especially if people have had weight loss or muscle wasting. "We encourage people to eat cold-water fish; lean meats, if they're eating red meat; and to use organic, grass-fed buffalo or wild game and lean, organic poultry," he says. People with muscle wasting and weight loss may also benefit from taking supplemental l-carnitine, an amino acid found in meat that aids energy production and helps preserve and build muscle mass. Research shows that it also helps maintain a normal white blood cell count. A usual dose is 6,000 milligrams a day, along with a good mix of dietary protein.

Number One: A High-Potency Multivitamin

Even with a healthy diet, Dr. Milkis still recommends taking a good high-potency multivitamin/mineral every day. That's because many nutrients maintain strong immunity, and your body needs every one of them, often in higher amounts than you would normally get from your diet.

Several studies have shown that people who have HIV/AIDS are deficient in many antioxidant vitamins and minerals, such as vitamins E, C, and selenium. In fact, the rate of progression from HIV to AIDS has been strongly correlated with selenium status. Research shows that having good amounts of these antioxidants helps your immune system work better; reduces viral load by slowing viral replication; helps your body produce its own important antioxidants, like glutathione; and helps protect your detoxifying organs—your liver and kidneys—from the effects of the virus and from the drugs you need to take.

"Any good multivitamin is okay," Dr. Milkis says. "The really good ones require that you take more than one pill a day, and I prefer capsules to tablets because I think the ingredients are more easily absorbed." Your doctor should be able to help you pick out a brand that is good for you.

Fight Inflammation with Fish Oil

Fish oil does several things to help people with HIV/AIDS. It reduces the levels of pro-inflammatory biochemicals your body produces. That cuts down on tissue and organ damage and supports the immune system. The fats in fish oil can also help offset some of the damage caused by HIV drugs, especially protease inhibitors, which cause lipid disorders. (They interfere with how your body makes and stores fats, including cholesterol.) Fish oil increases levels of "good" HDL cholesterol and reduces triglycerides. (High triglycerides increase your risk for pancreatitis and heart disease.) In addition to getting more fatty fish such as salmon in your diet, take supplements. Start with 3 to 5 grams of fish oil a day.

Do the D-fense

Vitamin D is an important immunity nutrient, says Jared Skowron, ND, a clinic director at the University of Bridgeport, in Connecticut, and in private practice in Wallingford, Connecticut. "It seems to help reduce autoimmunity, where the body attacks itself. At the same time, it strengthens immunity, especially in the respiratory system," he says. Deficiency is associated with an increased risk for cancer, pneumonia, tuberculosis, and autoimmune disorders.

HIV drugs such as protease inhibitors are known to interfere with vitamin D metabolism, reducing the body's ability to produce the active form of the vitamin, Dr. Skowron says. One drug in particular, efavirenz, has been linked to severe vitamin D deficiency.

That's why he and Dr. Milkis check everyone with HIV/AIDS for vitamin D deficiency. Many of them are deficient and need large amounts to get back to normal. "A reasonable amount to take without medical supervision is 1,000 to 2,000 IU a day," Dr. Skowron says. But you may need 5,000 to 8,000 IU a day if you are found to be deficient. "I like to see them at about 55 ng/ml," he says. Dosages may need to be adjusted over time to maintain this level. Work with your doctor to find the best dose for you.

Protect Vital Organs with N-Acetylcysteine (NAC)

Both Dr. Milkis and Dr. Skowron use the amino acid NAC extensively with their HIV/AIDS patients. NAC helps your body make the powerful antioxidant glutathione, which helps protect the liver, kidneys, and brain—all organs that are at risk of damage when you have HIV or AIDS. "I have seen nothing repair organ damage better than NAC," Dr. Skowron says. "This supplement should be taken by everyone with HIV/AIDS." A usual dose is 1,000 milligrams two or three times a day. (Do not take with nitroglycerin.)

Build Up Nerves with Alpha Lipoic Acid

This vitamin-like antioxidant is in a class by itself. Research shows that it can block the reproduction of HIV by reducing the activity of an enzyme called reverse transcriptase, which is responsible for manufacturing the virus from the genetic material of blood-borne cells.

"Alpha lipoic acid is used to help prevent and treat HIV- and AIDS-related nerve damage," says Dr. Milkis. It's particularly effective at minimizing peripheral neuropathy—nerve damage to the hands and feet—and it even helps prevent HIV "brain fog." It reduces free radicals and removes toxic minerals from the body. It also raises levels of glutathione, vitamin C, and vitamin E. This supplement is available in health food stores. A usual dose is 200 milligrams two or three times a day.

Deploy a Tough Botanical Defense

As part of an HIV and AIDS treatment plan, a variety of botanical medicines have been shown to slow the spread of the virus in the body. They can be used to help maintain lower doses of antiretroviral drugs and to help keep the virus from becoming resistant to treatment, Dr. Skowron says.

He uses four botanicals: cordyceps, a Chinese fungus; schisandra, a Chinese berry also known as wo-wei-zi; salvia, a form of sage; and lemon balm. "All of these have strong research supporting their use as antivirals for AIDS," Dr. Skowron says. "We use them in my clinic and I see that they really work."

A usual dose of any of these botanicals is 500 to 1,000 milligrams a day of standardized extract. He starts his patients on two of these drugs, or all four if their viral load is high, and then rotates them from month to month and watches how his patients' symptoms and lab work (CD4 counts) change. "Rotating helps to keep the virus on its toes," he says. Viruses mutate frequently and can become resistant to the drugs—or herbs—being used to knock them out.

Also important: "These herbs do not interact with the antiretroviral drugs people are taking," Dr. Skowron says. (One herb that used to be used in HIV/AIDS, St. John's wort, was found to interfere with the effectiveness of HIV drugs.) Licorice isn't used much anymore as an antiviral, either, since its active ingredients, glycyrrhizin and glycyrrhetinic acid, can cause high blood pressure. (Deglycyrrhized licorice can be used for some things, but it is not effective as an antiviral.)

Milk thistle is another herb on both doctors' lists. It helps to protect and regenerate liver cells so, like NAC, it is especially helpful for patients who have both HIV and hepatitis C. A typical dose is about 1,000 milligrams a day.

Spice Up Immune Support

Both doctors also use curcumin extract, derived from the spice turmeric. Curcumin, an antioxidant, is also antibacterial and will help prevent the many opportunistic illnesses associated with HIV and AIDS, says Dr. Milkis. He prefers to use a form of curcumin that is coupled with phosphatidylcholine, called Meriva-SR Curcumin Phytosome, by Thorne Research. "This form is significantly better absorbed than regular curcumin," Dr. Milkis says.

impotence

If you're like most men, the very word *impotence* suggests a whole range of emotions that you'd rather deny, situations you'd prefer to forget, and issues you'd rather not face. Translated, that means fear, anxiety, and humiliation.

Here's a less loaded term, then: erectile dysfunction (ED). It means the same thing but doesn't have quite the same negative connotation that seemingly threatens the very fabric of manhood.

An estimated 10 to 15 million American men regularly suffer from erectile dysfunction, which is defined as the inability to achieve and maintain an erection long enough to have satisfactory sexual intercourse. Of those men, 15 to 25 percent are over age 65.

The most common cause of erectile dysfunction in men over 50 is clogged arteries in the penis. Frequently, what's behind this clogged-up situation is a buildup of cholesterol and fatty deposits inside artery walls. For other men, there are other possible causes. For those in their teens, twenties, and thirties, stress, depression, anger, fatigue, and performance anxiety are the most common triggers. Among the medical problems associated with erectile dysfunction are diabetes, thyroid problems, stroke, heart disease, and multiple sclerosis.

Otherwise helpful or beneficial medicines can also extract a hidden cost. Sometimes, erection problems are a reaction to blood pressure medications, tranquilizers, antidepressant drugs, or antihistamines.

Because erectile dysfunction could be a side effect of prescription drugs or a symptom of other health problems, see a doctor before you take any nutritional supplement. If you've been having trouble achieving or maintaining an erection for a period of more than 90 days, let your doctor know.

Alternative medicine practitioners believe that there are dietary and other natural measures that men can take to restore the ability to achieve erections. For starters, experts suggest that you get at least 30 minutes of aerobic exercise several days a week. Improving your heart health will boost your sexual virility.

Experts also say that you should eat a healthy-fats diet, including lots of fish, nuts, fruits, vegetables, whole grains, and legumes. Moreover, they say that men who smoke will just have to quit. Puffing just two cigarettes a day causes blood vessels throughout your entire body to constrict, reducing blood flow to the penis.

Alcohol is another roadblock to satisfying sex. Drink no more than two alcoholic beverages a day, says E. Douglas Whitehead, MD, associate clinical professor of urology at Albert Einstein College of Medicine in the Bronx and cofounder and director of the Association for Male Sexual Dysfunction in New York City.

Once you've adopted these changes, some practitioners believe that a combination of nutritional supplements can speed your progress toward sexual health and that certain herbs are potent enough to dramatically increase blood flow to the penis and boost your sex drive, says Thomas Kruzel, ND, a naturopathic doctor in Scottsdale, Arizona. Additionally, some vitamins and minerals provide the building blocks for sexual health.

Use L-Arginine to Restore Flow

This amino acid is a building block for nitric oxide synthase, an enzyme that the body uses to produce nitric oxide, a biochemical that causes the smooth muscles in blood vessels to relax. "The issue with ED is that the smooth muscle tissue doesn't relax, and that means the penis doesn't fill with blood," Dr. Kruzel says. "Viagra does the same thing. It relaxes those muscles and allows everything to fill up."

Research shows that taking high doses, 5 grams daily, of l-arginine improves sexual function in men with ED. Adding 40 milligrams of another supplement, pine bark extract (Pycnogenol,) three times daily may help the lower doses of the amino acid to work even better.

Dr. Kruzel likes to use a timed-release l-arginine product, Perfusia-SR, by Thorne Research. "You can use that every day, and use it long term," he says. If you have herpes, you will need to take lysine along with the arginine, to prevent breakouts. L-arginine is less likely than Viagra to cause low blood pressure when used with nitrites such as nitroglycerin, Dr. Kruzel says, but you will still need to be careful with l-arginine if you take these drugs or have low blood pressure.

Is DHEA for You?

DHEA is a supplement that acts as a hormone precursor. Your body can use it to make all sorts of things: cortisol (a stress hormone), testosterone, and estrogen. You won't want to take DHEA if you don't need it—doing so could cause higher levels of hormones than you need. But if a test shows that you are low—Dr. Kruzel says salivary DHEA testing is best for determining this—you might benefit from getting a little extra DHEA, he says.

Research shows that taking DHEA orally for 24 weeks seems to improve ED, orgasmic function, sexual desire, and overall sexual satisfaction in men with ED. DHEA seems to help men with ED secondary to high blood pressure or unknown causes, but it doesn't seem to improve ED related to diabetes or neurological disorders.

Dr. Kruzel uses saliva levels to figure out dosages for his patients. For men, a standard dose to try might be 25 milligrams a day for 2 to 3 months, followed by retesting to see if that amount is adequate. "That's a fairly safe dose for men," he says. "People do take it without medical supervision, but I would encourage seeing a doctor if you want to take DHEA," he says.

Yohimbine: Charge Up Your Sex Life

For centuries, people have used the bark from yohimbe, a West African tree, to boost sex drive. It contains an active ingredient, called yohimbine, that blocks receptor sites on tissues in the penis that cause restriction, so they allow blood vessels to relax and fill with blood. Experts say that it is better to take a prescription version of yohimbine (brand names include Yocon and Yohimex) than an over-the-counter bark or extract. That's because the prescription versions are purer and have fewer of the side effects sometimes associated with yohimbine, such as anxiety, increased heart rate, and hallucinations. You shouldn't take yohimbine if you have certain health conditions such as high blood pressure or heart disease or take it with certain foods and drugs. Be sure to discuss possible interactions and side effects with your doctor.

Other Herbs to Turn You On

Other herbal supplements are sometimes recommended by naturo-pathic doctors to treat ED. Ginkgo, a medicinal plant, is mainly used to improve blood circulation to the brain. Because it can improve blood flow throughout arteries and veins, it's been successfully used to treat many men whose impotence is caused by poor blood circulation, says Dr. Kruzel. Asian ginseng—also called panax, Korean, or Chinese ginseng—is an herb Dr. Kruzel will use to help men recover from illness such as cancer treatment, or from an injury. It does help restore vitality, boost energy, reduce fatigue, and improve physical performance, and traditionally, it's been used as an aphrodisiac. Research does seem to back up its reputation, showing that it can increase blood flow to the penis, says Dr. Kruzel. But because it is very stimulating, very expensive, and can cause liver damage if taken for a long period of time, Dr. Kruzel prefers Siberian ginseng, and only given during periods of recovery. "It helps ED indirectly by helping the other parts of your body to work better," he says. A typical dose is 15 to 30 milligrams daily, taken for up to 10 weeks. For longer periods of time, see your doctor for guidance.

For Prostate-Related Impotence

In rare cases, an enlarged prostate gland, known as benign prostatic hyperplasia (BPH), causes impotence. Located below the bladder and surrounding the urethra, the prostate gland is normally no bigger than a walnut. At some point in your late forties or fifties, though, it starts growing, and what was once walnut-size can balloon to the size of an orange, causing all sorts of problems.

If you've been diagnosed with BPH and it happens to be causing impotence, the herb horsetail may be what you need, says Dr. Kruzel. Although it hasn't been proven effective in clinical studies, he's seen it work in his practice.

Horsetail's anti-inflammatory properties can shrink the prostate gland to normal size and restore potency in some men, he says. "Horsetail is best used in men over age 60 who have BPH. For them, it can work very well," he comments. Saw palmetto and pygeum are two other herbs that help keep the male reproductive and urinary tract in shape. The amount of horsetail you should take depends on how much your prostate gland has enlarged. After a doctor examines you, he may prescribe a dose ranging from 400 to 800 milligrams of horsetail daily, Dr. Kruzel says.

(Also see Prostate Problems on page 558.)

Zinc and Other Vitamin Basics

The most important nutrient for overall sexual health is zinc. This trace mineral helps to balance levels of different forms of testosterone, the male hormone that's required for sexual development and potency. It also influences sperm motility—that is, the speed and mobility of sperm—which can be a factor in fertility.

Zinc has antibacterial and antiviral properties, says Dr. Kruzel. "The prostate has the highest concentration of zinc of any tissue in the body. It's abundant in semen and in the thin, milky fluid that the prostate gland secretes into the urethra just before ejaculation to prevent infections," he says.

Zinc picolinate, zinc citrate, and zinc monomethionine are the most absorbable forms of zinc. If you're experiencing impotence, Dr. Kruzel says that you can take 15 to 30 milligrams of zinc daily, but he advises that you talk to your doctor if you're considering taking more than 20 milligrams. If you don't see results after 4 to 6 weeks, Dr. Kruzel recommends that you see your doctor for a reevaluation.

He also recommends taking a high-potency multivitamin and mineral supplement in addition to the zinc to help keep your urinary tract in good working order and to lay the foundation for sexual health. "Vitamins C and E are also found in high concentrations in the prostate gland, so they can help speed your recovery from impotence," says Dr. Kruzel. He recommends 2,000 to 4,000 milligrams of vitamin C with meals and 400 to 800 international units of vitamin E daily.

indigestion

Indigestion is a general descriptive term for discomfort in the upper digestive tract. You might have belching and bloating after eating. Your stomach may be distended, and you may feel sick to your stomach or have heartburn. Or maybe you feel like last week's lunch is still sitting in your stomach.

If you have frequent indigestion or if it's causing you a lot of discomfort, you should see a doctor to make sure that you don't have a condition that needs medical attention. You could have gastritis (an inflamed stomach lining) or an ulcer. Or you might have *low* stomach acid, which can delay stomach emptying and promote the growth of inflammation-causing bacteria, such as *Heliobacter pylori,* in the stomach. Most conventional doctors don't even consider the possibility of low stomach acid, says Bernie Noe, ND, a naturopathic doctor in private practice in Montpelier, Vermont. In fact, they are likely to prescribe drugs that decrease stomach acid even more. "This relieves some symptoms, such as heartburn, but does not treat the underlying cause," he says.

It also helps to be tested for food allergies, but most conventional doctors don't do the kind of testing (serum IgG) that checks for delayed food allergies that can cause indigestion and irritable bowel syndrome, Dr. Noe says. "Once people get these foods out of their diets, their symptoms usually improve," he says.

Gluten (wheat protein) intolerance is more common than many people may realize. And bacterial overgrowth of the small intestine can be a real problem for people who've had to take several courses of antibiotics, as can a lack of digestive enzymes. Once those problems are properly addressed, lifestyle changes can help. So can some supplements that aid digestion.

Get Some Hydrochloric Support

Hydrochloric acid is corrosive stuff. Nevertheless, it is one of the most important secretions in the stomach. It helps in the digestion of protein and the absorption of some minerals and vitamins, plus it suppresses bacterial growth in the stomach.

Lack of this stomach acid is officially known as hypochlorhydria, and it's more likely to occur as you age, says Dr. Noe. Without it, you may have an upset stomach, a feeling of fullness, or a sense of discomfort or indigestion. Low stomach acid is also associated with some autoimmune diseases, and sometimes, with gastritis.

You can replace the stomach acid with a supplement called betaine hydrochloride. "I have them do a challenge protocol where they take one capsule with each meal for a day or two, and if that doesn't cause heartburn, then they go up to two capsules. And they just keep increasing the dosage until they feel some warmth or heartburn. Once they get that, I have them back off so that the burning goes away," Dr. Noe says. If you get burning after taking one or two capsules, you probably are making enough stomach acid, or else you have gastritis or some other condition that needs medical attention. "Most people with low stomach acid can take four to six betaine tablets before they feel burning," Dr. Noe says. One tablet has about 650 milligrams of betaine.

Add Pancreatic Enzymes

If indigestion really is your problem, your pancreas may be falling down on the job. It is this organ's duty to supply the digestive enzymes needed to break down fat, protein, and carbohydrates. When it doesn't do that, your food doesn't break down right, so bacteria have a field day in your gut.

It is possible to do a test for pancreatic function, Dr. Noe says. "But often I will just do a trial of pancreatic enzymes if I think that is the problem, based on someone's symptoms," he says. The pancreatic enzymes include lipase, amylase, and protease.

If your symptoms are being caused by low pancreatic enzymes, you will start to feel better as soon as you are getting enough replacement enzymes. Follow the directions on the bottle.

Stimulate Digestion with Bitters

Several herbs known as bitters, including turmeric, gentian, and ginger, are believed to stimulate the release of hydrochloric acid, bile, and gastric juices. "Bitters are really big in Europe for enhancing digestion," says Melissa Metcalfe, ND, a naturopathic doctor in Los Angeles. Most products contain gentian, manna, angelica, zedoary (a form of curcumin), aloe, rhubarb, senna, myrrh, camphor, and valerian. Bitters are designed to be stimulating, so they'll work for you if your digestive enzymes are low.

Out with the Bad Bacteria, in with the Good

Another cause of indigestion may be an overgrowth of yeast, or candida. Candida is a type of naturally occurring yeast that always grows in the gastrointestinal tract as part of what's called the gut's flora, or microorganisms. A bout of illness or a course of antibiotics can wipe out much of the other flora, however, leaving room for candida to thrive, says Dr. Noe. When the normal amount of yeast increases, it may contribute to malabsorption due to the inflammation it causes in the intestine, he says.

One way to help prevent the overgrowth of yeast after a course of antibiotics is to sow more good bacteria, called probiotics, in the gut. You can do that by taking a probiotic supplement. The best ones contain a mix of beneficial bacteria, such as *Lactobacillus acidophilus, Bifidobacterium bifidum,* and *B. longum.* Some also contain prebiotics, soluble fiber that the bacteria can feed on. That helps them to colonize your intestines and continue to multiply.

Look for a product that has several billion colony-forming units (CFU) per capsule and has been refrigerated in the store or is marked "heat-resistant." Commercially available prescription probiotics such as VSL#3 or Flora-Q, which are mixtures of several different bacterial species, are reputable brands that have been used for treating small intestine bacterial overgrowth and irritable bowel syndrome.

infertility

Conception is supposed to be a pretty simple process. The egg leaves the ovary to travel down the fallopian tube on its way to the uterus. Somewhere along the way, it encounters a swarm of sperm. Through sheer diligence, one of the tail-flailing sperm manages to make its way into the egg. The fertilized egg then implants itself into the cushiony, blood-lined wall of the uterus. Nine months later, if all goes well, there's a baby.

It's not that easy, however, for the 5.3 million American women and their partners who try for 12 months or more to initiate this close encounter of the first kind. Often, it's not clear why the initiation ceremony doesn't quite come off. When no cause can be found, some of these people are likely to seek out alternative therapies, says Jennifer Nevels, NMD, a specialist in reproductive health at East Valley Naturopathic Doctors in Mesa, Arizona. "There is a huge percentage of unexplained infertility in this country, and I think a lot of it has to do with chemicals in our environment," she says.

Besides helping people to clean up their diets and lifestyles, she does an environmental exposure assessment, looking at everything from the kinds of fish women are eating (some fish have high levels of mercury) to the types of beauty products they are using (some contain endocrine-disrupting chemicals such as phthalates and parabens). Plastics are a particular concern, she says, since they can contaminate foods with fertility-disrupting chemicals. "Even just switching from a plastic to a stainless steel water bottle can make a difference," she says. She likes women to be on a detoxification and dietary improvement program for 3 to 6 months before they attempt pregnancy.

Prenatal Multivitamins Are a Must

Dr. Nevels also puts her patients on a prenatal vitamin that has at least 800 micrograms of folic acid. "This is important not just to reduce the risk of devastating birth defects of the brain and spinal cord, but also to improve the quality of the egg and the ability of the egg to implant and divide properly," she says. Adequate folic acid and B$_6$ have also been associated with a reduced risk of miscarriage.

Even though folic acid is now added to fortified breads, rice, and cereal, it's not added to whole grains or whole-wheat flour. "So some women who are eating healthier diets by choosing whole grains may actually be getting less folic acid than they think," Dr. Nevels says.

A good prenatal vitamin will also contain antioxidants like vitamins C and E in amounts appropriate for pregnancy, she says.

Get Your Share of the Sunshine Vitamin

One nutrient a prenatal vitamin often does not contain enough of is vitamin D. "Vitamin D is really important. It is often low in women who are having trouble conceiving, and especially in women with polycystic ovary syndrome and ovulation disturbances. It plays a role in development of the uterine lining, which is important for proper egg implantation," Dr. Nevels says. Vitamin D deficiency is also associated with poor immunity, and women with a condition called bacterial vaginosis—a chronic bacterial infection of the vagina that can impair fertility—are often low in D.

Correcting a vitamin D deficiency quickly means taking doses of up to 10,000 IU a day. A dose that large should only be taken with medical supervision, Dr. Nevels says. It's best to get your blood levels of vitamin D to about 55 to 80 ng/ml, then cut back to a dosage that maintains that level, *before* attempting to get pregnant, she says. But the standard dose is 800 IU.

A Berry for Better Birthing

One botanical stands out for improving infertility in women: vitex, also called chasteberry.

Vitex has a long history of use for menstrual irregularities, premenstrual syndrome, and treatment of female infertility. Research suggests that taking vitex can increase the chances of getting pregnant for women who have a progesterone deficiency. It normalizes the luteal phase defects in the menstrual cycle—the part that comes after ovulation. It can restore hormone balance by counteracting estrogen and promoting progesterone levels, Dr. Nevels says, which helps a fertilized egg implant.

But vitex affects a number of hormones and neurotransmitters that may also help fertility, even though experts aren't exactly sure how. "I will use vitex after I have ruled out or treated polycystic ovary syndrome or thyroid problems, because both can cause irregularities in the menstrual cycle," Dr. Nevels says. If you do use vitex, be patient. Research shows that it can take 3 to 7 months of treatment to achieve pregnancy after taking it.

A Prenatal for Men?

Men may also benefit from taking a good multivitamin, says Glenn Finley, ND, a men's health doctor at the Brattleboro Naturopathic Clinic in Vermont. In one study, men who had previously had low fertilization rates were enrolled in an in vitro fertilization program and treated with vitamin E for 3 months. Fertilization rates increased significantly, from 19 percent to 29 percent, after 1 month of treatment with vitamin E. The vitamin improved sperm motility and reduced the number of deformed sperm. The usual dose to improve fertility is 200 to 600 IU a day. (Use d-alpha-tocopherol, not the synthetic vitamin E, dl-alpha-tocopherol.)

Another study showed that 1,000 milligrams a day of supplemental vitamin C improved sperm count by 140 percent. It also helped to keep sperm from clumping together, which impairs their motility. Research has found that when more than 25 percent of sperm are stuck together, the rate of fertility drops dramatically.

Zinc is another good nutrient for men because it can help increase sperm counts and improve sperm motility, Dr. Finley says. Low levels of zinc can decrease production of the male hormone testosterone, which can lead to impaired fertility.

Studies show that most men get between 10 and 15 milligrams of zinc a day, but Dr. Finley recommends anywhere from 20 to 50 milligrams a day, along with copper (1 milligram of copper per 8 milligrams of zinc) for infertile men. With your doctor's okay, you can take this amount until your partner becomes pregnant, or for up to 6 months.

Amino Acids for Men

Most men get all the amino acids they need from proteins in their diet, but men with fertility problems may not get enough. Dr. Finley supplements with the amino acids glycine, alanine, and glutamic acid to improve fertility. Glutamic acid is a precursor to carnitine, and some research indicates that carnitine can help infertility in men who have been taking nonsteroidal anti-inflammatory drugs for conditions related to prostatitis, epididymitis, or other inflammation of the reproductive tract. In one study, men who took 2 grams of L-carnitine and 1 gram of acetyl-L-carnitine a day improved their fertility.

insomnia

Insomnia is something that many of us have experienced at one time or another. Anyone can have a sleepless night or two—or three. Before you reach for that over-the-counter sleeping pill or a prescription-strength remedy, however, consider some dietary and lifestyle changes to help catch up on your rest. Sleep isn't just "downtime," as some of us might like to believe. "I tell my patients, rest is the key to 'restoration'—the healing of the 50-plus trillion cells that comprise the human body," says Chris Meletis, NMD, executive director of The Institute for Healthy Aging in Carson City, Nevada.

It's just common sense to eliminate caffeinated beverages and alcohol from your diet. Caffeine—whether from coffee, tea, or caffeinated soft drinks—is a nervous system stimulant that can keep you up at night. As for alcoholic drinks, they may seem like a shortcut to dreamland, but alcohol actually disrupts the chemical messengers that help initiate sleep. "Alcohol also decreases muscle tone and can worsen snoring and sleep apnea as well, which will contribute to disturbed sleep and decreased quality and depth of restorative sleep," says Dr. Meletis. A full bladder can also disrupt sleep. "I tell people not to drink any liquids for 1 hour or more before bed," he says.

Moderate aerobic exercise, as long as you time it right, is good for improving sleep. Try to get at least 20 minutes of exercise a day in the morning or afternoon, but not right before bedtime. This might be enough to help you quickly fall asleep and stay asleep throughout the night. Some research has found that yoga, for instance, can decrease the amount of time it takes to fall asleep, increase total sleep time, improve feelings of being well rested, and improve other sleep measures. Certain yoga poses are considered calming, while others are energizing, but a good book or a good teacher can help you find poses to aid sleep.

"Great sleep depends on physical and mental fatigue. If the body or mind is not ready for bedtime, sleep will be elusive," Dr. Meletis says. A truly dark room is essential, he adds. "Even the glow of a clock or night light can throw off your natural circadian (sleep-wake) rhythm and alter your body's ability to produce melatonin, the hormone produced by the pineal gland that is crucial for quality sleep."

Sleep apnea, a condition that causes you to stop breathing briefly while you sleep, is also an underlying cause of poor sleep that affects millions of Americans, Dr. Meletis says. "This condition causes underoxygenation of the body as you sleep and can actually trigger a heart attack or stroke while you sleep." If you or one that you love snores, getting screened for sleep apnea is a must. If you still have insomnia after taking these steps, you can try herbal and nutritional supplements. Herbal sedatives naturally calm your nervous system. Some relieve anxiety and serve as mild tranquilizers. Others, like magnesium and calcium, relax tense muscles and stimulate sleep-related brain chemicals. There is also a hormone supplement that works with your body's own natural sleep-wake cycles.

When Stress Makes You Toss and Turn

Lots of people who have trouble sleeping are under stress and, as a result, have unregulated levels of the stress hormone cortisol, says Thomas Kruzel, ND, in private practice at the Rockwood Natural Medicine Clinic in Scottsdale, Arizona. "Instead of rising in the morning, their cortisol levels peak between midnight and 3 a.m.," he says. "That wakes them up and they have trouble falling back to sleep." To check for this problem, he has patients measure their salivary cortisol levels at night.

To "reset" the circuitry that controls this important hormone, Dr. Kruzel uses a supplement called phosphatidylserine. "It resets the hypothalamus-adrenal-pituitary axis and basically dampens that spike in cortisol at night," he says. "If they take 200 milligrams at night, they will sleep through the night."

Relax Your Mind with Melatonin

Melatonin is a supplement with a reputation for aiding sleep, helping people recover more quickly from jet lag, and helping people who do changing shift work to maintain a more normal sleep schedule.

This hormone helps reset your body's internal clock, its circadian rhythm, by acting on the pineal gland, a pea-size gland in your brain that helps control periods of sleepiness and wakefulness. Your pineal gland is sensitive to light and dark, and that's the way it normally sets itself to release melatonin. At night, your body produces more melatonin, while the stimulus of light inhibits production. Between 2:00 and 4:00 a.m., production peaks. Then, toward dawn, it tapers off.

Taking 0.5 to 3 milligrams of melatonin about 45 minutes before you want to go to sleep may help, Dr. Kruzel says. But it doesn't help everyone, he notes. "I live in Arizona now, and I just don't use it much, because it doesn't seem to work here, where most people get plenty of sunshine," he says. "When I lived in Oregon, where there were lots of gray days and some of my insomnia patients had seasonal affective disorder, I used melatonin a lot."

This supplement is for short-term use only. "Although melatonin works very well as a sleep aid, you shouldn't take it indiscriminately," says Dr. Meletis. "Melatonin can interact with some drugs, and it has many other effects on the body. While some may be good, other potential side effects are just plain unknown for long-term use," he says.

5-Hydroxytryptophan (5-HTP)

Since it was introduced to the market, 5-HTP has been called one of the next best alternatives to the hormone supplement melatonin.

This supplement is a precursor to the amino acid tryptophan. Tryptophan is used by your body to make an important neurotransmitter, serotonin. Low levels of serotonin are usually involved in depression, and many antidepressants help serotonin stick around longer in your brain. In some people, depression also brings on bouts of sleeplessness, and this is where 5-HTP can be helpful, Dr. Kruzel says.

Studies show that 5-HTP can shorten the time it takes to nod off and reduce middle-of-the-night awakenings. It is reported to increase the time you spend in REM sleep (the dream state) and in the deep sleep stages that you need to feel fully rested in the morning.

To fall asleep shortly after your head hits the pillow, take 25 to 50 milligrams of 5-HTP 1 hour before bedtime on an empty stomach, or take it at least 2 hours after dinner, says Dr. Meletis.

Even though 5-HTP can help some symptoms of depression, you shouldn't take it if you are taking an antidepressant. That combination could cause dangerously high levels of serotonin. Taking 5-HTP also appears to relieve pain and help people with fibromyalgia sleep better.

Valerian for Steady Sleep

Long before over-the-counter and prescription sleeping pills became available, herbal sedatives were widely used to help people get some slumber. One of nature's more popular herbal sedatives is valerian. Research does show that this herb can allow you to fall asleep faster and have better quality sleep. What's more, you won't wake up as often during the night, nor will you feel fatigued and drowsy in the morning. Valerian's active ingredients, found in the roots, include a group of compounds called valepotriates. Research shows that these components attach to the same brain receptors as two types of pharmaceutical tranquilizers. Unlike the pharmaceuticals, however, valerian produces few side effects, and it doesn't carry the risk of dependency.

"Valerian root is a great herbal sleep aid because it sedates the central nervous system," says Dr. Meletis. It's a good choice if occasional anxiety, muscle tension, or muscle spasms are keeping you awake. A small amount, as recommended by the manufacturer or your health-care provider, may be all you need, he adds. Don't overdo it.

You should avoid valerian if you're taking sleep-enhancing or mood-regulating medications such as diazepam (Valium) or amitriptyline (Elavil).

Magnesium and Calcium: A Snoozer's Duo

If tense muscles are keeping you up, pop some magnesium and calcium. Taken together, these two minerals act as mild muscle relaxants, says Dr. Meletis.

Some research suggests that people who get less than 200 milligrams a day of magnesium can sleep more lightly and have more nighttime awakenings. These patterns of insomnia sometimes show up among people who have reduced their calorie intakes or started on weight-loss diets.

Even if your magnesium intake is normal, certain medications (such as diuretics for high blood pressure, which reduce water retention) cause the kidneys to excrete excessive amounts of the mineral. The Daily Value for magnesium is 400 milligrams from food and supplements, and this amount should be enough to prevent sleep problems. If you still have trouble sleeping, take 500 milligrams of magnesium and 500 milligrams of calcium, along with a carbohydrate like milk, within 1 hour of bedtime, says Dr. Kruzel.

Lavender Can Lull You

Finally, Dr. Kruzel suggests a simple trick to get you to sleep with absolutely no side effects: Spray a little lavender oil on your pillow, or put a few drops of essential oil on a cotton ball and lay it on your pillow. You can also put it in a diffuser or a room humidifier. Research shows that lavender really does have some sleep-promoting properties. It increases slow-wave sleep, the very deep slumber in which the heartbeat slows and muscles relax. In studies, people who've used it report sleeping more soundly and feeling more energetic in the morning. Use a fresh, good-quality essential oil, not lavender perfume.

intermittent claudication

If the arteries in your legs are clogged by cholesterol deposits, chances are good that your legs will eventually seize up when you walk. When your leg muscles don't get enough oxygen-rich blood for the amount of activity they're being asked to do, the result is pain and muscle spasms. That condition is called intermittent claudication.

The pain of intermittent claudication is severe when you walk. In addition, poor circulation in your legs can cause related problems, such as skin breakdown and poor wound healing.

Treatment for intermittent claudication addresses the cause: poor circulation. If you smoke, are overweight, or have high blood pressure or diabetes, you will need to get those conditions under control as well in order to improve leg circulation.

You'll probably need a controlled walking program or some other form of exercise that gradually trains your leg muscles to make the most of their limited oxygen supply. "I also find that older people really benefit from yoga or tai chi for this problem," says Decker Weiss, NMD, director of the Weiss Institute for Naturopathic Excellence in Scottsdale, Arizona, and author of *The Weiss Method: A Natural Program for Reversing Heart Disease and Preventing Heart Attacks*.

In addition, Dr. Weiss and other alternative medicine doctors use herbs and nutritional supplements. If you've been diagnosed with intermittent claudication, talk with your doctor about trying these remedies.

Arginine and Magnesium Can Open Up Arteries

The amino acid arginine is involved in the production of nitric oxide, a chemical released by the cells lining the artery walls. Nitric oxide allows blood vessels to relax and open up, Dr. Weiss says.

A standard dose is 500 milligrams up to three times a day. If you've been infected by the herpes virus, though, you should use arginine only with medical supervision, Dr. Weiss says. "In people harboring the virus, high doses of arginine can cause severe outbreaks."

Along with arginine, Dr. Weiss recommends magnesium, an essential mineral. Magnesium is known for its ability to relax the muscles that wrap around blood vessels, so it can help dilate arteries that have been clogged by cholesterol deposits.

You might have a deficiency of magnesium if you are taking drugs meant to help heart problems, such as diuretics. Some people have deficiencies if they're taking commonly prescribed digitalis heart medications, such as digitoxin. Signs of magnesium deficiency include muscle weakness, nausea, and irritability.

Most people can safely take up to 350 milligrams of supplemental magnesium, Dr. Weiss says. He recommends it in the form of magnesium orotate or glycinate.

B Vitamins Give You a Leg to Stand On

Researchers now realize that an amino acid by-product, homocysteine, can harm the insides of blood vessels, setting the stage for the cholesterol deposits that cause intermittent claudication. In one study, researchers were able to reduce high homocysteine levels using 5 milligrams of folic acid, 400 micrograms of vitamin B_{12}, and 50 milligrams of vitamin B_6. "I recommend these B vitamins to all my patients with heart or circulatory problems as part of a high-potency multivitamin or, if they have absorption problems, as injections or under-the-tongue supplements," Dr. Weiss says. This therapy should be done only under a doctor's supervision, he adds.

Ginkgo Gets You Going

Ginkgo has a reputation for improving circulation in the brain, but it also has bodywide effects that make it useful for all sorts of circulatory problems, including intermittent claudication, Dr. Weiss says. It helps to stimulate the growth of new blood vessels and improves the use of oxygen and blood sugar (glucose), the main form of energy for muscle cells.

Ginkgo also helps to reduce the stickiness of clotting components, called platelets, in the blood. When the platelets become less sticky, harmful clots are less likely to form, especially in areas where blood flow is hindered.

Ginkgo has been tested in several studies of intermittent claudication, and it has worked at least as well as pentoxifylline (Trental), a drug that is commonly prescribed for this problem. Many people in the studies found that they could walk much farther without experiencing pain when they were taking ginkgo. The supplement also improved blood flow to the limbs, which was measured using a noninvasive technique called Doppler ultrasound.

Herbalists often recommend 120 milligrams of ginkgo in divided doses of 40 milligrams three times a day. In some studies, however, people have used 160 milligrams a day with good results.

Dr. Weiss's recommendation is lower. He prefers to use a standardized liquid extract of ginkgo, prescribing 20 drops four times a day for at least 6 months.

Antioxidants Act on Arteries

People with intermittent claudication usually do better in general if they are taking antioxidant nutrients such as vitamins E and C, which may help prevent the early stages of atherosclerosis (hardening of the arteries), Dr. Weiss says.

Vitamin E has a long history of use for intermittent claudication. In one study, conducted in Sweden, researchers found that they could reduce symptoms if they gave people supplementation with 300 international units (IU) a day.

For smokers, however, supplementation with vitamin E doesn't seem to reduce the symptoms of intermittent claudication. It's quite possible that the vitamin can't entirely overcome the harmful effects that smoking has on your circulatory system, Dr. Weiss says. Breaking the habit comes first: Often, when people stop smoking, intermittent claudication disappears with time.

Dr. Weiss gives many of his patients with atherosclerosis 400 to 800 IU of vitamin E and 1,000 to 3,000 grams of vitamin C a day. Vitamin E helps prevent the oxidation of harmful LDL cholesterol, a first step in cholesterol blockage. Vitamin C regenerates vitamin E and also helps the cells lining the blood vessel walls to produce nitric oxide, which keeps blood vessels open and dilated.

For vitamin E, you should use natural d-alpha-tocopherol and mixed tocopherols, says Dr. Weiss.

Take Ginger and Pineapple

"Ginger can be a wonderful addition to a treatment program for intermittent claudication, especially if you also have arthralgia, or pain in your joints," Dr. Weiss says. Like ginkgo, ginger helps keep platelets from getting too sticky, so it keeps your blood flowing smoothly. "It's also a slight vasodilator and a warming herb," Dr. Weiss says, so if you have cold feet, it might provide additional benefits.

Most research studies with ginger use about 1,000 milligrams a day of powdered gingerroot, which is about what you'd get from a ¼-inch slice of fresh root. Ginger is safe to take long-term, Dr. Weiss says.

Another common food—pineapple—also offers some relief in supplement form. The same ingredient in pineapple that prevents gelatin from setting can help the arteries in your legs stay open, Dr. Weiss says. It's an enzyme called bromelain, which helps keep blood from clotting too readily and may also help existing clots dissolve.

"I might use this if someone with circulatory problems also has had clotting problems in their legs, such as thrombophlebitis," Dr. Weiss says. "Since bromelain also helps to reduce inflammation, I find it's good to use after surgery or injuries," he adds.

Take bromelain between meals; otherwise, it will be used up digesting your meal. Common daily doses used in studies range from 60 to 160 milligrams. Dr. Weiss usually recommends much more to his patients—500 milligrams twice a day, for as long as needed. With your doctor's supervision, take note of how your body reacts.

irritable bowel syndrome

In the scary world of intestinal tracts, the most common ghost—unfortunately—is a mysterious disease that travels under the code name IBS. These three sinister initials are shorthand for irritable bowel syndrome, and up to 15 percent of people report that they have it.

People with IBS tend to have alternating constipation and diarrhea, bloating, unformed stools, gas, and sometimes cramps followed by an urgent need to have a bowel movement.

Unfortunately, there is no good way to diagnose IBS, so symptoms that mimic IBS must first be ruled out: infections by parasites, yeast, or pathogenic bacteria; diverticular disease (see Diverticulitis, page 394); inflammatory bowel disease, such as ulcerative colitis or Crohn's; celiac disease; and lactose intolerance.

The good news is that naturopathic medicine has much to offer people with IBS, says Bernie Noe, ND, a naturopathic doctor in private practice in Montpelier, Vermont, who specializes in IBS and other bowel problems.

Check for Food Allergies and Sensitivities

"From my perspective, food allergies or sensitivities are very clearly the number one cause," says Dr. Noe. "Conventional doctors will check for immediate food reactions, but they don't tend to believe that delayed food reactions are the cause of IBS, and they don't do the tests that might detect such allergies," he says.

The test most likely to detect a delayed food allergy is serum IgG, he says. This blood test can easily check about 100 foods. It looks for antigens, which are part of the immune system's response to allergies. High levels mean that you're allergic to a specific food. This takes the guesswork out of figuring out which foods are problems for you. "Once people stop eating their problem foods, their symptoms tend to clear up," Dr. Noe says.

The most common foods that have been linked to IBS are dairy products, wheat products, beans, caffeine, and foods containing fructose or sorbitol, citrus, soy, eggs, and even chocolate, as well as many others.

Rebalance Your Microflora

The *American Journal of Gastroenterology* recently reported that 78 percent of people with IBS have excessive levels of pathogenic bacteria in their lower intestines. These organisms are not the usual ones that conventional doctors might check for, Dr. Noe says. "They tend to cause mild disease and can be there for a long period of time," he says. The most common is yeast overgrowth as a result of antibiotic therapy, but other organisms, such as *Citrobacter freundii* and *Klebsiella oxytoca,* can also cause problems and are not usually detected by conventional doctors, Dr. Noe says.

Stool analysis can tell you if you have a current yeast overgrowth in your bowel and it is the only test that can tell you if you have bacteria or parasites. Sometimes drugs are necessary to knock out these organisms for good, Dr. Noe says. With yeast, for instance, "you need to stop eating all the foods that yeast feeds on," Dr. Noe says. "This includes not just white sugar, but also white flour, most other grains, potatoes, and alcohol," he says. (See Yeast Infections, page 621.)

There are many botanicals used to help treat chronic yeast overgrowth. Some of the more popular are grapefruit seed extract, caprylic acid, oregano oil, garlic, olive leaf extract, pau d'arco, berberine, goldenseal, and Oregon grape. All of these have mild antiyeast properties and may help keep things under control, says Dr. Noe.

Probiotics, the friendly bacteria found in live-culture yogurt, can also help maintain proper microorganism balance in the intestines, especially if they are taken after a course of antibiotics, Dr. Noe says. Strains of bacteria most likely to be beneficial are *Lactobacillus* and *Bifidus*. One prescription brand, VLS#3, has been found to reduce bloating associated with IBS. It contains *Lactobacillus, Bifidus, and Streptococcus* strains of bacteria. If the product you are taking is working right and you are eating right and can avoid antibiotics, you should only need to take it for a few months, Dr. Noe says.

Make Sure You're Digesting Properly

Some people don't have enough digestive enzymes in their GI tract, which allows bacteria to create gas, bloat, methane, and sulfur—gases that come out as off-putting, to say the least.

To treat this problem, Dr. Noe may use a product called betaine hydrochloride to replace digestive enzymes. With this supplement, he has patients do a challenge protocol where they take one capsule with each meal for a day or two, and if that doesn't cause heartburn, then they increase it to two tablets, and keep increasing the dosage by one a day until they feel some warmth or heartburn. Once they get that, he has them back off so that the burning goes away. "Most people with low stomach acid can take four to six betaine tablets before they feel burning," he says. One tablet has about 650 milligrams of betaine.

An inability to digest foods may also mean that you're not secreting adequate amounts of pancreatic enzymes, which are needed to break down fat, protein, and carbohydrates. When this vital organ isn't doing its job right, bacteria in your gut have a picnic, and in the process, they create gas and toxins.

It is possible to do a test for pancreatic function, Dr. Noe says. "But often I will just do a trial of pancreatic enzymes if I think that is the problem, based on someone's symptoms," he says. The pancreatic enzymes include lipase, amylase, and protease.

If your symptoms are being caused by low pancreatic enzymes, you'll feel better as soon as you are getting enough replacement enzymes.

What about Fiber?

Getting enough fiber is often recommended as helpful for IBS. "I will definitely use it if constipation is a symptom," Dr. Noe says. "But it can be hit or miss if someone with IBS doesn't have constipation."

For constipation, try foods like prunes, oat bran, beans, and carrots. A popular fiber supplement is ground psyllium seed, a nontoxic bulk laxative sold as Metamucil or Konsyl. You can take as much as you need to have regular bowel movements and to feel like your colon has emptied completely. A usual dose to achieve that is 1 tablespoon, twice a day, with 8 ounces of water. Drinking eight glasses of water a day is important if you take a water-soluble fiber supplement, and it can help relieve constipation on its own, too.

Dr. Noe also likes to use prebiotics, the fibers that probiotics feed on. Prebiotics help to establish long-term colonies of healthy bacteria in the intestines. One popular prebiotic is inulin, made from chicory, which promotes the growth of *Bifidus*. It's added to some yogurts and some probiotics, and it's available separately as an over-the-counter supplement. Take 1 teaspoon daily.

Herbal Remedies Can Relieve Symptoms

Herbs can help relieve some symptoms of IBS. Peppermint, for instance, can inhibit colon contractions and spasms, and also relieves gas. It's important to take enteric-coated peppermint capsules or tablets. The coating releases the peppermint only after it enters the small intestine. Regular peppermint and peppermint tea can increase symptoms of heartburn because they relax the upper sphincter muscle in your stomach, and that muscle is what prevents the contents of your stomach from entering your esophagus.

Chamomile tea is also helpful for relieving overactivity in the GI tract, Dr. Noe says, as are fennel seed, ginger root, valerian, and lemon balm.

Soothe Your Guts

For mild inflammation in the GI tract, which may come from bacterial overgrowth or food allergies, Dr. Noe suggests a demulcent, an herb that coats and soothes the tissues lining the gut. Slippery elm, aloe vera gel, marshmallow root, and deglycyrrhizinated licorice are all demulcents that can soothe IBS. Just follow the product directions.

kidney stones

The pain of passing a kidney stone has been compared to the pain of childbirth. With childbirth, there's a sweet reward. With a kidney stone, there's nothing but the production of a granular object.

Men are more likely than women to get kidney stones (sometimes called calcium stones), and genes play a role as well. Because of that genetic factor, if your parents or grandparents had kidney stones, you're at higher risk for getting them yourself.

Some people have a tendency to excrete high levels of calcium oxalate and calcium phosphate. If all goes well, you get rid of these calcium salts every time you urinate. Sometimes, however, the salts hang around the kidneys like bad leftovers. Eighty percent of all kidney stones are composed of these calcium salts.

But a small percentage of stones are formed from uric acid crystals, the same stuff that causes gout, and some are composed of cystine. Try to find out what kind of stones you're prone to; it will make a difference in what you need to do to prevent future episodes. Some drugs also increase the risk for kidney stones, including certain diuretics like calcitriol and probenecid.

Diet is important if you're trying to avoid kidney stones. If your stones are formed from calcium oxalate, stay away from foods such as spinach, beans, parsley, tea, and coffee. Although some of these items are thought of as healthy foods, they are rich in oxalates and may contribute to stone formation, says Anne McClenon, ND, a naturopathic doctor at the Compass Family Health Center in Plymouth, Massachusetts. If you have a problem turning oxalates into a form that your body can use, they remain in your urine. "They may precipitate as a stone," she says.

Kidney stones can't be ignored, and there's no way to treat them yourself. If you have a stone, you may have severe pain, blood in your urine, and a fever. Any of these symptoms should tell you to see a doctor as soon as possible. "It can be a medical emergency. The pain can be excruciating," says Dr. McClenon.

Sometimes, a small stone will pass on its own—with that childbirth-type pain mentioned earlier. If you have a stone that's too big to pass, your doctor will probably recommend an ultrasound procedure that breaks it up without surgery.

There are a few strategies and supplements that might help you avoid forming another kidney stone from calcium salts. First, however, you should see your doctor and have a blood test and chemical analysis of your urine and stones to determine if calcium is really your problem. Other types of stones can form because of a urinary tract infection, gout, or a hereditary kidney disorder. For example, if you tend to form uric acid or cystine stones, you should follow an antigout diet that's low in purine-containing foods and alcohol. (See Gout, page 422.)

If you're prone to getting calcium stones, here are some tactics and supplements to help prevent them.

Drink Up

Water, that is. It's a simple bit of advice, but it makes a lot of sense when you consider that stones come from dissolved solids, says Leon Hecht, ND, a naturopathic doctor at North Coast Family Health in Portsmouth, New Hampshire.

The reason for this advice is similar to the rationale behind adding more and more water to soup that's too salty. The objective is to keep the saltwater solution in the kidneys extremely diluted so that a concentration of stone-forming salts doesn't get stuck there. Water causes the concentration of chemicals in the urine to decrease, making them more soluble and less likely to form stones.

Drink at least eight to 10 full 12-ounce glasses of water each day. Don't drink juice or soda or milk—just water, says Dr. Hecht. (Salt and sugar can raise the level of calcium in your urine.) "You should drink enough so that you're urinating every couple of hours," he adds.

Stonewall with Magnesium

Having high levels of calcium oxalate and calcium phosphate in your urine isn't a problem as long at you excrete those salts. For that to happen efficiently, they need to hook up with other essential chemicals in the urine.

Otherwise, they'll clump together, form crystals, and precipitate out like sugar settling to the bottom of a glass of iced tea.

That's where magnesium comes in. It binds with the calcium salts so they stay dissolved in the urine.

Magnesium is a regulator of calcium, says Michael Gazsi, ND, a naturopathic doctor in private practice in Danbury, Connecticut. "You excrete it rather than having it settle out in the kidney," he explains. "If you keep the magnesium ratio in the urine high, there's less chance of forming a stone."

If you have a predisposition to calcium stones, Dr. Gazsi suggests that you take 500 milligrams of magnesium a day. The most absorbable forms, which are least likely to cause diarrhea at higher levels, are magnesium chelates such as citrate, glycinate, or malate. "Taking magnesium is the single best thing you can do to prevent these types of stones," Dr. Gazsi says.

B$_6$ Boosts Protection

For added insurance, you can take a vitamin B$_6$ supplement, since B$_6$ reduces the production of oxalate, says Dr. Hecht.

He recommends taking 25 to 50 milligrams of vitamin B$_6$ daily along with a magnesium supplement. "Magnesium alone decreases the likelihood of kidney stones, but when you put it with vitamin B$_6$, it has an even greater effect," he says.

leg cramps

Baseball players coined the term *charley horse* more than 100 years ago to describe the cramps they got in their tired, overworked leg muscles.

Whether you're running the bases or lying in bed, nerves send signals to the muscles to tell them when to contract and relax. When these signals get scrambled, the muscle responds by cramping.

What mixes up the messages? The first suspected cause is a mineral imbalance, says Jacqueline Jacques, ND, a naturopathic doctor and specialist in pain management in Portland, Oregon. That's not the only possibility, though. Cramps can also be caused by strenuous exercise, dehydration, and excess salt loss from sweating. Even sitting or standing too long can bring on leg cramps.

When you get a cramp, stretch and gently massage the muscle immediately. This should relax the muscle and provide you with some much-needed relief. If you find that you're having muscle cramps every night, your doctor might prescribe quinine, but only for a limited time. This often-used treatment for leg cramps can quickly build to toxic levels in the blood and can cause nausea, vomiting, ringing in the ears (tinnitus), and deafness. It can even damage your eyesight.

A safer way to eliminate that knot of pain in your muscles is to try a combination of vitamin, mineral, and herbal supplements, say natural healers. (See also Muscle Soreness, page 520, and Restless Legs Syndrome, page 566.)

A Trio of Supplements for Nighttime Cramps

If you're getting a nightly wake-up call from your leg muscles, you probably need to get more magnesium and calcium, says Mark Stengler, ND, a naturopathic doctor in Beaverton, Oregon, and author of *The Natural Physician: Your Health Guide for Common Ailments*. Both of these minerals are involved in relaxing nerve impulses and regulating muscle activity. Calcium is needed to contract the muscle, and magnesium is needed to relax it. An imbalance in this dynamic duo can irritate and confuse the muscle.

Since the calcium in bone provides a nearly inexhaustible mineral supply to replenish the relatively tiny amount that you need in your blood, you're more likely to be low on magnesium, says Dr. Jacques. If you're like most people, you probably get only 75 percent of the Daily Value (DV) for magnesium, which is 400 milligrams from food and supplements.

Mix In Magnesium

Start with a dose of 250 milligrams of magnesium glycinate or chelated magnesium twice a day, says Dr. Jacques. These amino acid–based mineral supplements are easier to absorb than magnesium oxide. The more you absorb, the less likely it is that you'll have diarrhea, a common problem with magnesium supplements.

To help relieve cramps that interrupt your nightly Zzzs, take your second dose of magnesium right before you go to bed. If you don't get relief in 3 to 5 days, increase the dose to 500 milligrams twice a day, says Dr. Jacques. Stay at that level for another week to allow the tissue levels of the mineral to build up.

A Time for Calcium

If cramps are still a problem at that dosage, it's time to add 500 milligrams of calcium to the regimen. The average adult absorbs only about 30 percent of the calcium consumed.

To maximize absorption, Dr. Jacques gives her patients calcium citrate instead of calcium carbonate, the form commonly found in antacid tablets.

Make sure you're also getting enough vitamin D, since this nutrient is essential to ensure that calcium and magnesium are available to be used by your body. Most people don't get optimal amounts of vitamin D, and experts are now recommending 1,000 to 2,000 IU a day or more. Ask your doctor to help you determine a dose of vitamin D that will keep your blood levels above 50 ng/ml year-round, recommends John Cannell, MD, director of the Vitamin D Council.

If you're taking both calcium and magnesium, keep in mind that they work best when they are taken in certain ratios. The two ratios recommended by naturopathic doctors are either equal doses of calcium and magnesium or twice as much calcium as magnesium. "A lot of it is a guessing game, particularly with something like leg cramps," says Dr. Jacques. "You have to find out what ratio works best for you."

Try the 1:1 ratio first, taking 500 milligrams of calcium and 500 milligrams of magnesium twice a day, Dr. Jacques says. If that doesn't give you the results you want, shift to a 2:1 ratio by reducing the magnesium to 250 milligrams.

The E Potential

Some patients with nighttime cramping have success with vitamin E, says Dr. Stengler. Although it has had mixed results in clinical trials, early studies suggest that you'll improve arterial blood flow and reduce leg cramping at night if you take vitamin E.

In one of the largest studies, 123 of 125 people who suffered from nighttime leg and foot cramps reported complete relief after taking vitamin E supplements. To see if it works for you, take 400 to 800 international units (IU) a day of natural vitamin E, d-alpha tocopherol, says Dr. Jacques. To boost vitamin E naturally (and deliciously), eat a handful of walnuts every day.

Are You Lacking Potassium?

Potassium is another mineral that helps regulate muscle contraction, says Dr. Stengler. Deficiencies of this crucial electrolyte aren't normally a problem if you eat a variety of fruits and vegetables. If you change your diet drastically, however, you might become deficient. This is a potential problem if you are on one of the high-protein weight-loss diets that some experts advocate.

"When people go on high-protein diets, they begin to develop leg cramps. I see it repeatedly," says Dr. Jacques. She believes that such diets are related to potassium deficiency. (They can also be related to dehydration, since people lose lots of early water weight with these sorts of diets.)

When protein makes up more than 30 percent of your daily calories, potassium levels may fall far short of the DV of 3,500 milligrams, according to Dr. Jacques. If you're eating eight or nine servings of fruits and vegetables, you'll get enough potassium to meet the DV, but the shift to a high-protein diet makes this significantly more of a challenge.

Cramps are more prevalent when you first start a high-protein diet, Dr. Jacques has observed. After a few months, they normally disappear on their own. Don't bother trying to relieve them with over-the-counter potassium supplements. By law, supplements can't contain more than 99 milligrams per tablet—about the amount in a bite or two of banana. The banana tastes better.

If you are taking diuretics, which can deplete potassium, magnesium, and other minerals, tell your doctor about your leg cramps and ask her to check your potassium levels. Don't take extra potassium without clearing it with your doctor first.

Little Players That Loosen Your Legs

When you get leg cramps, the first suspects are naturally the big minerals that we've already discussed—calcium, magnesium, and potassium. But maybe those cramps are due to an imbalance of trace minerals, especially if the pain is triggered by overexertion, says Dr. Jacques. "Muscle and nerve function are electrical, and we need the right mix of minerals for that to happen. There are a lot of little players in there."

You can deplete levels of trace minerals as you perspire. The best way to restore trace minerals is with a varied diet that includes lots of seeds, nuts, root vegetables, dark leafy greens, and even herbs like parsley and spices like cinnamon. You can also take a trace mineral supplement that contains copper, manganese, zinc, selenium, and chromium, says Dr. Jacques.

Evie Katahdin, ND, a naturopathic doctor specializing in sports medicine at AthletiZen, in Costa Mesa, California, likes to use Spaz-Out by Metabolic Maintenance. It has calcium, magnesium, potassium, and vitamin C, plus some trace minerals required for energy metabolism in muscle cells.

Although trace mineral supplements vary in content, don't exceed the dosage guidelines on whatever product you choose. "Trace" means a little goes a long way, so you do not want to go overboard.

If you get leg cramps when you walk, see your doctor to rule out other conditions such as intermittent claudication, which is caused by poor blood flow to the legs.

Soothing Spasms

Herbal extracts offer a natural way to soothe and relax spastic muscles. One of the most valuable is black cohosh, says Dr. Stengler. Also known as black snakeroot and bugbane, black cohosh root contains active substances called triterpene glycosides, antispasmodics that act as natural muscle relaxants.

When muscles seize up with pain, take a 500-milligram capsule of the root powder or 30 to 60 drops of a tincture in warm water every 1 to 2 hours.

For acute cramps, two or three doses should be sufficient for a therapeutic effect, says Dr. Stengler. Don't use black cohosh during pregnancy, though, or for more than 6 months at a time.

Bilberry contains chemicals called anthocyanins, a type of flavonoids that have muscle-relaxant properties. Bilberry also helps to improve circulation in the extremities. To reduce muscle cramping, take 80 milligrams three times a day of an extract standardized to contain 25 percent anthocyanidin. You should take it for at least a couple of months, but you can continue indefinitely if necessary, says Dr. Stengler.

"Ginkgo is also useful, since it improves circulation through the extremities by dilating the arteries that feed the leg tissue," he says. While cramps are a problem, Dr. Stengler gives patients 60 milligrams three times a day of an extract containing 24 percent ginkgoflavonglycosides and 6 percent terpene lactones. If you have circulation problems, you can probably use ginkgo on a long-term basis.

lupus (SLE)

A painful and potentially life-threatening illness, lupus occurs when your immune system turns renegade and attacks your body's own tissues, causing inflammation and damage. The skin, kidneys, blood vessels, eyes, lungs, nerves, joints—just about any part of the body—can be involved. At the same time, your immune system sometimes ignores its normal duties of fighting infection, so you end up being prone to all sorts of illnesses.

The exact causes of lupus aren't known for sure, but research has shown that genetic and environmental factors are involved. There is no cure. Conventional treatment generally involves controlling the symptoms with drugs, including anti-inflammatories such as ibuprofen, analgesics such as acetaminophen, and corticosteroids (hormones) such as prednisone. Some people are also treated with immune suppressants—that is, medications that suppress the action of the immune system.

Alternative practitioners believe that their treatments can reduce inflammation, increase the body's production of certain hormones, and strengthen immunity. Naturopathic doctors may also treat what they think are possible underlying causes of lupus. They believe that diseases of this kind, called autoimmune diseases, may be associated with environmental toxin exposure, digestion problems, food allergies, and weakness of the adrenal glands.

A naturopathic doctor will usually do tests to determine whether any of these underlying problems exist, says Jody Noe, ND, a faculty member at the University of Bridgeport College of Naturopathic Medicine and in private practice at Natural Family Health and Integrative Medicine, in Westerly, Rhode Island. Once the possible causes are identified, there are a number of alternative treatments that may help.

"It's important to try to figure out the cause of this disorder," she says, "and to work out a treatment plan based on each person's symptoms." Supplements often play a role in alternative treatments, but you should get your doctor's approval before taking supplements to treat lupus. You'll also need to consult a holistic physician or naturopath to determine the dosages best suited to you.

Knocking Out Free Radicals

When inflammation occurs, the body produces more free radicals, the unstable molecules that can harm cells. One of the first lines of defense that a naturopathic doctor uses against inflammation is extra amounts of nutrients that neutralize the free radicals. These nutrients, called antioxidants, are vitamins E and C, beta-carotene, and selenium. They also include zinc, which has antioxidant activity, and phytochemicals such as bioflavonoids, which are found in plants and herbs, Dr. Noe says.

Dr. Noe recommends that her patients take a mixture of antioxidant nutrients daily with food, as part of a good multivitamin/mineral supplement. She suggests 1,000 to 3,000 milligrams of vitamin C in divided doses, 400 to 600 international units (IU) of vitamin E, 200 to 400 micrograms of selenium, and 15 to 30 milligrams of zinc in the form of zinc picolinate or citrate.

She also recommends 1 or 2 milligrams a day of copper and 5 to 15 milligrams of manganese. Both help the body make its own antioxidants. These trace minerals should be taken only in these recommended doses to avoid getting toxic amounts.

Essential Fatty Acids Fight Inflammation

You can reduce levels of inflammation-generating biochemicals in your body by changing the kinds of fats you eat, Dr. Noe says. Meat and other animal products provide your body with something called arachidonic acid, which is used to make pro-inflammatory biochemicals. On the other hand, fish oils, which contain eicosapentaenoic acid (EPA) and docosahexaenoic acid (DHA), and certain plant oils, which contain gamma-linolenic acid (GLA), follow a biochemical pathway that reduces production of these biochemicals.

In studies of animals that spontaneously develop a lupuslike syndrome, diets high in fish oil reduced inflammation and improved kidney function and immunity.

One study found that people with the most common type of lupus showed a reduction in free radical chemical "markers" and increased amounts of antioxidants in their blood after undergoing therapy with the omega-3 fatty acids EPA and DHA. Researchers surmise that fish oil, which is high in omega-3s, might be helpful for people with lupus. Other research shows that people with impaired kidney function, a side effect of lupus, who get high-dose omega-3s experience less of a decline in function than people not getting these oils.

"In my practice, I've seen that most people with an autoimmune disease benefit from getting omega-3 fatty acids," Dr. Noe says. "These oils are good for everyone with chronic inflammation."

Dr. Noe recommends that people with lupus take 1,500 to 2,000 milligrams a day of EPA and 500 to 700 milligrams a day of DHA. Get these from a good, pharmaceutical-grade fish oil, such as Nordic Naturals. "Fish oil really is the best because your body does not have to convert the fat to EPA or DHA," she says. "The oil is already in a form your body can use."

Make Sure You're Getting Enough Vitamin D

Since sun exposure can inflame the skin of people with lupus, those who have it often avoid the great yellow orb in the sky. But they do need something the sun provides—vitamin D. Many people with this condition have been found to be severely deficient in this vitamin.

Now, though, researchers are finding out that vitamin D is more important than ever for people with lupus and that they may need to be taking a lot more than was previously recommended.

Research has found that vitamin D deficiency may actually induce some of the immune problems associated with autoimmune diseases like lupus, rheumatoid arthritis, multiple sclerosis, scleroderma, and others. In animals, adding vitamin D reverses immunologic abnormalities characteristic of lupus.

"Recommendations for dosages of vitamin D have really increased," Dr. Noe says. The new standard recommendation for vitamin D is 800 IU daily. If you feel like that isn't working, you can ask your doctor to test your vitamin D blood levels. "I like to see blood levels of vitamin D (25-hydroxy vitamin D) at least 50 ng/ml, and even up to 100 ng/ml," she says. Work with your doctor to determine what dose would help you reach those levels. "I'd rather see people take a smaller daily dose than a large weekly dose," says Dr. Noe. (Some experts think taking one large weekly dose can interfere with parathyroid hormone function. These glands regulate calcium levels in the body.)

DHEA—And What Sex Has to Do with It

Lupus is influenced by hormone fluctuations in the body. In some people, an imbalance of the estrogenic (female) and androgenic (male) hormones can make lupus symptoms worse. While scientists don't quite understand why this happens, they do have some clues, says Philip Mease, MD, a rheumatologist at Minor and James Medical Center and clinical associate professor of medicine at the University of Washington Medical School, both in Seattle. Lupus may first appear during pregnancy, for instance, when there are changes in the hormone balance, according to Dr. Mease. Stress can also precipitate an outbreak, Dr. Noe says.

Animal studies also indicate a link between the balance of male and female hormones and lupus. Female mice with lupus tend to have more severe symptoms than male mice do, according to Dr. Mease. Scientists found that the female mice's symptoms improved considerably when they were given male hormones.

In two studies at Stanford University Medical Center, researchers looked closely at the effects of DHEA to find out whether it could be helpful in treating lupus. DHEA—short for dehydroepiandrosterone—is a hormone that sets off a chain reaction when it arrives in certain tissues. At the end of that chain reaction, the body produces sex hormones—either testosterone (in male organs) or estrogen (in female organs). Thus, when taken as a supplement, DHEA leads to increased production of sex hormones.

The Hormone in Action

One study of DHEA involved 28 women who had mild to moderate lupus. Most of the participants were already taking doses of prednisone, a corticosteroid drug, to relieve their symptoms. Fourteen of the women were given pills that contained 200 milligrams of DHEA. The other 14 took pills that looked exactly the same but were inactive (placebos). At the end of a 3-month trial period, the women who were receiving DHEA showed a marked improvement and were able to reduce their dosages of the prednisone. Women in the placebo group showed little improvement.

In another study, 10 women with lupus were given 200 milligrams of DHEA for 3 to 6 months. Three of the women had protein in their urine, which is a sign of kidney damage resulting from lupus. At the end of the trial period, 8 of the 10 women felt that their overall well-being had improved, and those with signs of kidney damage had less protein in their urine, indicating that they were getting some protection.

Two hundred milligrams is a large dose for women, Dr. Noe says, and adds that it can cause side effects, such as acne and facial hair growth. Also, the side effects of taking a large dose for a long time are not known. Although these large amounts have been used in some research studies, you should not take a dose this large without knowledgeable medical supervision, and even then, not for more than a few weeks before cutting back to a much smaller maintenance dose. Some doctors recommend that even a maintenance dose of 20 milligrams once or twice a day should be medically monitored. It's best to take DHEA only with knowledgeable medical guidance.

DHEA is available over-the-counter. Many naturopathic doctors prefer an under-the-tongue form of DHEA, which seems to break down and be absorbed faster. You mix it with saliva for about 20 seconds, and then swallow it. Fifteen to 20 milligrams of DHEA twice a day will replace physiologic levels in women. Lower doses may be helpful with a comprehensive nutritional program, but again: Take DHEA only under a doctor's care.

"People who need to take corticosteroid drugs, namely prednisone, to control their symptoms can usually reduce their drug dosage if they take DHEA," Dr. Mease says. Being able to reduce the dosage of steroid drugs is a benefit because these drugs cause bone loss, suppress immunity, and have other side effects, he adds.

Support Your Adrenal Glands

Low DHEA is often one early sign of exhausted adrenal glands, Dr. Noe says. Long-term chronic stress can lead to high, then, over time, low levels of the hormones that help the body react to stress. If saliva tests show low DHEA, Dr. Noe will also offer herbs and nutrients that help the adrenal glands recover. These include an Ayurvedic (Indian) herb, ashwagandha. "This herb is an adrenal tonic, anti-inflammatory, and has secondary effects that influence the thyroid gland, so if you have Hashimoto's thyroiditis, ashwagandha would work really well for that," Dr. Noe says. It also seems to have a good safety profile.

Nettle is another reliable old standby, she says. "It's anti-inflammatory and can stabilize mast cells (which cause allergic reactions) and, if you eat it, you get all kinds of good nutrients, including trace minerals like silica, zinc, and manganese," she says.

Licorice root is the classic adrenal support herb because it helps to keep cortisol from breaking down and, in doing so, allows the adrenal gland a "break" at producing more of it. But because it has a number of potential side effects, especially high blood pressure, it is best used with knowledgeable medical supervision. One cup a day of pure licorice tea or about 200 milligrams of licorice root extract may be all you need and is a fairly low, safe dose for people with normal or low blood pressure.

Plugging a Leaky Gut

Some alternative doctors and practitioners who have studied cases of autoimmune diseases, especially certain types of arthritis, believe that these conditions might be associated with a special kind of intestinal problem. They call the condition increased permeability or, more commonly, leaky gut.

The theory proposes that if the walls of the intestines are leaky, molecules derived from incompletely digested foods or from bacteria are able to seep through the intestinal lining and get into the bloodstream. There, they set off an immune response that can result in immune cells going haywire, ultimately triggering attacks on the body's own cells. Whether or not this happens in some cases of lupus isn't certain, says Dr. Noe. "Autoimmune diseases probably have a variety of causes, and leaky gut is just one of them," she says.

Tests are available that some experts claim can detect a leaky gut. Dr. Noe says that she orders certain blood, urine, and saliva tests to reveal whether someone is having an immune reaction that could cause lupus. Among the tests that she might order are tests for antinuclear antibodies (ANA) and other antibody tests that indicate that your body is attacking itself; C-reactive protein; a 24-hour urine test to measure for protein and cell casts normally filtered out by the kidneys; and saliva tests for cortisol and other hormones, which may help to determine your course of treatment. The Lupus Foundation of America Web site has a good list of tests your doctor may do. (See www.lupus.org.)

Nutrients to Restore Bowel Health

In addition to eliminating foods identified as contributing to the problem, such as wheat gluten, corn, and dairy products, Dr. Noe recommends nutritional supplements that nourish and rebuild the intestinal lining and restore good bacteria to the bowel. If there are enough good bacteria there, they will crowd out the bad types that can contribute to digestive problems.

"I also may recommend enzymes that help break down food for proper digestion if tests suggest that someone's pancreas is not producing enough for normal digestion," she says. The following supplements are among those that Dr. Noe recommends.

- 500 to 750 milligrams of the amino acid glutamine
- 100 to 300 milligrams of gamma oryzanol, a component of rice bran oil
- 50 to 150 milligrams of butyrate
- 50 to 100 milligrams of fructooligosaccharides (FOS), naturally occurring sugars that promote the growth of friendly bacteria in the intestines

She suggests taking all of these two or three times a day between meals. She notes that these substances are safe to take on a continuous basis as long as you remain under a doctor's supervision while taking them.

All of these supplements except FOS are broken-down forms of amino acids, fats, or sugars that can be absorbed directly by the intestinal cells, bypassing digestion. FOS promotes more friendly flora by providing food for intestinal bacteria. Although there are no studies to show that supplements are effective for lupus, some alternative doctors use them in an attempt to decrease intestinal permeability.

To restore friendly bacteria and improve digestion, Dr. Noe suggests the following supplements.

- One or two capsules two or three times a day of a product that contains various forms of lactobacillus and other so-called friendly bacteria—*Lactobacillus acidophilus, L. rhamnosus, L. casei, L. plantarum, Bifidobacterium bifidum, B. longum,* and *B. breve*—with 2 to 5 billion active organisms in each capsule. (If you can't find some of these bacteria in supplements at a health food store, you may need to ask a naturopathic or holistic doctor to get them for you.)

• 500 to 1,000 milligrams of 10X USP of digestive enzymes. (10X USP is a measure of strength and is listed on the bottle.)

• A mixture of other enzymes derived from plants, including 12,500 to 18,000 USP of protease, 2,675 USP of lipase, 12,000 to 27,000 USP of amylase, and 175 CU(2) of cellulase.

Dr. Noe says that these supplements are safe to take on a continuous basis as long as you get your doctor's approval to take them and remain under medical supervision.

Indian Spice Eases Aches

Turmeric, an Indian spice used in traditional Ayurvedic medicine, contains an anti-inflammatory and antioxidant compound called curcumin that might be helpful for people with conditions, such as lupus, that involve inflammation, says Andrew Rubman, ND, director of the Southbury Clinic for Traditional Medicine in Connecticut and consultant to the Office of Complementary and Alternative Medicine at the National Institutes of Health.

"In animals, curcumin has excellent anti-inflammatory and antioxidant effects, without any toxicity," Dr. Rubman says. When curcumin is present, the body is much less likely to form the compounds that are instrumental in causing inflammation, he explains. "Plus," he adds, "it may stimulate the body's own anti-inflammatory mechanisms by interacting with the adrenal glands and preventing the breakdown of cortisone in the body." Indeed, research is proving that curcumin has powerful anti-inflammatory properties.

The problem with curcumin, even as a concentrate or extract, is that it can be hard for your body to absorb enough to do any good. In traditional Indian cooking, it's mixed with oil and heated up before other foods are added to a dish, and this can improve its absorption.

There is also a new liposomal form of curcumin, usually just labeled liposomal curcumin or phytosome curcumin, that is much more absorbable than the traditionally used form. There are several brands on the market. Just follow the label directions to determine the correct dosage.

macular degeneration

What would life be like if you had macular degeneration? Well, for one thing, reading these words would be difficult or even impossible, because macular degeneration affects the macula, a tiny part of the back wall of the eye that's responsible for clear straight-ahead vision.

Loss of sight due to this disease affects more than 1.5 million Americans. Officially, it's called age-related macular degeneration (AMD) because your risk for developing macular degeneration rises substantially after your 60th birthday. In fact, it is the number one cause of blindness in people age 60 and older. Smoking and poorly controlled diabetes are the other two top reasons for AMD.

One form of the disease, known as wet macular degeneration, makes vision deteriorate rapidly because tiny, delicate blood vessels start to grow under the macula, all the while leaking blood and fluid. For some lucky people with this type, laser treatment can destroy the new blood vessels. They won't recover the vision they've lost, but at least the deterioration won't get any worse.

The dry form is more common, affecting 90 percent of those with macular degeneration. In this type, light-sensing cells in the eye are slowly broken down. Scientists still don't know what causes this breakdown, although the free-roaming, unstable molecules called free radicals are partially to blame. There's a lot of chemical activity among oxygen molecules in the eye, and wherever those oxidative processes occur, cells are damaged by free radical action.

Even though sight loss is slower with the dry type than with the wet type, it seems to be an irreversible process. As of now, there's no medical treatment that can help.

Supplements may help slow the progression of AMD. Research suggests that taking a number of vitamins, minerals, and other nutrients can help. They include beta-carotene; DHA (a component of fish oil); folic acid;

Bilberry for Night Blindness

Macular degeneration isn't the only eye problem that can alter your vision for the worse. If you find that your day vision is about the same but you're having more trouble seeing at night, you may have a condition that's called, logically, night blindness.

As the name suggests, night blindness primarily affects vision in low-light situations. When you're driving after dark, for instance, you may find that you're momentarily blinded by the glare from headlights, or you may find that your eyes are slow to adjust when you move from a brightly lit room into a dim one.

Blame these difficulties on a chemical called rhodopsin. Produced in the rods of the eye—the photoreceptors that help us see in low light—rhodopsin is necessary for distinguishing things that are poorly lit. If you lack rhodopsin, your night sight will be less than perfect.

As the story goes, British pilots during World War II began eating bilberry jam—made from a type of northern European blueberry—to help counteract night blindness. Searching for the active component in these dark berries, scientists found chemical substances called anthocyanins. "Blueberries, elderberries, huckleberries, and red grapes also contain this pigment," says Robert Abel Jr., MD, clinical professor of ophthalmology at Thomas Jefferson University in Philadelphia and author of *The Eye Care Revolution.* In the body, Dr. Abel says, anthocyanins benefit the eyes by converting to rhodopsin.

You probably won't be able to find bilberries or bilberry jam in your local supermarket. You should be able to locate bilberry capsules at your local health food store or drugstore, though. Take 100 to 500 milligrams of bilberry twice a day. "Try it right before you go out at night," says Dr. Abel. "You should notice an effect within 20 minutes or so." You may take this for a month or two and see how it works for you. If you find that it's working, you can continue to take one dose of 100 milligrams before you go out at night.

lutein and zeaxanthin (both pigments found in vegetables and fruits); vitamins B_6, B_{12}, C, and E; and the trace mineral zinc.

Eat to Save Your Eyes

That saying about carrots being good for your eyes is right. Beta-carotene, one of the many carotenoids found in carrots and lots of other vegetables and fruits, is consistently associated with a reduced risk of AMD. One study found that taking 15 milligrams of beta-carotene along with 500 milligrams of vitamin C, 400 IU of vitamin E, and 80 milligrams of zinc (a large dose you'll want to get a doctor's okay on first) reduced the rate of progression of AMD by 25 percent in people with advanced disease. But other carotenoids are involved in eye protection, too, so your best bet is to eat a mix of colors in fruits and vegetables every day, including oranges, yellows, greens, and reds. This will get you a healthy dose of all the antioxidants that protect your eyes, says Mark Lamden, ND, a naturopathic doctor and adjunct faculty member at Bastyr University in Kenmore, Washington.

If you take supplements, look for those that contain "mixed carotenoids" and for lutein and its related compound, zeaxanthin. (Kale is a good source, providing about 25 milligrams per cup, raw or cooked.) These two have a special association with the macula: They form the visible yellow color that your doctor can detect when he examines your eyes with an ophthalmoscope.

"There is lutein actually present within the eye," says Robert Abel Jr., MD, clinical professor of ophthalmology at Thomas Jefferson University in Philadelphia and author of *The Eye Care Revolution*. Eyes affected by macular degeneration may be lacking this lemon-colored luster. The pigment protects your retina from harmful blue light by filtering it out. A good dose is the equivalent of that cup of kale—25 milligrams a day.

B Vitamins Protect Eyes

Research also shows that taking 50 milligrams a day of vitamin B_6, along with 1,000 micrograms of vitamin B_{12} and 2,500 micrograms of folic acid, reduces the risk of developing AMD. Women over age 40 with a history of or risk factors for heart disease who took this combination for an average of 7.3 years had a 34 percent reduced risk of developing AMD and a 41 percent reduced risk of AMD serious enough to impair their vision compared to women taking placebos.

These B vitamins help to reduce blood levels of homocysteine, a metabolic by-product that can hurt the tiny blood vessels in the retina of the eye and cause leakage or impair blood flow, researchers say. You'll need to take supplements to get these doses.

Fish Oil Sharpens Vision

Fish oil, especially the portion known as DHA, also supports the health of your retinas. In fact, these omega-3 fatty acids make up 30 to 50 percent of the retinas' photoreceptor cells—the nerve cells that actually send the signals that translate into "vision" in your brain. Since the DHA that's been shown to help eyes has come from foods, especially fatty fish, there is no known dosage to take to treat AMD, but some eye experts recommend between 500 and 1,000 milligrams a day of DHA from fish oil.

Try an Herbal Antioxidant

Antioxidants of all kinds, including vitamins C and E, are very effective at protecting cells from free radical damage. When it comes to macular degeneration in particular, however, there is an herbal source of antioxidants that stands out. Ginkgo, besides improving blood flow to the brain, is a macula-protecting antioxidant. Look for capsules containing standardized ginkgo extract and take 40 milligrams three times a day, says Dr. Lamden.

menopausal changes

The changes that arise around the time of menopause may be predictable, but that certainly doesn't make them comfortable. Hot flashes and night sweats are just the beginning. Women may also experience vaginal dryness, loss of sex drive, mood swings, depression, and a host of related problems.

If you're experiencing uncomfortable menopausal changes that prompt you to see a conventional doctor, he is not likely to quickly recommend the usual hormone replacement therapy (HRT) these days, now that research shows that it may actually be harmful to your heart health (although its short-term use to reduce hot flashes is fairly low risk for women in their fifties). Some women, however, fear the increased risks of breast cancer that go along with HRT, or find the side effects, such as breast tenderness, headaches, and swelling, intolerable.

Alternative practitioners, both medical and naturopathic doctors, take a different approach. They address lifestyle changes that can make the transition smoother and help reduce the risks of heart disease and osteoporosis that increase after menopause. Among these strategies are exercising (including weight training); keeping coffee, alcohol, smoking, sugar, and salt consumption to a minimum; eating lots of fruits and vegetables; and cutting down on stress.

They're also likely to recommend a number of supplements, including phytoestrogens (plant estrogens), herbs, vitamins, and minerals. Sometimes they'll prescribe hormones that more closely match a woman's own, such as progesterone, DHEA, Bi-Est, a combination of estradiol and estriol, or estriol alone applied topically for vaginal dryness. Some of these hormones are available only by prescription. (And some states do not allow naturopathic doctors to write prescriptions.) And even though some are available over-the-counter, a practitioner can help individualize your treatment to maximize your results.

Some of these recommendations address the whole range of menopausal discomforts, while others take aim at specific problems such as vaginal dryness or low sex drive. Here's an overview of what these supplements can do and what we know about how they work.

Hormone Enhancers

Estrogen levels fluctuate during perimenopause—the 5 or so years prior to menopause. At menopause, estrogen levels drop quickly, and then they slowly drop further as you age. It's that drop in estrogen that triggers the hot flashes, osteoporosis, vaginal dryness, and other symptoms associated with menopause. A natural "HRT" can be found in plant (phyto-) estrogens, compounds in some foods and herbs. These versions of estrogen are weaker than typical HRT but can still do the trick, says Lorilee Schoenbeck, ND, in private practice at the Vermont Women's Center in Burlington and a coauthor of *Menopause: Bridging the Gap Between Natural and Conventional Medicine*.

Soy is a good source of phytoestrogens, although it's not quite as popular as it used to be. "It can be hard to digest," Dr. Schoenbeck says. Soy or red clover isoflavone supplements aren't as popular now either, she says. "There is a lot of controversy, and there are unanswered questions, about the benefits and risks of these supplements," she says. For a commonsense approach to soy, she suggests that if you like eating soy, have a serving or two a day of natural soy foods, like edamame, soy milk, or tofu. That way, you get both the heart benefits of soy protein and the hot flash–cooling, bone-boosting estrogenic benefits of isoflavones. A cup or two of red clover tea at night is also okay, she says. (If you've had an estrogen-positive cancer, though, check with your doctor first regarding soy and red clover.)

Ground flaxseed is also a favorite among natural-leaning doctors. It provides essential fatty acids (like linolenic acid), some of which can convert to EPA, an anti-inflammatory component of fish oil. Flaxseed also contains lignans, another form of phytoestrogens. It has lots of fiber, so it can substitute for something like psyllium (found in Metamucil or Konsyl), a bulk laxative. It has a nice, nutty taste and is easy to get down. A suggested dose is 2 tablespoons a day of freshly ground flaxseed. (You can grind it in a coffee bean grinder and store it in the freezer to keep it fresh.)

Several herbs are also popular for treating symptoms of menopause. One that's found in almost all menopause formulas is black cohosh, which can reduce hot flashes. The most consistent results with black cohosh seem to be with quality brand name extracts, such as Remifemin, (from Phytopharmica/Enzymatic Therapy). This extract is standardized to contain 1 milligram of black cohosh's active ingredients, triterpene glycosides, per 20-milligram dose. (There is considerable variation among different preparations.) The benefits of black cohosh are comparable to a popular prescription hormone, an estrogen patch known as Estraderm.

"I like to use black cohosh, along with sage, which is great for hot flashes, night sweats, even mood," says Jennifer Nevels, NMD, with East Valley Naturopathic Doctors in Mesa, Arizona. She'll make up a tincture of these two (the amounts used vary with a woman's symptoms). "I might add maca, which is good for low libido, hot flashes, and mood swings, and for depression and anxiety associated with menopause," she says. Dong quai, a Chinese herb, is another all-around favorite. "I tend to use a combination of herbs because they seem to have a synergetic effect that's better than single herbs," Dr. Nevels says. One over-the-counter product with a good combination of herbs, she says, is Menocaps, by Wise Woman Herbals.

If you are taking black cohosh alone, a good dose is 20 milligrams, twice a day, of the standardized extract. It can take 2 to 4 weeks to see an effect. Some doctors recommend taking it long term for 6-month periods, with a month off in between.

Do You Need Adrenal Support?

After menopause, the adrenal glands take over more than 50 percent of a woman's hormone production, Dr. Nevels says. "I will often use black cohosh, sage, and an adrenal support herb, because anyone who is going through menopause is going to see her adrenal glands being taxed," she says. "If they have insomnia, anxiety, and stress, and are not sleeping well when they do manage to nod off, their adrenals don't have a chance to regenerate at bedtime."

Her choice for this is pure licorice root extract in a tincture. Licorice balances estrogen levels while also increasing progesterone levels. And it inhibits the breakdown of an important stress hormone, cortisol, which can help—but sometimes hurt, as well. That's why it's best to work with a holistic doctor if you want to take licorice and have your blood pressure and side effects monitored. (A form of licorice, DGL, has the ingredients that cause side effects removed, and it's a good choice for people with stomach ulcers, but it does not help during menopause.)

Ashwagandha, an Ayurvedic herb, also has a long list of active ingredients but is often said to be a safer herb than licorice for adrenal support. Its main use is to help the body withstand and recover from physical and mental stress. It also has antianxiety and immune-stimulating effects. People typically use 1 to 6 grams daily of the whole herb in capsule or tea form. The tea is prepared by boiling ashwagandha roots in water for 15 minutes and allowing it to cool before drinking. The usual dose is 3 cups daily. If you'd prefer a tincture or fluid extract, take 2 to 4 milliliters three times per day.

"I'll use licorice, in varying amounts, for a few months, and then switch for a while to a different adrenal support herb, such as ashwagandha," Dr. Nevels says. "That helps to avoid any side effects."

Any time you're thinking "adrenal support," you should also be taking these vitamins and minerals vital to proper immune function, Dr. Nevels adds: vitamin C, all the B vitamins (especially pantothenic acid, or B_5), and magnesium.

Replenishing Progesterone

Progesterone is the flip side of estrogen. Like estrogen, it drops after menopause, says Samantha Brody, ND, a naturopathic doctor specializing in women's health in Portland, Oregon.

Progesterone is the hormone that affects the endometrial lining—that is, the tissue that lines the inside of the uterus. Before menopause, this hormone plays a role during ovulation, helping to prepare the endometrial lining to receive the egg.

Progesterone levels drop off sharply once ovulation stops, Dr. Brody says. "That's one reason some women start taking supplemental progesterone during perimenopause," she says. "Progesterone can also help stop hot flashes and improve mood. Taken sublingually or orally, it can help you fall asleep."

And if you're taking estrogen, even its natural forms, you should be taking progesterone to reduce your risk for endometrial cancer. The only form of natural progesterone widely accepted to reduce your risk of endometrial cancer is an oral form of micronized progesterone, called Prometrium, that's available by prescription.

Over-the-counter progesterone creams are not considered a reliable choice to protect against endometrial cancer, experts say. That may be because of dosage or absorption problems, or because some products just don't contain enough. Still, women may use them to help reduce hot flashes.

Good brands, like Emerita's Pro-Gest body cream and Life-Flo Progesta-Care have "USP" progesterone, which means that their active ingredient really is what the label says it is. Good brands will also state the amount of progesterone in a dose, sometimes have a pump bottle with a measured dose, and have an expiration date on the tube or bottle.

Many over-the-counter creams, especially those that say "yam extracts" and "yam creams," do not contain progesterone, and the ingredients they do contain cannot be converted to progesterone. Save your money and skip them.

Cool Down with Hesperidin

Maybe you've heard of citrus bioflavonoids. They are usually combined with natural forms of vitamin C, like rose hips or what is sometimes called vitamin C complex. One of these forms, called hesperidin, is used for hot flashes, and it is safely used in women who've had an estrogen-positive cancer, Dr. Nevels says.

Hesperidin alone, or in combination with other citrus bioflavonoids, is most often used for vascular conditions such as hemorrhoids and varicose veins. Hesperidin seems to work by improving tone in blood vessels, making tiny capillaries less "leaky," and improving both blood flow and lymph drainage.

In one study, women who took 900 milligrams of hesperidin plus another bioflavonoid, diosmin, had an 87 percent reduction in hot flashes. "That's as good as any herb or drug can do," Dr. Nevels says. "This is something you can take by itself."

You can find vitamin C with citrus bioflavonoids at a health food store, or a hesperidin-based product online, such as Hesperidin Complex Powder by Life Extension, or Hesperflav by Ultra Life. Follow product directions for dosing.

mitral valve prolapse

Things react differently to pressure, but they always react. Squeeze a toothpaste tube, and toothpaste squirts out. Put pressure on a balloon, and it pops. Push hard against a mitral valve, and you've got a case of mitral valve prolapse. This is not due to high blood pressure, however. It happens because there is something wrong with the connective tissue of the valve.

The mitral valve is located between the two left chambers of the heart. Usually it works fine, letting blood flow from chamber to chamber when the heart compresses, then shutting off like a clever trapdoor when the heart muscle expands. In some people, however, misshapen connective tissue causes real problems. When the heart compresses, the valve pops upward, almost like a parachute being snapped in the wind.

Although you may not feel the difference, a doctor can detect that slight popping sound with a stethoscope. It means that one of the fibrous cords holding the valve in place has stretched too far or that one of the two leaflets that make up the valve has become elongated, thickened, or floppy. Often it's an inherited disorder.

The valve problem may be accompanied by mood and body changes such as jumpiness, irritability, and muscle stiffness. These symptoms seem to be associated with hyperactivity in the body's autonomic nervous system, says Sidney M. Baker, MD, a physician in Weston, Connecticut. The autonomic nervous system works without conscious control and governs the glands, the heart muscle, and the tone of smooth muscles, such as those of the digestive system, the respiratory system, and the skin, Dr. Baker says. "People with mitral valve prolapse may have a hard time adjusting to changes in their environment. They may be sensitive to noise and light, for instance."

To treat mitral valve prolapse, doctors want to reduce pressure on the valve, which is best done by keeping blood pressure normal or slightly below normal, says Decker Weiss, NMD, director of the Weiss Center for Naturopathic Excellence in Scottsdale, Arizona, and author of *The Weiss Method: A Natural Program for Reversing Heart Disease and Preventing*

Heart Attacks. They also caution people to avoid stress as a way to help the heart work as efficiently as possible. Treatment may also relieve symptoms of irritability and anxiety.

Pharmaceutical drugs can help with all of these approaches, but natural remedies can have fewer side effects, Dr. Weiss says. If you've been diagnosed with mitral valve prolapse and want to try supplements, talk to your doctor about the following treatment options.

Magnesium—A Mineral for All Symptoms

Several studies indicate that many people with mitral valve prolapse are low in magnesium. Moreover, in one study by researchers at the University of Alabama School of Medicine in Birmingham, people with mitral valve prolapse who took 250 to 1,000 milligrams of magnesium daily had a 90 percent decrease in muscle cramps, a 47 percent decrease in chest pain, and a definite decrease in blood vessel spasms.

This study revealed other benefits, too. People had fewer heart palpitations, the rapid or irregular heartbeat that's accompanied by a fluttering sensation. Magnesium also helped to regulate heartbeat in those with a type of arrhythmia called premature ventricular contraction. People taking magnesium also reported fewer migraines and less fatigue.

It's reasonable for people to take 350 milligrams a day of magnesium, Dr. Weiss says. You have your choice of mixtures. If magnesium citrate or gluconate tends to cause diarrhea, you can take the glycinate or orotate form instead. "I've recommended as much as 1,500 to 2,000 milligrams a day to some people with severe symptoms" he says.

Magnesium has a bodywide calming effect, Dr. Weiss says. "In addition to being jumpy and irritable and nervous, many people with mitral valve prolapse also have muscle fatigue and stiffness throughout the body, and magnesium helps with all those things."

People who are going to respond to magnesium generally do so fairly quickly, within a week or less. If you have heart or kidney problems, check with your doctor before taking supplemental magnesium.

More Pump Power with CoQ_{10}

Along with magnesium, Dr. Weiss always recommends coenzyme Q_{10} (CoQ_{10}) for mitral valve prolapse. This vitamin-like substance is made in the body, and provides an energy boost to the heart muscle.

If you get additional CoQ$_{10}$, it seems to pour even more energy into the muscle cells. That means that the heart contracts more effectively, Dr. Weiss says.

CoQ$_{10}$ also seems to help reduce stiffening of the muscle, says Peter Langsjoen, MD, a Tyler, Texas, cardiologist who has been using the substance in his private practice to treat heart disease since 1985.

The diastolic, or filling, phase of the cardiac cycle actually requires more energy than the systolic, or contraction, phase, Dr. Langsjoen notes. "This stiffening of the heart muscle returns to normal with supplemental CoQ$_{10}$, and many of my patients have less fatigue, irregular heart rhythm, and chest pain."

How much you need to take depends on your symptoms. Dr. Weiss starts with a minimum dose of 120 milligrams a day, divided into three 40-milligram doses. To aid absorption, he suggests taking CoQ$_{10}$ with omega-3 and omega-6 fatty acids.

Dr. Langsjoen starts people on twice that much, 240 milligrams a day, and he may go as high as 360 milligrams a day divided into three doses if symptoms are severe. CoQ$_{10}$ is expensive, so you'll want to stay with the lowest dose that relieves your symptoms, but there are no apparent side effects or toxicity related to the supplement, says Dr. Langsjoen.

Because blood and tissue levels build slowly, it takes 4 to 6 weeks to notice improvements. "In a month, most people can tell if they're wasting their money or not," says Dr. Langsjoen. "Improvement in stamina is usually very obvious to the person and does not require any fancy testing or blood work."

CoQ$_{10}$ is a fat-soluble supplement, and gelcaps are more easily absorbed than tablets. If you do opt for the tablets, chew them with a fat-containing food such as peanut butter or essential fatty acids to maximize absorption.

Heart-Smart Fats

Dr. Weiss recommends that you cut back on the fats that can harm your heart—saturated and hydrogenated fats—and get more of two essential fatty acids that help to protect your heart. You'll need some omega-3 and omega-6 fatty acids, which are found in various proportions in fish oil, flaxseed oil, borage oil, and cold-pressed safflower or sunflower oil.

People with mitral valve prolapse should get 1,000 to 3,000 milligrams a day of a mixture of these two fats, says Dr. Weiss, which are available as gelcaps.

Hawthorn Helps Hearts

When someone's heart is additionally weakened by cardiovascular disease or congestive heart failure, Dr. Weiss may add hawthorn, an herb long known for its heart-strengthening effects. Hawthorn contains bioflavonoids, compounds that, like vitamins C and E, act as heart-protective antioxidants.

Although hawthorn is relatively safe, you should take it under medical supervision, especially if you have low blood pressure or are under doctor's orders to take other heart medications, Dr. Weiss says. The amount you'll need depends on your symptoms and the type of hawthorn you're using. For capsules, a typical dose would be 150 milligrams three times a day.

morning sickness

Not every expectant mother goes through morning sickness, of course, but those who do tend to list it among their worst experiences. Not only do they have to endure the daily bouts of nausea, they have to be very protective of the fetus that's prompting the disturbance. That means that they can't do much, particularly in the way of pharmaceuticals, to quell the nausea.

For women in this pickle, doctors may recommend some very basic procedures to settle their stomachs. For starters, eat five or six frequent meals that combine carbohydrates and proteins, says Barbara Silbert, DC, ND, a chiropractor and naturopathic doctor in Bethel, Vermont.

For breakfast, for example, she recommends plain crackers or toast rather than a sugar-laden doughnut. Combine your plain carbs with protein such as cheese, peanut butter, or yogurt. She also recommends kefir (a type of liquid yogurt usually found in health food stores). "The key here is to always have easily digestible food in your stomach," she says.

Chewing gum might also help quell feelings of nausea, says Willow Moore, DC, ND, a chiropractor and naturopathic doctor in Owings Mills, Maryland.

If you still need some extra help sparing your stomach while you nurture your baby, reach for some safe, time-tested natural remedies.

A Vitamin to Settle Your Stomach

"Vitamin B_6 is the primary supplement I suggest for morning sickness," says Dr. Moore. Studies from as early as the 1940s suggest that B_6 provides effective morning sickness relief. In studies since then, researchers have found that pregnant women who take between 10 and 25 milligrams every 8 hours get varying degrees of relief from their morning sickness.

In a more recent study, researchers from Columbia University's department of obstetrics and gynecology and the university's Center for

Complementary and Alternative Medicine Research in Women's Health evaluated all available evidence for every type of alternative remedy for morning sickness. They concluded that acupressure, vitamin B_6, and ginger are currently the most effective.

Try taking 50 milligrams of B_6 twice a day, says Dr. Silbert. "I think the activated form of vitamin B_6, called P5P, works best." Take the supplement first thing in the morning, even before you get out of bed. Then take a second dose around lunchtime, Dr. Silbert advises. You should feel relief after the first few doses.

It might seem logical to take the vitamin as a preventive before you go to bed, but Dr. Silbert warns against it. "Several of my patients have complained of having nightmares when they took a dose of B_6 before going to bed," she says. "Just to be on the safe side, get your two doses in before the sun goes down."

Some women's nausea is so bad that they can't keep the capsule down, says Dr. Moore. Such women may need a vitamin B_6 injection. The injection has to be given by a doctor, of course, but you may not have to go back repeatedly. One injection is usually sufficient to get things under control enough so that you can start taking the supplement orally, Dr. Moore says.

The Ginger Cure

Ginger is another great nausea fighter. One study showed that 940 milligrams (about ½ teaspoon) of ginger worked as well for relieving motion sickness as the common over-the-counter remedy dimenhydrinate (Dramamine). The results of a British study suggest that ginger works as well as drugs for relieving the nausea and vomiting sometimes induced by general anesthesia and showed that it didn't have as many side effects as antinausea drugs.

One theory is that ginger works to prevent the gastrointestinal tract from relaying messages to the brain that trigger nausea and vomiting. Whatever the reason, it's worth a try.

While ginger ale or ginger tea might help, the most effective form of ginger is the powder in a supplement capsule, says Dr. Silbert. You can follow the dosage directions on the bottle, but do not exceed 250 milligrams four times a day. Ginger contains some mutation-causing compounds and may not be safe at dosages higher than 1,000 milligrams a day.

multiple sclerosis

In multiple sclerosis (literally, "many scars"), the immune system acts like a troublemaking mouse living in the walls of your home. For reasons that are unknown, the immune system will attack various spots on the covering of nerve cells in the brain and spinal cord, like a mindless mouse chewing away at the vinyl coating on electrical wire.

When the fatty material that normally protects nerve endings (called myelin) is damaged or completely worn away, nerve signals sputter and sometimes go dead. Depending on where the random damage occurs, multiple sclerosis (MS) can lead to various symptoms, including blurred vision, fatigue, loss of movement, memory problems, numbness, and trouble with bowel, bladder, and sexual functions.

MS is an autoimmune disease, meaning that the body attacks itself, and as with other autoimmune diseases, no one is quite sure what causes it. "There are probably multiple causes," says Jody Noe, ND, a faculty member at the University of Bridgeport College of Naturopathic Medicine and in private practice at Natural Family Health and Integrative Medicine in Westerly, Rhode Island.

Among the possible culprits are infectious diseases, such as the organism *Chlamydia pneumoniae* (now recognized as a cause of pneumonia, pharyngitis, bronchitis, and several chronic diseases, such as reactive arthritis and coronary artery diseases). These are all medical conditions that, like MS, are characterized by ongoing inflammation.

Other possible causes include sensitivities to foods such as gluten (wheat protein), which can affect the brain; leaky gut syndrome, which can lead to autoimmunity as allergens in the GI tract that normally wouldn't get into the bloodstream leak in and trigger reactions by the immune system; and environmental toxins, including mercury fillings, which act as neurotoxins.

One of the newest findings is that the selective membrane that forms the blood–brain barrier may be "leaky" in people with MS, allowing in substances that set off inflammation in the brain.

The standard medical approach is to give a person with MS drugs that suppress the over-revved immune system. Holistic doctors look for causes, such as leaky gut and environmental toxins. They also treat symptoms, using therapies that may naturally regulate a self-destructive immune response. None of these treatments promises to provide a cure, but in some cases, they seem to help control the symptoms of MS. Quite possibly, they can also help heal damaged and inflamed myelin.

Make Sure You're Getting Healthy Fats

A cornerstone of alternative treatments for MS is reducing pro-inflammatory fats in the diet and supplementing with fats that reduce inflammation, says David Perlmutter, MD, a neurologist in Naples, Florida, and author of *LifeGuide*. Dr. Perlmutter has devised an entire protocol of diet and supplements for people with MS.

The best way to avoid pro-inflammatory fats? Eat a mostly vegetarian diet, also avoiding dairy products and eggs, unless they are omega-3–enriched eggs. Wild, cold-water fish are good, too. "Nuts, seeds, and dark green leafy vegetables, all rich in essential fatty acids, should be emphasized," Dr. Perlmutter says. "Alcohol should be eliminated since it enhances the formation of inflammatory biochemicals." Refined sugars need to go, too.

Supplement with fish oil, making sure you get a product that is free of toxins (pharmaceutical grade) and that you are getting at least 500 milligrams of DHA a day, Dr. Noe says. That's the component of fish oil that has a special affinity for brain cells. Most fish oil has an EPA to DHA ratio of about 3:1, so you'll also be getting about 1,500 milligrams of anti-inflammatory EPA with this dosage.

You might also want to take a form of omega-6 fatty acids, such as flaxseed or borage oil. In that case, aim for about 300 milligrams a day of gamma linolenic acid (GLA.) Keep these oils fresh in the refrigerator.

Additional nutrients to reduce the formation of inflammation-producing biochemicals include vitamins B_3, B_6, and C, as well as the minerals zinc, selenium, and magnesium. You can get all of these through a healthy diet and a multivitamin.

Focus on Vitamin D

Traditionally, doctors who treat MS do make sure their patients get some supplemental vitamin D, but research now suggests that they may need much more than has usually been prescribed, Dr. Noe says. In fact, in one study, high daily doses of vitamin D dramatically cut the relapse rate in people with MS.

In the study by researchers at the University of Toronto, those who took an average of 14,000 IU a day of D experienced significantly fewer relapses than those who took only 1,000 IU (the usual recommended dose for people with MS). Also, people taking high-dose vitamin D suffered 41 percent fewer relapses than they did in the year before the study began, compared with 17 percent fewer relapses in those taking typical doses.

Vitamin D appears to suppress the autoimmune responses thought to cause MS, researchers say. In MS, haywire T lymphocytes—the cellular "generals" of the immune system—order attacks on the myelin sheaths that surround and protect the brain cells. In people given high-dose vitamin D in the study, T cell activity dropped significantly.

The researchers also measured the concentration of 25-hydroxyvitamin D in the blood, considered the best indicator of a person's vitamin D status. It appeared that MS patients did best if levels reached 100 ng/ml, which is relatively high.

"New vitamin D research is really changing our thinking about what is a high dose of vitamin D," Dr. Noe says. "We're seeing now that these higher doses are doing a lot of good and not causing the toxic effects some feared." She gives her patients with autoimmune diseases a dose of vitamin D3 (the active form) that maintains their blood levels at 50 to 100 ng/ml. Work with your doctor to find the optimal dose for you.

Maximize Protection with Vitamin E

Like vitamin D, vitamin E is fat-soluble and supports the regeneration of other brain antioxidants like vitamin C and glutathione (a powerful antioxidant made in the body). "Adequate supplementation with vitamin E is mandatory, especially when you are taking essential fatty acids like fish oil," Dr. Perlmutter says. These oils are easily oxidized, a process that renders them useless. Vitamin E helps prevent that. He recommends 400 IU a day.

Add Alpha Lipoic Acid

"Alpha lipoic acid is emerging as one of the most powerful brain antioxidants available," Dr. Perlmutter says. Because it is both water soluble and fat soluble, it can readily get into the brain, where it assists in the regeneration of other brain antioxidants. In animals, alpha lipoic acid produced a significant reduction in demyelination and reduced the infiltration of inflammatory T cells across the blood–brain barrier. In human studies, it has also interfered with T cell migration into the central nervous system. "Alpha lipoic acid is a key nutrient in our protocol for MS," Dr. Perlmutter says. The recommended dosage is 200 milligrams a day.

Get Ginkgo Biloba

"Ginkgo is useful in virtually all the neurodegenerative conditions due not only to its ability to reduce the activity of free radicals, but also because of its potent effects enhancing neurotransmission, the process by which neurons are able to communicate with each other," Dr. Perlmutter says. For MS patients, he recommends 60 milligrams a day.

Boost Glutathione with N-Acetyl-Cysteine (NAC)

NAC is a key supplement in MS and all other neurodegenerative conditions because it enhances the production of glutathione, one of the most important brain antioxidants, Dr. Perlmutter says. Taking 400 milligrams a day at bedtime has been shown to help you sleep better, too.

Prevent Breakdown with B$_{12}$

Vitamin B$_{12}$ has been used by some doctors to treat patients with MS. Although the symptoms of B$_{12}$ deficiency mimic those of MS, the amount of the vitamin used to treat MS is far greater than the amount required simply to correct a deficiency.

The question, however, is how to take it and how much to take. Dr. Perlmutter believes that injections are necessary. "In order to achieve therapeutic blood levels, our patients are trained to self-administer 1,000 micrograms once a week," he says. Since you need a prescription for this, you'll need to ask your doctor to let you try this therapy. B$_{12}$ is considered a very safe nutrient, even at high levels. Since this is an injection that goes into muscles, it is easy to learn how to do it yourself.

Help Nerves Communicate with Phosphatidylserine (PS)

Lecithin has for decades been part of complementary treatment programs for MS, and with good reason, Dr. Perlmutter says. "Lecithin is one of the important building blocks for neuronal membranes, the real business end of brain cells where cell-to-cell communication takes place."

Deficiencies of intracellular communication are the ultimate functional flaws in MS. "Newer research has revealed that perhaps the most important component of lecithin is phosphatidylserine," Dr. Perlmutter explains. "Adequate amounts of phosphatidylserine are required not only to preserve, but also to enhance the ability of nerves to transmit information." He recommends 100 milligrams a day.

Queue Up for Coenzyme Q_{10} (CoQ_{10})

CoQ_{10} plays a critical role in energy production in cells, and low levels hamper the fundamental process of cellular energy production and enhance the damaging effects of free radicals, Dr. Perlmutter says. Although CoQ_{10} has not been investigated specifically for the treatment of MS, it is generally recognized as safe, well tolerated, and potentially useful in the treatment of neurodegenerative disorders. Dr. Perlmutter recommends at least 60 milligrams a day.

muscle soreness

A little muscle soreness after a good workout isn't so bad—it lets us know we earned our stripes by stressing our muscles. And the saying, "no pain, no gain" has some truth to it. The stress we put on our muscles by pushing them as we exercise causes microscopic damage, and it's the repair process that actually builds and strengthens muscles. That's the deal—balancing the stress of muscle-building with the pain it takes to do that. But none of us want so much pain from our activities that we stop doing them.

Nonsteroidal anti-inflammatory drugs (NSAIDs) are the usual go-to med when your muscles cry out. These drugs do work: They reduce the biochemicals we produce in our bodies that cause postexercise muscle soreness and inflammation.

But there are natural substances that reduce inflammation, too, and sometimes with fewer side effects than NSAIDs. And other natural products help reduce muscle soreness in other ways that no NSAID can, such as by improving energy metabolism in muscles, promoting relaxation in muscles, and improving blood flow to tired, tense muscles.

CoQ$_{10}$ for Less Pain and Better Performance

Japanese researchers have found that coenzyme Q$_{10}$ supplements may boost physical performance and reduce feelings of tiredness associated with exercise. Both fatigue and recovery times were decreased as a result of 300 milligrams of CoQ$_{10}$ for 8 days.

CoQ$_{10}$ has properties similar to vitamins, but since it is naturally synthesized in the body it is not classed as such. The level of CoQ$_{10}$ produced by the body begins to drop after the age of about 20, and the coenzyme is concentrated in the mitochondria—the power plants of the cells. "It plays a vital role in the production of chemical energy by participating in the production of adenosine triphosphate (ATP)—the body's so-called energy currency," says Evie Katahdin, ND, a naturopathic doctor specializing in

Stop Statin-Induced Muscle Pain

The use of cholesterol-lowering statin drugs is also a major culprit in muscle pain, says Jacob Schor, ND, a naturopathic doctor in Denver and president of the Oncology Association of Naturopathic Doctors. Statin drugs deplete muscles of CoQ_{10}, which can lead to muscle tissue breakdown and muscle soreness.

In one study, taking 100 milligrams of CoQ_{10} for 30 days was found to significantly reduce statin-induced muscle pain. Another study, though, found that 12 weeks of 200 milligrams of CoQ_{10} didn't work.

How much CoQ_{10} it takes to work for you may depend on the type of statin you take, the dosage, how depleted you are of CoQ_{10}, and how active you are, says Peter Langsjoen, MD, a cardiologist in Tyler, Texas, who has been studying and using CoQ_{10} for many years. "People absorb it differently, too," he says. A good trial to see if CoQ_{10} will work for your statin-induced muscle pain is 200 milligrams a day for about a month, he says. If it doesn't help, try doubling the dosage to 400 milligrams a day for another month. If it is going to work for you, you will see results by then.

sports medicine at AthletiZen, in Costa Mesa, California. "It also acts as a potent antioxidant. The coenzyme plays an important role in preserving levels of vitamin E and vitamin C," she says. "I am using it more and more, as research confirms its benefits."

She recommends 100 to 300 milligrams a day of CoQ_{10} during heavy training or on an intense day (such as a race day), and then for 5 to 7 days after, or as long as muscle soreness continues. "It depends on how intense the activity is," she says. "You probably won't need this for a 5K, but you would for a marathon, half-marathon, or triathlon."

Drink Sour Cherry Juice

"This is my top recommendation now for exercise-induced muscle soreness," says Jacob Schor, ND, a naturopathic doctor in Denver and president of the Oncology Association of Naturopathic Doctors. "It works really well and it tastes really good." Research shows that marathon runners who drank a cup of cherry juice three times a day for 3 weeks prior to racing and every hour during the race reported less of an increase in pain after the race than people drinking a fruit juice cocktail.

Sour cherries are loaded with all sorts of goodies: vitamin C, vitamin A, alpha-linolenic acid, and traces of vitamin E, beta-carotene, folate, and thiamin, as well as varied antioxidants including kaempferol, quercetin, and melatonin. A preliminary study suggests that compounds found in the sour cherry may have anti-inflammatory effects that are 10 times stronger than those of aspirin, but without aspirin's side effects.

You can also get the effects with about 2 tablespoons a day of sour cherry juice concentrate, Dr. Schor says. This is available at health food stores, but you can get a highly concentrated extract online directly from cherry growers, too. The variety of sour cherry most studied for its anti-inflammatory effect is Montmorency.

Check Your D Levels

If you have a combination of unexplained muscle pain and weakness, or what doctors call "persistent, nonspecific pain" (i.e., "Hey, doc, I seem to hurt all over"), get checked for low levels of vitamin D. Doctors at the University of Minnesota examined patients with these symptoms and found that 93 percent were low in vitamin D—some severely low. (*All* of the patients under age 30 were deficient.) Some had been told their pain was "all in their head," researchers report.

Vitamin D deficiency promotes swelling in the tough connective sheath where muscle and bone meet, which puts pressure on muscles. Because it also influences both calcium and magnesium levels in the blood, not enough D in your system could also lead to chronically contracted muscles. (Both minerals are involved in muscle contraction and relaxation.) Leading experts in vitamin D are now recommending a dosage that maintains your blood level at 50 ng/ml or higher. Start out with 800 IU and work with your doctor if you think you need more.

Use the Curcumin Cure

Curcumin is a component of turmeric, the yellow spice found in curries. It reduces inflammation by inhibiting cyclooxygenase-2 (COX-2), prostaglandins, and leukotrienes—all inflammatory biochemicals your body cooks up that induce aches and pains.

The problem is that plain old curcumin is hard to absorb, Dr. Schor says. "We used to have all these ways of making it more absorbable, like mixing it with coconut oil and taking it between meals," he says. In fact, in Indian cooking, that's often what's done with curry and turmeric. The spices are mixed in with hot oil before food is added to a dish.

But now there are new forms of curcumin—and drugs—that increase absorption dramatically. In the case of curcumin, it is attached to phosphatidylcholine, a form of lecithin that acts as an emulsifier. Then it's subjected to ultrasonic vibration, which breaks it up into tiny spheres, with the curcumin on the inside, coated by the phosphatidylcholine. "The intestinal cells suck it right in," he says. "It's a really smart way to do things." It increases absorption several hundredfold. At the health food store or online, just look for liposomal curcumin or Curcumin Phytosome.

"For acute muscle pain, where we want to prevent or reduce swelling right away, we might start someone on as high a dose as 3 to 4 grams a day," he says. After a few days of that, he'll cut back to 1 to 2 grams. Low-dose curcumin is safe to take regularly, but talk to your doctor first if you are taking any kind of anticoagulant, since curcumin can increase anticoagulant activity. It can also cause gallbladder contractions.

Do Some Damage Control

Even before your muscles seize up, you can get a jump on the healing process with proteolytic enzymes. These are enzymes that help to dissolve and clean up microscopic bits of broken-down proteins from acute exercise or a muscle or joint injury, as well as reduce inflammation and pain. They are the "clean-up crew" of your immune cells, and they attack inflammation-causing circulating immune complexes.

Because these enzymes do not affect prostaglandin synthesis, they are thought to be free of many of the side effects associated with nonsteroidal anti-inflammatory drugs (NSAIDs), such as gastric bleeding.

There are a number of these enzymes, and Dr. Schor likes to use a mix of them. One popular brand, Wobenzym, contains pancreatin, trypsin, chymotrypsin, bromelain, papain, and rutoside. Just follow the label directions.

Dr. Katahdin likes to use Traumeric (made by Ortho Molecular Products), a product that contains both enzymes and herbs. "You use it two or four times a day, on an empty stomach, while you have pain, and I tell people to stop using it once the pain is gone," she says. Some people get a

Warm Up and Cool Down

You can prevent sore muscles by warming up before you exercise and cooling down afterward, advises Dr. Schor. Include at least a few minutes of movement with each of the major muscle groups—the calves, thighs, hips, back, abdomen, chest, and arms.

Once the damage is done, says Dr. Schor, you can treat the muscle with alternating hot and cold–water baths, alternating every 1 to 3 minutes, for 10 to 15 minutes. The contrast in temperatures works like a pump to increase the flow of oxygen and nutrients in the muscle. It also provides a flushing action to remove lactic acid, a by-product of energy metabolism when muscles are running low on oxygen.

stomachache from taking proteolytic enzymes, though, Dr. Katahdin says. If you're one of them, your body is telling you to stay away from these enzymes, she says.

Tread Gingerly

Ginger's been used as a remedy for muscle soreness and inflammation for a long time, and it does work, but not as well as some other, new products like liposomal curcumin, Dr. Schor says. "I'll suggest ginger if someone just hates taking curcumin," he says. Ginger inhibits a number of inflammatory pathways in the body. As a supplement, you can take ginger in tincture or capsule form. If you're in acute pain, take six 500-milligram capsules of the concentrated extract per day, says Dr. Schor. Ginger can interact with some anticoagulant drugs, so talk with your doctor first if you are taking coumadin, Plavix, or similar drugs.

Dr. Katahdin likes to use products with a mix of anti-inflammatory herbs and other botanicals, such as ginger, boswellia, quercitin, cayenne, and lemon bioflavonoids. "One I've been using lately is Inflavonoid Intensive Care by Metagenics," she says.

What about Antioxidants?

Large doses of antioxidants like vitamins C and E used to be recommended to reduce postexercise muscle soreness, but new research has found that antioxidants don't seem to do much for this sort of pain and that high-dose antioxidants can impair gains in strength-building. "Exercise, especially the kind that makes your muscles hurt, does cause oxidative damage to muscle tissue. But that damage is what triggers your body to build new muscle so you get stronger," Dr. Schor says.

The trick is to find a balance that works for you, especially as you get older. If you feel like you do need to take antioxidants, for whatever reason, do not take them close to the time that you exercise, he suggests. For example, if you're exercising in the morning, take them at night. "Separate them by as much time as you can," Dr. Schor says.

osteoarthritis

Just like age, osteoarthritis can creep up on you. It starts out quietly, with some occasional stiffness. Later, you may begin to feel some occasional joint pain. Human nature tells you to ignore it, but maybe you shouldn't. It's true that many people develop osteoarthritis (OA) by age 70, but for many, it's possible to prevent or manage the condition so it doesn't become debilitating. Still, arthritis is the leading cause of disability among Americans over age 15. Osteoarthritis, the most common form, affects 20.7 million people. While there aren't any miracle cures, there's a lot you can do to minimize the damage.

Doctors who treat OA with nutritional therapy view it as a metabolic disorder—a breakdown in the body's ability to regenerate bone and cartilage. Although they concede that the breakdown is partly the result of aging and injury, they also believe that providing the proper nutrients can help stop deterioration and reduce pain and swelling. Early, aggressive treatment is best. Joint-specific supplements can maintain healthy cartilage, restore joint-lubricating synovial fluid, and keep bone structure under the cartilage healthy, which helps keep that cartilage in tip-top shape.

The Basics of Care

First, doctors suggest that you maintain a healthy weight because people with osteoarthritis are more likely to be overweight. Research shows that losing weight can significantly reduce the risk of developing OA. In a large study done in Framingham, Massachusetts, women who lost an average of 11 pounds were much less likely to get arthritis of the knee over the next 10 years than women who didn't shed the pounds.

Exercise is another essential. Low-impact activities like brisk walking, swimming, and biking are best at strengthening muscles and are easy on your joints. Stronger muscles help protect your joints by providing support and added stability.

526

Exercise also helps the joints absorb fluid and needed nutrients. Unlike muscle or bone, cartilage doesn't get its nutrients from blood. It soaks them up like a sponge from the fluid surrounding the joint. The more you exercise, the more you force fluid in and out of the joint.

Aspirin and other similar drugs called nonsteroidal anti-inflammatory drugs (NSAIDs) focus on nursing arthritis pain, but that pain relief isn't in your long-term interest, according to doctors. While NSAIDs are easing the pain, they can actually speed up joint deterioration. Natural measures attempt to slow the progression of the disease and preserve cartilage and bone by providing the proper nutrients in the right amounts.

A Steady Supply of Building Materials

One arthritis treatment that has hit the spotlight is the supplement combo glucosamine and chondroitin. These are two substances that your body makes to help build and protect cartilage. (See Molecules on the Bestseller List, on pages 528–529.)

Glucosamine is synthesized by cartilage-producing cells, called chondrocytes, to produce joint cartilage. In OA, glucosamine synthesis is defective, and supplementation with glucosamine can help the body make the components of cartilage by stimulating various joint-building processes. It also inhibits enzymes that destroy cartilage.

Like glucosamine, chondroitin stimulates the production of cartilage and has the ability to prevent enzymes from dissolving cartilage. Chondroitin also inhibits free radicals that degrade joint cartilage and collagen. It improves blood circulation to joints, which enables antioxidants and glucosamine to enter inflamed joints to actually stimulate joint repair.

In a study conducted by Amal Das, MD, an orthopedic surgeon at Hendersonville Orthopedic Associates in North Carolina, people with osteoarthritis were given two tablets containing 500 milligrams of glucosamine hydrochloride and 400 milligrams of chondroitin sulfate in the morning and evening. For people with mild to moderate arthritis, the supplements decreased pain and allowed them to decrease the amount of anti-inflammatory medication they used. They did not help people who already had severe arthritis in a joint—that is, bone rubbing on bone.

In another study done in Europe, 200 people with active osteoarthritis of the knee took either 400 milligrams of ibuprofen or 500 milligrams of glucosamine sulfate twice a day. Although the people in the ibuprofen

Molecules on the Bestseller List

Glucosamine is a word that's made up of two other words that may be familiar from biology or chemistry—glucose and amine. Glucose is just blood sugar, the energizing "food" that your body uses in its cells. As for amine—well, it's not an everyday word, but in chemistry it means that nitrogen and hydrogen are glued together in the same molecule. Put it all together, and you have a word that describes a simple molecule—one that combines the stuff of blood sugar, nitrogen, and hydrogen.

Despite its simple components, this molecule is a complex contributor to your body's health—especially joint health. That's where the osteoarthritis connection comes in. One theory holds that osteoarthritis results from the body's inability as we age to make enough glycosaminoglycans, the major molecules that give cartilage its ability to bear weight, notes Amal Das, MD, an orthopedic surgeon at Hendersonville Orthopedic Associates in North Carolina. "Your body has a hard time making glucosamine," says Dr. Das. "It would be a lot easier if your body could get that glucosamine somewhere else—say, from a supplement."

The second substance that may play a role, chondroitin sulfate, is actually built up from glucosamine. "If glucosamine is the two-by-four used to build a house of cartilage, then chondroitin sulfate is an entire wall," says Dr. Das.

group got immediate pain relief, 35 percent of them experienced adverse reactions such as upset stomachs. Glucosamine took a little longer to work—about 2 weeks—but none of the group reported any side effects.

Two to the Rescue

Although researchers aren't sure why, the two supplements seem to work best together, says Dr. Das. Because the pair works best by preserving the cartilage you have left, don't wait until you're in agonizing pain to start on a supplement program, advises Dr. Das. If you've been diagnosed with arthritis, get your doctor's approval first, then take 500 milligrams of glucosamine and 400 milligrams of chondroitin sulfate twice a day, he says. From the time you start the double dose, allow from 2 weeks to 4 months for the supplements to do their work. You can continue to take them indefinitely.

Chondroitin sulfate is a long chain of glucosamine molecules. According to Dr. Das, it helps promote water retention in the cartilage, which is necessary for shock absorption. There's a big difference in the way your body absorbs chondroitin sulfate, however. Studies show that if you take a supplement of chondroitin, your body absorbs less than 8 percent of it. By comparison, you absorb about 90 percent of glucosamine sulfate from a pill or capsule.

Although we produce our own supplies of glucosamine and chondroitin sulfate, our aging bodies can always use some help from supplements, says Dr. Das. The glucosamine in supplements comes from chitin, a compound that forms crab shells. Chondroitin sulfate is found in cartilage. Although cow cartilage is usually the source, it doesn't matter what animal the cartilage is from.

Apart from their absorption rates, another difference between glucosamine and chondroitin sulfate may lie in how they go about the business of saving cartilage from destruction. Whereas glucosamine may help with the rebuilding of cartilage to keep up with its breakdown, chondroitin may actually decrease the breakdown, says Dr. Das.

Although the patients in Dr. Das's study took glucosamine hydrochloride, many naturopathic physicians typically recommend taking glucosamine sulfate because it is the type that has been tested most thoroughly in clinical trials.

Add Methylsulfonylmethane (MSM) and Fish Oil

MSM is a natural source of sulfur, which helps maintain protein structures in your body. Research shows that MSM can modestly reduce the pain and swelling of OA, especially when taken in combination with glucosamine. For OA, between 500 milligrams three times a day and 3 grams twice a day has been used in studies. Don't take any more than that, as high doses can cause nausea. Don't take MSM if you are allergic to sulfur.

Although the powerful anti-inflammatory fish oil is more likely to be used for rheumatoid arthritis, some research suggests that it can help treat people with moderate-to-severe hip or knee osteoarthritis, and it also helps boost glucosamine's effectiveness. For treatment of OA, take 3,000 milligrams a day.

Other Natural Anti-Inflammatories

There are two other natural anti-inflammatories that can relieve OA pain: curcumin and green tea extract. A component of the yellow spice turmeric, curcumin inhibits the secretion of collagenase, hyaluronidase, and elastase, all pro-inflammatory enzymes that are linked to the breakdown of cartilage that happens in osteoarthritis. And compounds found in green tea, like epigallocatechin gallate (EGCG), also inhibit inflammatory biochemicals that cause cartilage breakdown in arthritic joints.

For green tea, a commonly recommended dosage is the equivalent of about three cups of brewed tea a day, or 240 to 320 milligrams of EGCG. For curcumin, it's about 900 milligrams a day. If you use a liposomal version of curcumin, which is much more absorbable than the usual kind, only take 100 milligrams a day.

Double Up on D

Results from the famed Framingham Osteoarthritis Cohort Study showed that people with low dietary intakes and blood levels of vitamin D were three times as likely to experience bad OA symptoms compared to those who got more of the sunshine vitamin. Not getting enough D appears to increase cartilage loss, and the vitamin is also necessary for proper calcium absorption and bone structure, which are crucial to proper joint functioning. Experts today say that you may need up to 2,000 IU or more of vitamin D. If you want to find out more about your D levels, ask your doctor to check your blood levels and help you find a dosage that keeps those levels at 50 to 80 ng/ml year-round.

Antioxidant Relief

Antioxidants—especially vitamin C, vitamin E, and beta-carotene— are another means of preventing your cartilage from wearing away.

"Arthritis is known to increase free radical production, so your need for antioxidant nutrients increases," says Lauri Aesoph, ND, a health-care consultant in Sioux Falls, South Dakota, and author of *How to Eat Away Arthritis*. Those free radicals are free-roaming, unstable molecules that can set off a chain reaction in your body, aging cells prematurely and sometimes harming your genetic material. While the healing powers of antioxidants may seem somewhat mysterious, the process is crucial when it comes to protecting your joints.

If you have arthritis, antioxidants can protect joints from damage caused by oxidative stress, a process that speeds up cartilage breakdown. Joints damaged by osteoarthritis release the unstable free radical molecules that are missing an electron. Like scavengers, these highly reactive compounds look for a place from which to snatch an electron in order to stabilize themselves. They usually attack the nearest healthy molecule, which then becomes a free radical itself.

Antioxidants help break this chain reaction and stop cell damage by offering up their own extra electrons. No one is sure exactly how this process occurs in the joints, but research has shown that diets high in antioxidants help reduce pain and cartilage deterioration.

Three Protectors

Researchers in the Framingham osteoarthritis study evaluated the diets of 640 people to see if there was a link between their osteoarthritis and their intake of vitamins C and E and beta-carotene, the highly pigmented component that is converted to vitamin A in the body. The results showed that the trio of antioxidant nutrients won't prevent you from getting osteoarthritis, but it may keep it from getting worse.

After reviewing knee x-rays of the participants over a 10-year period, researchers concluded that people who had the most vitamin C in their diets were three times less likely to experience progressive deterioration of the joint. They also were less likely to develop knee pain. Vitamin E and beta-carotene also helped ailing joints stay healthier.

The benefits of vitamins C and E extend beyond their antioxidant properties. Together, they enhance the stability of components called proteoglycans, which help to protect your cartilage, according to Jody Noe, ND, a faculty member at the University of Bridgeport College of Naturopathic Medicine and in private practice at Natural Family Health and

A Devilish Pain Reliever

Devil's claw gets its odd name from the woody fruits of the plant, which look like clawlike hands. The active substance, a compound called harpagoside, is found in the tuberous roots. The bitter compound is used primarily by herbalists as an appetite stimulant and as a supplemental treatment for arthritis and rheumatism.

Extracts of the root are available in supplement form as capsules, tablets, tinctures, and ointments.

Integrative Medicine, in Westerly, Rhode Island. Vitamin C helps to form the structural protein known as collagen, the single most important protein in connective tissues.

To protect your cartilage and quell those aches and pains, take 1,000 milligrams of buffered vitamin C three times a day, says Ruth Bar-Shalom ND, a naturopathic doctor in Fairbanks, Alaska.

Studies show that vitamin E offers relief from inflammation. In research conducted by German scientists, people with osteoarthritis who took 600 international units (IU) of vitamin E every day for 6 weeks had significantly less pain. They also had better range of movement and were able to take fewer pain relievers. To get these benefits, include 600 IU of vitamin E and 10,000 IU of beta-carotene in your daily antioxidant regimen, says Dr. Bar-Shalom.

Crucial Cartilage Nutrients

If you're not getting the right nutrients, your body cannot make and maintain cartilage. In addition to antioxidants, trace minerals and B vitamins play important roles. Studies show that low intake of selenium, manganese, copper, and zinc is associated with an increased risk for OA. These minerals are involved in bone hardening, cross-linkage of collagen fibers, protein metabolism, natural antioxidant production, and a host of other chemical reactions that influence the body's ability to heal itself. Most diets these days are low in trace minerals, which are found in whole grains, nuts, and seeds. Your best bet is a good multivitamin/mineral supplement, so look for one with about 200 micrograms of selenomethionine (the most bioactive form), 2 milligrams each of copper and manganese, and 20 milligrams of zinc (best as picolinate or orotate).

Cartilage also needs pantothenic acid to grow. Studies have found that supplements of this B vitamin relieved arthritis symptoms, and research with animals has shown that a profound deficiency of pantothenic acid stops cartilage growth. It's usually thought that people get plenty of this vitamin from foods. Still, getting more than you'd get from a normal diet seems to help joints, and Dr. Bar-Shalom recommends 12.5 milligrams of pantothenic acid plus 50 milligrams of vitamin B_6 daily to encourage your body's ability to regenerate cartilage.

Gentle Pain Relief

Supplementing with the herb devil's claw can sometimes relieve joint pain, says Dr. Bar-Shalom. Studies have shown that this herb provides some relief from pain and inflammation. (See "A Devilish Pain Reliever.")

In a German study of 54 people with chronic back pain, 9 became completely pain free after taking 800 milligrams of extract three times a day for 1 month. In a comparable group that didn't take the extract, just one person showed the same recovery. The study suggests that devil's claw may work when traditional pain relievers fail. Most of the people had experienced back pain for 15 years, even while taking conventional painkillers.

The active substance at work is harpagoside, a compound found in the tuberous roots of the plant. It reduces inflammation in the joints and helps stimulate cortisol, your body's natural version of pain-relieving cortisone. A sensible dose to start with is 400 milligrams of dry, standardized extract three times a day, says Dr. Noe. Do not use devil's claw, however, if you have gastric or duodenal ulcers.

Although better known for its power to defuse migraines, feverfew also inhibits an enzyme that causes inflammation, says Betzy Bancroft, a professional member of the American Herbalists Guild in Washington, New Jersey.

To control joint pain, take 125 milligrams of standardized extract containing at least 0.2 percent parthenolide or 1 to 3 milliliters of tincture daily, says Dr. Noe.

osteoporosis

We're all at risk for bone loss as we age, but women are hit the hardest. That's because bone density is strongly influenced by the amount of estrogen in a woman's body.

For about the first 5 years after menopause, when a woman's body stops producing much estrogen, the rate of bone loss may be as high as 2 to 5 percent a year. The people who are most at risk are thin, small-boned women who are fair-skinned and of northern European or Asian descent, says Lorilee Schoenbeck, ND, in private practice at the Vermont Women's Center in Burlington and a coauthor of *Menopause: Bridging the Gap Between Natural and Conventional Medicine.*

Don't wait until you *have* osteoporosis to do something about it, Dr. Schoenbeck says. Natural medicine can only prevent, not cure, osteoporosis. "Prevention really is by far the best medicine for this potentially crippling condition," she says.

Along with a healthy diet, you should be doing regular, weight-bearing exercise, such as walking or running. "And pay attention to your posture," she adds. "Women who allow themselves to stoop forward may put additional stress on their spines, and that leads to microfractures and fusion of vertebrae." The result can be the permanent stooped-over posture called "dowager's hump." Stand up straight, and do exercises to strengthen your upper back muscles, Dr. Schoenbeck advises. Weight training can also help preserve strong bones. A few simple exercises with light hand weights a few times a week will also help protect your skeletal infrastructure. Need a place to start? Go to Prevention.com for some basic weight-bearing workouts.

Nutrients are the key to building and keeping bone, but most women don't get enough of the nutrients they need to prevent osteoporosis from diet alone, she adds. That's where supplements come in. Nutritional supplements can help you get some of the nutrients you need to maintain strong bones throughout your lifetime. Those suggested here all work together, so consider them a package deal.

Calcium: The "Nonnegotiable" Nutrient

"Calcium is a nonnegotiable part of every regimen I set up to help women avoid or slow the rate of osteoporosis," says Dr. Schoenbeck.

Postmenopausal women who do not take calcium supplements lose about 2 percent of bone per year. Taking 1,000 to 1,600 milligrams a day decreases this rate to 1 percent and cuts the rate of fractures by 50 percent. Supplements need to be taken long term, since calcium's effects on bone mineral density are largely lost within 2 years of discontinuing the supplements.

Most women get about 500 milligrams of calcium a day from food, says Dr. Schoenbeck. Much of that comes from dairy sources. If you happen to be lactose intolerant and therefore avoid most dairy products, you're probably getting even less than the average. In any case, you should probably have two or three times as much calcium as you're getting from food.

Dr. Schoenbeck recommends 1,000 milligrams a day for women who haven't gone through menopause and for men of all ages. Women who are pregnant should plan on taking around 1,200 milligrams a day. Women who are in menopause or have passed through it should take 1,500 milligrams every day.

Calcium citrate, aspartate, and malate are the most absorbable forms of calcium, but they are bulky and taking them means six capsules a day, Dr. Schoenbeck says. "Most women just don't take as much as they need with these forms," she says. "If that is a problem, just take calcium carbonate." It's a more compact form, so one or two tablets or capsules may provide all you need.

Don't Forget the Vitamin D

Calcium can't work its bone-building magic alone: It needs vitamin D, which helps maintain adequate blood levels of calcium, control calcium absorption in the gut, and (it's not done yet!) stimulate stem cells in bone to mature into bone-building osteoblasts. Getting more than 400 IU a day of vitamin D can cut the risk of hip fracture by 50 percent, but even higher amounts are often needed to get and keep your blood levels of vitamin D in the range Dr. Schoenbeck likes to see—55 to 80 ng/ml. "My patients may be taking 3,000 to 5,000 IU a day of vitamin D_3, to get them into a healthy range," she says. Then, they may be able to cut back to 1,000 to

2,000 IU a day. You don't need to take vitamin D at the same time of day as calcium, but you do need to take *both* for either to be effective.

Key In on Vitamin K

Vitamin K is known as the clotting vitamin because it's what stops your body from bleeding. But it is also critical for the formation of a strong bone matrix. "It is responsible for the activation of osteocalcin, a protein produced by osteoblasts, which helps attract calcium to bones," Dr. Schoenbeck says. Without it, the protein scaffolding of bones never mineralizes and hardens. Adequate vitamin K is linked to a reduction in fractures of the spine and hip. Aim for 100 micrograms or more each day, Dr. Schoenbeck says. Some multivitamins do not contain vitamin K, so you might need to take a separate supplement to get an optimal amount. But an even better way is to eat leafy greens such as kale, collards, or spinach, which all have about 1,000 micrograms per cup.

Max Out on Magnesium

Magnesium may play as much of a role in bone density as calcium does, research is finding. Magnesium acts as the "glue" that binds calcium and another important mineral, fluorine, to build bone. It also helps convert vitamin D to its active form in the body.

Even if you're getting calcium and fluorine in your diet, you may be simply excreting them unless you've got enough magnesium, and most people don't get enough.

For healthy bones, most experts recommend getting about 500 milligrams of magnesium for every 1,000 milligrams of calcium. The same leafy greens that give you vitamin K are also the best food sources of magnesium. Beans and seeds are other good sources.

More Mineral Magic

When calcium has other trace minerals (like boron, copper, zinc, and manganese) around, it does a better job at slowing bone loss in postmenopausal women than calcium does alone. Boron boosts blood levels of vitamin D. Copper helps to incorporate collagen and elastin, both proteins that give bones structure and flexibility. Zinc is a cofactor for many metabolic processes that affect bone health, and it also plays a role in the activity of bone-building osteoblasts. Manganese is needed to protect the proteins found in bone.

While a varied diet with lots of fruits and vegetables, nuts, seeds, and beans provides good amounts of these trace minerals, a good daily multivitamin/mineral supplement can make sure all of your bases are covered. Look for one that contains 2 milligrams of copper, 20 milligrams of zinc, 3 milligrams of boron, and 2 milligrams of manganese.

Favor the Phytoestrogens

Estrogen is needed to stabilize bone mineral density (which is why you see osteoporosis spike in postmenopausal women). But compounds called isoflavones in soy and red clover act like weak estrogens, so they can slow the loss of bone mineral density associated with a drop-off in estrogen levels. Eat two or three servings of soy foods a day, such as edamame or tofu, Dr. Schoenbeck recommends. (Talk to your doctor first if you've had an estrogen-positive cancer.) Some doctors suggest a cup or two of red clover tea a day, as an alternative.

Black cohosh may be a good substitute for women who can't take soy, Dr. Schoenbeck says. Research shows that postmenopausal women who take 40 milligrams of black cohosh a day have increased levels of a marker for bone formation, bone-specific alkaline phosphatase, after 12 weeks of treatment. However, it's not known if black cohosh can increase bone mineral density or decrease the risk of fractures. (High doses, though—1,000 milligrams—seem to suppress bone tissue formation, so don't assume that more is better.)

Sip a Cup of Tea

In studies that compare bone density with what people eat and drink, tea drinkers come out with high marks. Tea drinking is associated with increased bone mineral density in women ages 65 to 76 and with a lower risk of hip fracture in both men and women age 50 or older. In animal studies, some of the active components in green tea, polyphenols like EGCG, stimulated enzymes that promote bone growth and increased bone mineralization in osteoblasts, which also aids bone strength. The tea also inhibited osteoclasts, cells that break down bone.

It's hard to tell from these studies how much tea you need to drink each day for a bone-protecting effect. In studies that show improved health and longevity with green tea, a minimum of about three cups a day is required. If caffeine is a concern, it's possible to get decaffeinated green tea or take decaffeinated green tea extracts.

Put Fish on Your Plate

In population studies, people who have a higher intake of omega-3 fats from fatty fish like salmon and mackerel have higher bone mineral density. And in animal studies, fish oil has been linked to a significant increase in bone mineral density in the hip, compared to corn oil supplementation. The fish oil supplementation led to reduced levels of pro-inflammatory biochemicals called cytokines, which also reduced the activity of bone-disassembling osteoclast cells. Both of these actions are associated with reduced bone resorption and higher bone formation, the researchers conclude.

Most people need less corn oil (omega-6 fats) and more fish oil (omega-3 fats), so it's wise to cut back on grain-fed beef and most of the usual sources of fat in the diet and eat more fatty fish instead, Dr. Schoenbeck says. Wild salmon is a good source of omega-3s that is usually free of toxins like mercury or PCBs. If you want to take a fish oil supplement, look for a good brand—one that has been molecularly distilled and is free of contaminants—and take 1 to 3 grams a day.

overweight

If you're like many people, you're embroiled in a never-ending battle to lose weight and keep it off. The battle is often so tiresome and frustrating that advertisements about the latest magic pill that promises to melt away the fat and make you slim start to sound really good.

Unfortunately, there is no such thing as a miracle weight-loss pill, prescription or otherwise. If there were, we'd all be showing off our newfound physiques. Ninety-seven million American adults are overweight or obese, and carrying around these extra pounds is putting us at risk for developing diabetes, heart disease, and cancers of the breast, ovaries, uterus, prostate, and colon. The added weight is also affecting our emotional health.

To avoid these health problems, experts say that the best action plan is to achieve a healthy weight that's right for your age and build. But that process is much more complex than experts used to think, and it isn't just "calories in, calories out." Some people's metabolisms are very clever about conserving energy—refusing to burn excess calories. And people's genetic makeup may play a role in what type of weight-loss diet works best for them.

Still, given so many unknowns, common sense must prevail, which means that we still need to eat healthfully—and that means lots of fruits, vegetables, legumes, and whole grains, plus healthy fats like fish, nuts, and olive oil. And yes, exercise is a must. (Research shows that almost no one loses weight and keeps it off long term without exercise of some sort. Sorry about that!)

None of these measures is the equivalent of a magic potion, but taken together, they're reliable weight-loss strategies. Once you adopt them, however, you may find that supplements can also help you achieve your goals. Some nutritional and herbal supplements can help you stabilize blood sugar, feel full, reduce fat and carbohydrate absorption, help you preferentially burn fat as fuel, and slightly increase the rate at which you burn calories. When combined, those little things can give you the edge you need to move from gaining to losing.

Fill Up with Fiber

Just as fiber-rich fruits and vegetables can help you achieve that slender waistline, so can fiber supplements. "Once you take a fiber supplement, it expands in your stomach dramatically, filling you up," says Jennifer Brett, ND, a naturopathic doctor at the Wilton Naturopathic Center in Stratford, Connecticut. "When your stomach feels full, it sends a signal to your brain, telling it that you don't need to eat as much. The supplements diminish those hunger pangs." Fiber also reduces the roller-coaster ups and downs of blood sugar. Your blood sugar remains steadier, and you don't have the high highs—and then the low lows—that trigger hunger and carb cravings.

One study found that simply adding 14 grams of supplemental fiber per day (look for psyllium or guar gum, both available as nutritional supplements) led people to eat about 10 percent fewer calories. Just take 3 to 6 grams with water before each meal.

Get Lean with Chromium

Chromium is added to lots of weight-loss and diabetes-control nutritional supplements. The reasons for that are twofold. First, chromium helps your body turn carbohydrates and fats into energy. Second, it improves the effectiveness of insulin, the hormone that allows cells to pick up blood sugar and use it for fuel. As a result, blood sugar levels are kept under control. Your energy soars, you crave fewer sweets, and your body's sensitivity to insulin increases, which is key to successful weight loss, says Dr. Brett.

Even if weight loss isn't your goal, most people seem to benefit from getting more chromium than is found in the typical American diet.

Research shows that chromium picolinate, an easy-to-absorb supplemental form of chromium, can build muscle mass and reduce fat in people who exercise. The more muscle you gain, the more calories you'll burn each day.

In a study at the University of Texas Health Science Center, 154 participants were asked to drink two servings daily of a protein/carbohydrate drink. Fifty-five received plain drinks, 33 received drinks containing 200 micrograms of chromium picolinate, and 66 received drinks containing 400 micrograms of chromium picolinate. Body composition was measured before and after the study.

The study continued for 2½ months. In the end, researchers found no significant changes in body composition in those who received the plain drinks. Participants who received 200 or 400 micrograms of chromium picolinate daily showed significant increases in muscle mass and reductions in body fat.

Although this study suggests that chromium picolinate can be helpful as a weight-loss aid, other studies suggest that you also need to exercise regularly while taking the supplement if you want to reduce fat and improve muscle tone. Dr. Brett suggests taking 200 to 400 micrograms of chromium picolinate daily, as part of a multivitamin/mineral supplement that also contains the things that help chromium work: B vitamins and magnesium.

If you have diabetes, make sure you monitor your blood sugar carefully as you start taking chromium so you don't end up with hypoglycemia—low blood sugar. That's especially important if you are taking drugs that lower blood sugar. Check with your doctor before you start taking chromium.

Make Yours the Sunshine Vitamin

Vitamin D acts as a hormone in your body, and researchers are finding out it has a hand in a lot more biological processes than we'd previously realized, including weight loss.

In one diet study, for instance, every "point" increase in vitamin D blood levels was linked to ½ pound of additional weight loss. Researchers think that vitamin D may help weight loss by improving calcium absorption and decreasing fatty acid synthase, the enzyme that converts calories to fat. Vitamin D also seems to help normalize blood sugar and appetite. People with excess body fat tend to have low blood levels of vitamin D because this fat-soluble vitamin gets trapped in fat cells and can't circulate in the bloodstream.

As for how much to take, most experts now recommend taking an amount that keeps your vitamin D levels at about 50 to 80 ng/ml. It can take several thousand units a day to achieve those levels. (Experts now recommend a dose of at least 800 IUs.) If weight loss is a problem for you, ask your doctor to help you come up with a specific dosage for you.

Fat-Fighting Minerals

Both calcium and magnesium are important for weight loss. When the diet lacks calcium, there is an increase in fatty acid synthase, an enzyme that converts calories into fat. Diets low in calcium increase fatty acid synthase by as much as fivefold. Magnesium influences fat-regulating stress hormones that can deposit abdominal fat, and adiponectin, a hormone that controls fat cell activity. For weight loss, experts recommend getting about 1,200 milligrams of calcium and 600 milligrams of magnesium a day through food or supplements.

Tea, Please

Green tea extract is another ingredient often added to weight-loss products. Green tea does indeed have some modest weight-loss benefits, but researchers aren't sure yet if this is due to its caffeine, which raises your metabolic rate slightly and helps burn fat, or to other active ingredients in the tea, perhaps polyphenols such as EGCG.

Several studies on obesity have concluded that people who have been regular tea drinkers for more than 10 years showed lower body fat percentages than those who don't drink tea regularly. And overall, taking a caffeinated green tea extract of about 500 to 700 milligrams a day seems to give you a slight edge in weight loss, when compared to caffeine alone. Green tea has a wealth of other health benefits, so there's no harm in pouring yourself a cup or so.

The Fat You *Do* Need

If you're overweight, make sure you get enough fish oil, not just to protect your heart but because it could help you lose body fat. This is true even if your calorie intake remains the same.

In one study, French researchers examined a group of 27 older women with type 2 diabetes. Half of the group took 3 grams of fish oil a day for 2 months. The other half took a placebo. Their food intake remained constant. At the end of the study, the women taking the fish oil had 3.5 percent less body fat (that would be a 2.3-pound loss to a 200-pound woman with 30 percent body fat), and their fat cells were 6 percent smaller, compared to the placebo group. They had also reduced their risk for premature heart disease by lowering their triglycerides and reducing inflammation.

Researchers aren't exactly sure how fish oil works in this regard, but they have some ideas. In animal studies, fish oil affects fat-regulating genes, so it might help normalize levels of hormones like leptin and adiponectin, which are secreted by fat cells and that affect appetite and fat storage. Fish oil may also increase fat-burning for energy. Take 1 to 3 grams a day. For fish oil to work best, also cut back on pro-inflammatory saturated fats, corn oil, and trans fats.

Add a Fat-Burning Amino Acid

The nutritional supplement L-carnitine and its close twin, acetyl-L-carnitine, have some intriguing weight-loss properties. Carnitine, found in meats, is used by our bodies to transport fat from our blood into a cell's fuel-burning mitochondria to be used for energy. Carnitine also helps energize a failing heart, because the heart muscle relies on fat as a source of energy. Carnitine helps prevent muscle wasting during illness as well as age-associated muscle loss.

For weight loss, carnitine is thought to help mobilize fat from fat cells and burn it as fuel. It also helps you burn more fat during aerobic (cardio-vascular) and anaerobic (strength-training) exercise.

Experts recommend starting with 500 milligrams of L-carnitine, taken before both breakfast and lunch. If you're very overweight, start with 1,000 milligrams at each meal. Increase this dosage by 500 milligrams as needed to feel increased energy, but don't exceed 5,000 milligrams per day. L-carnitine can interfere with some drugs, so if you're on any medications, get your doctor's okay before you start taking it.

An Herbal Fat Burner

Kelp is one herb that may actually help whittle away extra pounds when combined with a low-fat diet and daily aerobic exercise, says Ellen Evert Hopman, a professional member of the American Herbalists Guild, a lay homeopath in Amherst, Massachusetts, and author of *Tree Medicine, Tree Magic*.

Kelp is a type of seaweed that's rich in antioxidant vitamins and iodine. It is believed to stimulate a hormone produced by the thyroid gland that's responsible for boosting metabolism. You can also get other kinds of seaweed in your diet by adding them to soups and salads, she says.

If you take kelp, follow the instructions on the bottle. While it's safe for most people, check with your doctor before taking it if you have a thyroid disorder, high blood pressure, or heart problems, says Hopman.

parkinson's disease

When doctors describe Parkinson's disease in clinical terms, they talk about symptoms like tremor, slowed movement, and muscle rigidity. These symptoms are far more than minor inconveniences. With Parkinson's, all of the little details that make us who we are—a jaunty gait, a sarcastically raised eyebrow—are slowly stripped away. Even a signature changes, since it becomes impossible to write with the usual flourish.

We don't know for sure what causes Parkinson's disease to affect some people and not others. It's clear, though, that symptoms are due to progressive destruction of cells deep inside the part of the brain called the substantia nigra, the area that controls movement. These cells normally produce dopamine, a chemical that transmits nerve signals to muscles. The death of these cells causes reduced dopamine levels, which in turn lead to the faulty muscle control that's characteristic of Parkinson's.

Many experts believe that Parkinson's disease comes from a combination of two malevolent forces—poor genes and a toxic environment. In some people, genetic messages carried from generation to generation allow them to detoxify cells—that is, dispose of any harmful components that might damage the cells. In someone who has a less-than-perfect ability to detoxify cells, nerve cells could be easily damaged.

Maybe that's not the whole story, however. There's also the possibility that certain toxins in the environment contribute to the problem. If we are overexposed to those toxins and they make their way to the cells, it's a recipe for progressive cell damage that leads to cell death.

Could the toxins contained in pesticides be adding to our susceptibility to Parkinson's? "The incidence of this disease is dramatically higher in farmers and other people who've had pesticide exposure," says David Perlmutter, MD, a neurologist in Naples, Florida, and author of *LifeGuide*. He has noted that in general, rates of Parkinson's are rising with rates of pesticide use around the globe.

You can reduce your risk for Parkinson's as well as slow its progression in two basic steps, Dr. Perlmutter believes. First, protect your brain cells from damage by taking antioxidants, then boost your body's ability to dispose of toxins. That can be done by taking supplements that target the liver and intestines as well as the brain, he says.

If you've already been diagnosed with Parkinson's, you should know that none of the remedies that follow are substitutes for any medication your doctor may prescribe. If they are started early enough, however, Dr. Perlmutter believes that they can help prolong the time before medication becomes necessary. If you're already taking prescription drugs, adding supplements like these is a safe and effective way to help keep your symptoms from getting worse, he says. Even so, be sure to inform your doctor about any supplements that you're taking, since some can interact with prescription medicines.

Antioxidants Are a Must

Free radicals—the free-roaming, unstable molecules that harm cells— and the damage they do are associated with Parkinson's in two ways. Excess free radicals may contribute to development of the disease in the first place. Then, once Parkinson's is under way, experts believe that the disease progression generates a wave of one kind of highly toxic free radical known as peroxynitrite.

Also, research has shown that Parkinson's symptoms are likely to be worse when there are not enough antioxidant nutrients in the body. "Studies on this topic have been done since 1984," says Dr. Perlmutter. "Using antioxidants to treat this disease is not new."

One study on antioxidants and people with early Parkinson's showed the result of high-dose supplementation with the high-powered antioxidants vitamin E and vitamin C. When people with early Parkinson's took those vitamins, their need for medication was delayed for up to 2½ years.

Another study published 2 years later looked at the effects of vitamin E alone, but this time there was no benefit from supplementation. Researchers believe they can explain the apparently contradictory results by the fact that antioxidants, particularly vitamins C and E, work much better in tandem.

Lipoic Acid Boosts Vitamin Power

When you're battling Parkinson's disease, you need to call in the big guns. According to Carl Germano, RD, a registered and certified nutritionist in New York City and coauthor of *The Brain Wellness Plan,* lipoic acid is just the weapon for the job.

Lipoic acid is a unique substance. It isn't really considered a vitamin because the body usually makes enough on its own, and what the body doesn't make, it can get from food. In certain crisis situations, however, supplements of this special antioxidant can add some power.

The other supernova antioxidant stars are vitamins E and C. Vitamin E is fat-soluble, while vitamin C is water-soluble. In other words, vitamin E travels in a medium of fat molecules, while vitamin C needs a water medium to move about. Because of that exclusivity, each of these vitamins has a limited way to travel, which in turn limits the tissues on which either of them alone can have an effect. Lipoic acid, on the other hand, is both fat- and water-soluble, giving it an edge when it comes to protecting brain tissue, which is made up of both fatty and nonfatty tissue, says Germano.

That's not all. Lipoic acid is also a "recycler" that keeps vitamins E and C in their active forms. It may also help raise levels of glutathione, according to a study by researchers at the University of California at Berkeley. This important substance is produced throughout the body, but people who have Parkinson's often have a shortfall.

The dose of lipoic acid that Germano recommends for people who have Parkinson's (200 milligrams daily) appears to be completely safe. In studies, no harmful effects showed up in people who took as much as 800 milligrams daily for 4 months. This supplement can be dangerous for people who are thiamin deficient, however. If your doctor determines that you have a thiamin deficiency, you should take a B-complex vitamin that contains thiamin whenever you begin taking doses of lipoic acid.

Experts who recommend supplements for Parkinson's agree that higher-than-normal amounts of these nutrients are often needed. Dr. Perlmutter recommends 4,000 milligrams of vitamin C a day. Since this vitamin doesn't stay in the body very long, you should take it in two separate doses of 2,000 milligrams each. Combine that with a once-daily dose of 800 IU of oil-based vitamin E, he suggests.

Put Ginkgo on Guard

Ginkgo, the popular "memory herb," boosts blood circulation to the brain, but it appears to have additional positive effects on gray matter. In particular, it may offer hope for people with Parkinson's.

Studies have shown that animals exposed to a neurotoxin called MPTP will develop symptoms that are identical to those of Parkinson's disease. When they are pretreated with ginkgo extract, however, they don't develop the symptoms, says Dr. Perlmutter.

Ginkgo performs its guardian gig through a process of membrane stabilization. By stabilizing nerve cell membranes, it helps prevent a breakdown of communication between the nerve cells. "It allows neurons to communicate with each other more readily," concludes Dr. Perlmutter.

Ginkgo has antioxidant properties that come in quite handy, as well. "Ginkgo blocks the formation of free radicals that would otherwise be stimulated into destroying brain cells," says Dr. Perlmutter. Take 60 milligrams of ginkgo extract twice a day, he suggests.

Call on Coenzyme Q_{10}

Coenzyme Q_{10} (CoQ_{10}) is a chemical with a dual personality. Not only does it help generate energy inside the microscopic cell bodies called mitochondria, it also functions as a powerful antioxidant.

CoQ_{10} is most often associated with treating heart disease, but people with Parkinson's should take note as well, says Germano. A study by Harvard Medical School researchers showed that CoQ_{10} protects certain neurons in the brain from the substance that produces Parkinson's damage, according to Germano.

In terms of its antioxidant ability, CoQ_{10} gives superhero vitamin E a run for its money. In fact, CoQ_{10} appears to go one step further than E, protecting not only the outer membranes of cells but their inner components, as well. In this way, it may be able to defend vulnerable DNA (cell genetic blueprints) from the oxidative damage that seems to cause Parkinson's, says Germano. He recommends taking 200 milligrams of CoQ_{10} once a day with a meal.

Lift Liver Function with a Helpful Herb

Parkinson's disease is often regarded as strictly a brain disorder, but addressing only the brain may mean missing out on other ways to ease the disease. "You need to look at the entire picture," says Germano. "There are many pathways to this disease." That means that there are many paths to healing, as well.

When the body is dealing with the negative effects of a possible overload of toxins such as pesticides, liver function is crucial. In fact, Dr. Perlmutter believes that healing the liver can bring dramatic improvement to people who have Parkinson's. "I have patients diagnosed with this disease in their thirties who respond beautifully to liver detoxification," he says.

One herb that's linked to liver health is milk thistle. This herb and the extract it yields, silymarin, are said to be powerful liver protectors. For anyone who regularly deals with pollutants like pesticides and who may thus be at higher risk for Parkinson's, milk thistle is one of several herbs recommended by Germano. Take up to 300 milligrams of standardized milk thistle extract daily, he says.

Be Free of Dangerous Debris with Fiber

The liver isn't the only organ that processes toxins. Properly functioning intestines are also very important for whisking unwanted, potentially dangerous substances out of the body, says Dr. Perlmutter.

Unfortunately, many people who have Parkinson's—who may have impaired detoxification abilities to begin with—also show signs of constipation, according to Jay Lombard, MD, assistant clinical professor of neurology at Weill Medical College of Cornell University in New York City and coauthor (with Germano) of *The Brain Wellness Plan.*

You could say that dietary fiber is like the whisk in the whisk broom, since it's the indigestible rough parts of fruits, vegetables, beans, and whole grains—and it does a pretty fair broom imitation. Ample fiber in your diet cleans out the colon. Waste products—and possibly pesticide residues—have less time to corrupt sensitive intestinal walls.

The Daily Value for fiber is 25 grams. To reach that amount, make it a point to eat more unprocessed foods, including fresh produce and whole grains. You may need to go one step further, though. "Almost every one of my Parkinson's patients is on some form of supplemental fiber," says Dr. Lombard. If you've increased your dietary fiber but are still experiencing constipation problems, ask your doctor about healthy fiber supplements like Metamucil or Citrucel.

phlebitis

Phlebitis is inflammation of a vein, usually caused by a clot that forms in the vein due to poor circulation. When the clot forms, blood flow is blocked, causing pain and swelling.

Often, someone who has phlebitis can actually feel a lump under the surface of the skin where the blood-distended vein is bulging. It may feel like a hard, painful knot or a sore, bruised spot. If the clot occurs very close to the surface of the skin, a red streak may be visible.

If you suspect that you have phlebitis, you need to get a medical diagnosis, followed by appropriate treatment. With the type called deep-vein phlebitis, there is a risk that the clot will dislodge and move to your heart, brain, or lung, where it can do extensive damage. Don't delay having it diagnosed, monitored, and treated by your doctor.

If you've had phlebitis in the past, however, there are ways to prevent a recurrence. Just moving around can help. So can elevating your legs when you sit down to rest, getting regular exercise, and wearing surgical pressure stockings.

If you're prone to phlebitis, you don't want to sit anywhere for very long. Sitting still for more than a couple of hours at a time can cause phlebitis in someone who's susceptible to the problem.

Along with those precautions, some supplements may help prevent phlebitis. They can reduce the tendency of your blood to clot, improve blood circulation in your legs, and help keep your legs from swelling with fluid. Just be sure to check with your doctor before trying these remedies.

Take Bromelain to Stop Clots

The blood-thinning and anti-inflammatory properties of bromelain, an enzyme derived from pineapple, work together to help prevent a recurrence of phlebitis, says Decker Weiss, NMD, director of the Weiss Center for Naturopathic Excellence, in Scottsdale, Arizona, and author of *The Weiss Method: A Natural Program for Reversing Heart Disease and Preventing Heart Attacks*. In a study of 73 people with a severe kind of phlebitis who took bromelain along with a pain reliever, researchers found that all symptoms of inflammation decreased, including pain, swelling, and elevated skin temperature.

"Bromelain is a potent inhibitor of platelets, components in blood that promote clotting," Dr. Weiss says. The enzyme prevents platelets from sticking together and also helps keep them from adhering to the sides of blood vessels.

Bromelain also declares war on fibrin, which is a protein at the core of the clotting process. By breaking down fibrin, the enzyme counteracts clot formation.

Dosages of bromelain typically range from 500 to 1,000 milligrams a day, says Dr. Weiss. To get the best effect, take a divided dose four times a day on an empty stomach, he advises. If it's taken with food, bromelain will simply act as a digestive enzyme rather than helping to prevent clotting.

Spices and Herbs as Add-Ons

Curcumin, a yellow pigment that comes from the Indian spice turmeric, acts as a strong natural anti-inflammatory and anti-clotting agent, says Dr. Weiss. Its anti-clotting properties resemble those of aspirin, which is commonly prescribed to help thin the blood and improve blood flow. "I like to use a mixture of curcumin and bromelain instead of aspirin with my patients," he says.

Dr. Weiss first prescribes a mixture of bromelain and curcumin, along with anticoagulants (blood thinners), to dissolve a clot. Once the clot is dissolved, he advises people to continue taking bromelain and curcumin. At the same time, he keeps them on an exercise program that includes yoga, and he prescribes hot and cold packs after the blood thinners have been discontinued. Usual doses of curcumin are 400 to 600 milligrams a day, which can be taken for up to 3 months without adverse effects, says Dr. Weiss. Do not take curcumin supplements if you are pregnant, however.

Ginger is another spice that can help prevent a recurrence of phlebitis. It also has strong anticlotting and anti-inflammatory powers, Dr. Weiss says. You can buy ginger in capsules. To reduce inflammation, you may need to take about 2,000 milligrams a day of dry powdered gingerroot, he says.

Vitamins to Help the Flow

Researchers now realize that an amino acid by-product called homocysteine can harm the insides of blood vessels, increasing the risk of atherosclerosis (hardening of the arteries). Homocysteine can also raise your chances of developing a blood clot, according to research.

In one study, researchers were able to reduce high homocysteine levels using 5 milligrams of folic acid, 400 micrograms of vitamin B_{12}, and 50 milligrams of vitamin B_6. "I recommend B vitamins to all my patients with heart or circulatory problems as part of a high-potency multivitamin," Dr. Weiss says.

The same antioxidant nutrients that are recommended to help prevent heart disease are also good if you have phlebitis, he adds. Vitamin E helps to reduce platelet stickiness, which means that you'll be less likely to have clotting. Studies suggest that reducing platelet stickiness with vitamin E could help treat people who have traveling blood clots, particularly those who have type 1 (insulin-dependent) diabetes and thus are at higher risk for clotting problems.

Vitamin C is essential because it helps to regenerate vitamin E, and both vitamins also help to reduce inflammation. Dr. Weiss recommends 400 to 800 international units a day of vitamin E and 1,000 to 3,000 milligrams a day of vitamin C in divided doses. Before you take that much vitamin E, however, you should check with your doctor, particularly if you are taking anticoagulants or aspirin.

PMS and menstrual problems

We're not going to wax poetic here about cycles of the moon, red tents, and all that. It's true, though, that being able to respect your body's cycles and the possible need for some downtime helps many women through that time of month, including the days preceding it, when mood swings and irritability may flare.

Whatever your concerns during this time, making some lifestyle changes can help, especially if those changes are coupled with herbs, minerals, and other supplements to rebalance your hormones, reduce bloating, and help you relax.

Defense Tactics

To help defuse PMS symptoms, cut down on or steer clear of coffee, chocolate, soda, and sugar-laden foods, says Barbara Silbert, DC, ND, a chiropractor and naturopathic doctor in Bethel, Vermont. Instead, experts recommend that you go for a diet that's full of fruits, vegetables, and fiber. Fiber helps move excess estrogen out of your body, instead of recirculating it back into your body via bile reabsorption. Regular exercise can also go a long way toward curbing PMS.

If you're having any kind of menstrual problems, it's always important to keep your physician informed, says Dr. Silbert. She cautions that supplements can't take the place of a doctor's care. If your cramps or blood flow are excessive enough to disrupt your life, be sure that your doctor knows about your symptoms before you start taking supplements.

A Hormonal Balancing Act

One possible cause of cramps and heavy bleeding during periods is an unbalanced ratio of estrogen to progesterone, says Jennifer Nevels, ND, a practitioner with East Valley Naturopathic Doctors in Mesa, Arizona.

These are the two hormones that play the biggest part in regulating the female reproductive system. Usually, women who experience problems with their periods have too much estrogen and not enough progesterone in the 1 to 2 weeks before their periods. This imbalance can set the stage for painful cramping and heavy flow, along with other unwelcome symptoms such as headaches and mood swings.

Supplements that balance estrogen and progesterone can make a big difference in how you feel before and during your period, says Dr. Nevels. Along with a high-fiber diet and herbs that help detoxify the liver and break down excess estrogen, she recommends vitex, or chasteberry. "It's something every woman I see with PMS gets," she says.

Research does show that vitex can help some symptoms of PMS, including breast pain and swelling, fluid retention, constipation, irritability, depressed mood or mood swings, anger, and headache. Its benefits have been attributed to its indirect effects on hormones and neurotransmitters such as dopamine, acetylcholine, and opioid receptors—the brain's pleasure centers. It also seems to help restore what's called the "luteal" phase of the menstrual cycle, the second half of the cycle, after ovulation. This may help restore normal estrogen-progesterone balance, Dr. Nevels says.

The dosage of chasteberry depends on the formulation you use and can vary considerably, from 4 to 20 milligrams per day, so it's best to follow the directions on the product you choose. One product Dr. Nevels recommends is PMS Support by Vital Nutrients. In addition to vitex, it contains dong quai, passionflower, vitamin B_6, and other herbs. The dosage is one or two capsules twice a day.

Black cohosh is another hormone-regulating herb that's often used for women's health problems. In one study, researchers analyzed the effects of a standardized black cohosh extract that's been used in Germany for more than 40 years. They found that it reduced depression, anxiety, and mood swings in women with PMS.

If you take black cohosh, follow the dosage directions on the package you buy. A typical dose would be 20 milligrams in the morning and 20 milligrams in the evening.

The Chinese Solution

Dong quai is an herb that's long been used in traditional Chinese medicine for various women's ailments. One of its primary benefits is its ability

Find Relief with Chasteberry

Chasteberry, or vitex, has been used since Greco-Roman times, most frequently to treat women's ailments. The berries come from a tree that is native to the Mediterranean region. As you might guess from its name, it was also once used to suppress sexual urges.

Today, chasteberry extract is popularly used to help relieve symptoms of PMS, along with menopausal discomforts and certain menstrual problems, such as the absence of periods. It's especially helpful during the time of perimenopause, when you may have stopped ovulating but are still having periods. This is when you are most likely to have an estrogen-progesterone imbalance.

Chasteberry isn't for everyone, however. Women with hormone-sensitive conditions should avoid chasteberry. Some of these conditions include breast, uterine, and ovarian cancer, and endometriosis and uterine fibroids.

And if you are taking birth control pills, try a different remedy, since chasteberry may counteract the effectiveness of oral contraceptives.

to relieve cramps by helping the uterus relax. Dong quai can also help reduce menstrual blood flow.

If you'd like to try dong quai, it's available in most health food stores. Just follow the dosage directions on the package you buy. (A typical dose might be one or two 550-milligram capsules twice a day.) Practitioners usually recommend taking it from 14 days after a period begins until the start of your next period. Do not take dong quai while menstruating, as it can increase blood loss.

Clearing Up Cramps

"Cramps are very common among menstruating women," says Samantha Brody, ND, a naturopathic doctor specializing in women's health in Portland, Oregon. Fortunately, you may not have to resort to over-the-counter pain relievers to get them under control.

One of the first things you should do is back off on consuming chocolate, coffee, soda, and anything else that contains caffeine. Menstrual cramps have also been associated with sugar and refined carbohydrates, adds Dr. Brody. After making these dietary changes, consider trying some of the best cramp relievers around—magnesium, calcium, vitamin B_6, and feverfew. (Take them with plenty of water and they will work even better!)

Calcium works wonderfully to relieve some women's cramps. According to a study at Metropolitan Hospital in New York City, 73 percent of women who took 1,000 milligrams of calcium a day for at least a month experienced fewer PMS symptoms than they had previously. The research suggests that the calcium helped reduce breast tenderness, headaches, and abdominal cramps. Researchers think that these benefits stem from calcium's ability to relieve muscle contractions. A good daily dose is 1,000 milligrams, says Willow Moore, DC, ND, a chiropractor and naturopathic doctor in Owings Mills, Maryland.

Like calcium, magnesium helps relieve muscle contractions, says Dr. Moore. Some studies have found lower levels of magnesium in women who have PMS. Other studies suggest that increasing magnesium can ease or eliminate PMS symptoms.

Taking 500 milligrams of magnesium a day may help ease the pain, says Dr. Brody. Too much magnesium, though, can cause diarrhea. If that happens, reduce your intake to a level that your body can tolerate or take a form that is more easily absorbed than magnesium carbonate, such as magnesium glycinate or citrate.

Do You Need B_6 and Feverfew?

Vitamin B_6 is a good supplement to take because it works together with magnesium to reduce cramps and relax muscles, says Dr. Silbert. She recommends 50 milligrams twice a day, with breakfast and lunch. (Taken at bedtime, B_6 is reported to sometimes cause "vivid dreams.") And she prefers a kind of B_6 called P5P, short for pyridoxal-5-phosphate, because it is the active form of B_6. (Some people have trouble converting B_6 to its active form.) P5P can be found at health food stores and online.

Many antispasmodic and anti-inflammatory herbs are also used to relieve cramps, says Dr. Silbert. She often recommends feverfew. Some research suggests that this herb helps lessen pain by preventing the formation of prostaglandins, chemicals that are a critical part of the chain that creates the sensation of pain.

Take the amount indicated on the package on the days that you experience cramping, says Dr. Silbert. A typical dosage of feverfew is 125 milligrams three times a day.

Fish Oil to the Rescue

At least eight studies have found that women who get good amounts of the omega-3 fatty acids found in fish oil have an easier time of it when that time of the month rolls around. Fish oil is well known to decrease levels of inflammatory prostaglandins that contribute to pain. In one study, women who took about 2 grams a day of fish oil reported significantly less menstrual pain. Fish oil is also a good choice if moodiness or depression is part of your monthly scenario, since it seems helpful for both stabilizing mood and lifting depression. It is safely used with antidepressants and even seems to help them work better. It can take a few months of use before you begin to see the full benefits of fish oil.

Supplements for Heavy Bleeding

Life is busy enough without having to worry about embarrassing accidents. Luckily, there are a lot of supplements that you can try, individually or in combination, to stem heavy menstrual flow. A few of these are yarrow, shepherd's purse, iron, vitamin C, and bioflavonoids.

Yarrow and shepherd's purse are two herbs that can help stem bleeding. But how do you decide which one to take?

Yarrow works best for women who have bright red blood flow, says Matthew Wood, a professional member of the American Herbalists Guild in Minnetrista, Minnesota, and author of *The Book of Herbal Wisdom*. It also tends to be more effective in women who have strong, robust constitutions, he says. Shepherd's purse, on the other hand, is best-suited for women whose flow is more clotted and who have milder temperaments.

Both are astringents that promote rapid blood clotting to slow or stop excess blood loss. Two clinical studies suggest that shepherd's purse is an effective remedy for heavy menstrual bleeding. Whichever remedy you decide to try, you'll need to take it every day, says Wood. But he cautions against using shepherd's purse if you have kidney stones.

"You'll know within 6 weeks if it's working," he says. If you don't see any results in that time, switch to another remedy or consider seeing a doctor. Since concentrations vary by product, Wood recommends using a tincture and following the dosage instructions on the label.

Iron Things Out

Iron is probably the most important mineral you can take to help control menstrual blood loss, says Dr. Brody. Heavy menstrual flow can deplete your body's iron stores, and some researchers also believe that chronic iron deficiency may cause heavy bleeding.

In one study, 75 percent of women who supplemented with iron had decreased menstrual blood flow compared with only about 33 percent in a group that took inactive substances (placebos). Thus, iron might just be the answer to your heavy bleeding problems. Do not take more than the Daily Value of iron (18 milligrams) without medical supervision, though, says Dr. Brody. You must be tested for iron deficiency before supplementing with higher doses.

Get a C-Plus

Two other supplements for heavy bleeding are vitamin C and bioflavonoids, says Liz Collins, ND, a naturopathic doctor and co-owner of the Natural Childbirth and Family Clinic in Portland, Oregon. Vitamin C can significantly increase iron absorption, so it goes in tandem with an iron supplement, but the combination of vitamin C and bioflavonoids is better yet, according to Dr. Collins.

If you're prone to excessive menstrual bleeding, it might be the result of fragile blood vessels. Vitamin C and bioflavonoids may strengthen those blood vessels and make them less susceptible to damage. In one study, for example, 14 out of 16 women who supplemented with 200 milligrams of vitamin C three times a day along with bioflavonoids found relief from heavy bleeding.

Dr. Collins recommends taking 500 to 1,000 milligrams of vitamin C three times a day and 500 to 1,000 milligrams of bioflavonoids once a day.

prostate problems

Many men start to experience some prostate gland problems by the time they reach their late forties or early fifties. Hormonal changes associated with aging, poor diet, and an accumulation of abdominal fat all cause this walnut-size gland found below the bladder to swell, a condition called benign prostatic hyperplasia (BPH). The process involves inflammation and stagnation of fluids and can set the stage for infection.

What BPH is most famous for is its effect on a man's ability to urinate. You may feel the urge to urinate more often, your bladder may still feel full after you've finished urinating, your stream may be weak, or you may find it difficult to get things going and keep things flowing.

Although BPH is not a sign of cancer, it's still a good idea to use natural means to get BPH under control, since some of the same hormonal imbalances and nutritional problems that cause BPH are also risk factors for prostate cancer. Natural treatments address these risks at their root cause—something BPH drugs can never do. Even if you end up having to use drugs, you'll probably feel better with a combination of drugs and supplements than you would if you just relied on BPH drugs alone.

But guys—make sure you work with your doctor. Get properly diagnosed, which will include a PSA test and possibly a prostate gland ultrasound and/or biopsy. Make sure BPH really is what you have. Once you're sure of that, here's what you can do to treat BPH naturally.

Foods to Favor

Eating the right foods (and avoiding the wrong ones) can help improve the hormones that affect BPH. "Eating *only* hormone-free meats and dairy products is really important, as is avoiding environmental toxins, especially in plastics, that act as hormonal mimics," says Glenn Finley, ND, a men's health specialist at the Brattleboro Naturopathic Clinic in Vermont. And even if you only eat hormone-free meats, limit red meat consumption to once or twice a week to minimize your intake of saturated fats.

In addition to avoiding red meat, make sure you get more healthy fish in your diet, including wild salmon, sardines, herring, and mackerel. And load up on lots of vegetables, especially detoxifying cruciferous vegetables, which help break down excessive hormones, and fill up on lots of fiber, which helps your body eliminate toxins and hormones by absorbing bile. You can have some soy, but don't overdo it. "I prefer men to use beans that are a little less estrogenic than soy, such as black beans and adzuki beans," Dr. Finley says.

Even beer can be a problem, since it is made with hops, which are a rich source of phytoestrogens, says Thomas Kruzel, ND, a naturopathic doctor at the Rockwood Natural Medicine Clinic, in Scottsdale, Arizona. And guys who are trying to lose the beer belly by drinking "light" beer only make their prostate problems worse, since light beers use more hops than regular beers do, Dr. Kruzel says. "I tell guys to stick with the good stuff, the regular stuff, and just drink less of it."

Shrink with Saw Palmetto

One of the most widespread herbal medicines used to reduce the size and irritating symptoms of an enlarged prostate is saw palmetto extract, usually in combination with other ingredients, such as nettle. Studies show that up to 60 percent of men with mild to moderate BPH experience some relief from all major symptoms—frequent urination, hesitancy, urgency, and perineal heaviness—within the first 4 to 6 weeks of treatment with this herb.

Research shows that saw palmetto can work in a number of ways. Studies with a specific "fat-friendly" (liposterolic) extract of saw palmetto berries showed that it reduced the uptake by prostate tissue of both testosterone and dihydrotestosterone (DHT) by more than 40 percent, suggesting it blocks activity of male hormones. The extract also inhibited binding of DHT to its receptor sites on prostate tissue and blocked the conversion of testosterone to DHT by inhibiting the activity of 5-alpha-reductase. That's exactly the same therapeutic action as the most commonly prescribed drug for BPH, finasteride (sold as Proscar). The berries also inhibit two biochemicals that cause inflammation: cyclooxygenase and 5-lipoxygenase.

If you decide to try saw palmetto, you should work with your doctor to choose a high-quality brand. Researchers think that one reason not all studies show a benefit is that the quality of saw palmetto products can vary widely. It's the *fats* in saw palmetto that provide the active ingredients, so look for a lipophilic extract containing 80 to 90 percent fatty acids. (It should say it contains a liposterolic extract.)

If you have mild to moderate BPH, take 160 milligrams twice a day with meals until your symptoms improve, says Dr. Kruzel. Then, he suggests, continue taking at least 160 milligrams daily as a maintenance dose. The capsules should contain 85 to 95 percent liposterolic extract. Most clinical studies have used a liposterolic extract of saw palmetto berry containing 80 to 90 percent free fatty acids. The brand used in studies showing positive results is Permixon, which is a prescription-only product in Europe. However, its formulation is similar to Super Saw Palmetto (by Enzymatic Therapy), Standardized Saw Palmetto Extract (by Nature's Way), and others, which are all available over-the-counter.

Help from Tree and Weed

Two other botanical medicines that are widely used to treat prostate enlargement are *Pygeum africanum* and nettle. Although neither has been as widely studied as saw palmetto, they are still considered good choices by complementary medicine experts.

P. africanum is an evergreen tree native to Africa that contains compounds that have anti-inflammatory properties. Several clinical trials involving more than 600 men have shown that pygeum extract is effective at reducing BPH symptoms.

In a study in which 263 men were given 50 milligrams of pygeum in the morning and evening for 60 days, 66 percent of the men reported that they had fewer problems urinating. During the same study, a similar group of men with similar problems was given pills that contained no pygeum (placebos); among that group, only 31 percent showed any improvement.

As for nettle, this herbal supplement is best used during the early stages of BPH, says Dr. Kruzel. Researchers believe that extracts of nettle root reduce BPH symptoms by blocking inflammatory chemicals within the prostate tissue or by inhibiting the action of a sex-hormone-binding protein.

Because nettle and pygeum relieve BPH symptoms differently, they're often used in combination with one another or with saw palmetto for the best results, says Dr. Kruzel. One combination product that he uses has 160 milligrams of saw palmetto, 320 milligrams of pumpkin seed oil, and

20 milligrams of pygeum. Take two capsules twice a day until your symptoms improve, he suggests, then take one capsule twice a day to maintain prostate health. For men with mild BPH, he also suggests taking two 300-milligram doses of nettle twice a day until symptoms improve, then taking one capsule once or twice a day to maintain prostate health.

Zinc: A Highly Influential Mineral

Getting enough zinc can help rebalance hormones and prevent the progression of BPH, Dr. Kruzel and other natural health practitioners say. "The prostate has one of the highest concentrations of zinc of any tissue in the body," says Dr. Kruzel. Adequate amounts of zinc help to prevent testosterone from converting to its stronger version, DHT, which stimulates prostate enlargement.

Many people, especially vegetarians, don't get enough zinc. Forms of supplemental zinc that are most absorbable are protein chelates, such as zinc picolinate, which means you may be able to take less of those forms. If you have BPH, consult your doctor for the appropriate zinc dosage. Doses higher than 20 milligrams daily should be taken only with medical supervision. The current safe upper limit is 40 milligrams, and amounts higher than 100 milligrams a day cause an increase in prostate cancer risk. Since zinc interferes with copper absorption, it's good to take 1 milligram of copper for about every 7 milligrams of zinc supplementation.

Fatty Acids for Prostate Maintenance

The fats you get in your diet make a big difference in the kinds of inflammatory biochemicals you make in your body. They also affect hormone production. Most people get too much of saturated fats and polyunsaturated fats called omega-6 fatty acids. What they don't get enough of are omega-3 fatty acids, which are anti-inflammatory in your body. So alternative medical practitioners recommend getting more omega-3s and less of the bad fats to reduce inflammation bodywide—and that includes inflammation in your prostate.

You can easily get omega-3s by taking fish oil supplements, Dr. Kruzel says. Take 1 to 3 grams a day of a good, molecularly distilled brand. That process removes mercury and other toxins from the oil. Check with your doctor before taking fish oil capsules if you take any kind of blood-thinning medication.

Dr. Finley also likes his prostate patients to use ground flaxseed, the same stuff recommended to postmenopausal women to help smooth things out. "Flaxseed is a good source of healthy fats, and it helps to balance out both estrogen and testosterone," he says. He recommends 1 to 2 tablespoons a day. It's fine to take both fish oil and flaxseed, especially if you are otherwise on a fairly low-fat diet.

Amino Acids for Symptom Relief

The combination of the amino acids alanine, glutamic acid, and glycine has been shown in some studies to relieve many symptoms of BPH. "There are many amino acids that are present in the prostate gland, but these three, in particular, are key in developing and maintaining prostate health," says Dr. Kruzel.

In one study, 45 men were given this combination of supplements. At the end of the study, researchers saw a reduction in nighttime bathroom visits in 95 percent of the participants. Eighty-one percent said they didn't have the urge to urinate as often, and 73 percent made fewer daily trips to the bathroom.

For symptom relief, Dr. Kruzel suggests taking combination products that contain herbs and vitamins as well as 50 milligrams of alanine and glycine and between 50 and 100 milligrams of glutamic acid. He suggests taking two capsules twice a day for 10 to 14 days and then reducing the dose to one capsule once or twice a day as a maintenance dose.

You may need to get this specific formula from a holistic practitioner, but similar products are available commercially. Dr. Kruzel recommends talking to your doctor before you begin taking these amino acids.

raynaud's disease

If you have Raynaud's disease, your hands overreact to cold and your feet may, too. Stepping outdoors on a wintry day, you feel as if all your fingers or toes go numb instantly. Odder still, the numbness can assault your fingers even if you're just rummaging around in the freezer for a package of frozen carrots. When you look at your numb toes or fingers, they appear dead white, as if all the blood had left them. Even after you've rescued your hands or feet from the arctic temperatures and tried to warm them up, the numbness can linger.

It's thought that people who have Raynaud's disease have something slightly awry in the way their nervous systems function. The nerves that are connected with the muscles that control blood flow somehow get their wires crossed so that their messages don't get to the right places.

The sympathetic nervous system is responsible for expanding or shrinking blood vessels in response to temperature. Normally, if your body gets cold, the blood vessels that lead to your arms and legs will open up, allowing warm blood to flow to fingers and toes. In Raynaud's disease, blood vessels get the wrong message and constrict, instead, sending already cold fingers to the deep freeze. Smoking, by the way, constricts blood vessels in the extremities. If you have Raynaud's and you smoke, just quitting may clear up your symptoms.

Women seem to have Raynaud's more often than men do. Someone with Raynaud's may have other problems as well that seem to be associated with the disease, such as migraines, carpal tunnel syndrome, or mitral valve prolapse, a condition that occurs when one part of a heart valve malfunctions.

Raynaud's can also be associated with lupus, a disease related to a defective immune system, or scleroderma, a problem of abnormally thickening skin. All of this suggests to scientists that there may be a genetic link between some of these other conditions and Raynaud's. (For more information, please see Scleroderma on page 581.)

While Raynaud's is usually not much more than an annoying problem, some of the related conditions mentioned above are serious. If you think that you may have Raynaud's, you should see your doctor to get a proper diagnosis.

Doctors recommend a variety of different procedures for helping alleviate the symptoms of Raynaud's. You might start by learning relaxation techniques and biofeedback, which will help you teach your body to send more blood to your fingers and toes even when your jumpy nervous system is telling the blood vessels to slam shut.

Some doctors also recommend warm-water exercises. If you periodically submerge your hands in a tub of warm water while standing in a cold room, you can retrain your body to warm up rather than cool down when it's exposed to a cool environment. Your doctor can give you more information about the conditioning procedures that sometimes prove effective.

Whether or not you try a conditioning regimen, there are some supplements that may also help. The ones that are most likely to be beneficial are those that relax and open blood vessels. Here are some natural ways to support proper circulation.

Try Magnesium for Relaxed Blood Flow

The mineral magnesium is known for relaxing smooth muscle, which is the kind that lines the insides of blood vessels. "Magnesium can counter the inappropriate activation of the sympathetic nervous system," says Jay Lombard, MD, assistant clinical professor of neurology at Weill Medical College of Cornell University in New York City and coauthor of *The Brain Wellness Plan.* Instead of shutting down, the blood vessels may be encouraged to open up when they're under the influence of magnesium.

Take 1,000 milligrams of magnesium a day, Dr. Lombard recommends. One form that he suggests is magnesium gluconate, which won't give you the diarrhea that may be caused by other forms. Avoid magnesium oxide or magnesium chloride, he advises.

Turn Up the Heat with Niacin

Niacin is a supplement with side effects. The most noticeable one is what's referred to as "flushing," a sensation of heat and tingling that comes from high doses of the pure form of the nutrient. It's just this side effect that can be helpful in Raynaud's disease, says Ross Hauser, MD, director of Caring Medical and Rehabilitation Services at Beulah Land Natural Medicine Clinic in Thebes, Illinois.

Doses many times higher than the Daily Value of niacin make the capillaries dilate. That's what causes the famous side effect, says Dr. Hauser. While the feeling can be uncomfortable or even frightening if it happens unexpectedly, a controlled niacin flush can help bring warmth to frigid digits, he notes.

Niacin has two chemical structures, but only one, nicotinic acid, causes flushing. Nicotinamide or niacinamide, the form of niacin usually found in multivitamins, won't cause the desired effect, says Dr. Hauser. To see if niacin helps, you'll need to find pure niacin or nicotinic acid. Check labels to be sure.

Before taking supplements, you should check with your doctor. With your doctor's consent, you can start with 100 milligrams of nicotinic acid a day, suggests Dr. Hauser, although he sometimes recommends higher and more frequent doses to some patients. He recommends that you see your doctor for re-evaluation after 2 months of this treatment.

restless legs syndrome

If you have restless legs syndrome, you may not know it, but your bed partner probably does. When you—and your legs—are ready to rest, restless legs are ready to run. Sensations of jumpiness, itchiness, burning, aching, or twitching are all common in people with restless legs.

"It's often an unrecognized cause of insomnia," explains Jay Lombard, MD, assistant clinical professor of neurology at Weill Medical College of Cornell University in New York City and coauthor of *The Brain Wellness Plan*. You may think that you "just can't sleep," but in fact, it's the annoyance of your overactive limbs that is robbing you of your rest.

Calming restless legs can require some patience. If you're a pregnant woman, your legs will probably feel better after you've had your baby. Smokers with restless legs should quit smoking to give their leg circulation a chance to flow full-force. For some people with severe restless legs, a trial of medication may be in order. Then, there are also some leg-soothing supplements that are definitely worth trying.

A Mineral Trio to Calm Cranky Muscles

A combined deficiency of three minerals could be responsible for the annoying jumpiness of restless legs syndrome, according to Ross Hauser, MD, director of Caring Medical and Rehabilitation Services at Beulah Land Natural Medicine Clinic in Thebes Park, Illinois. "A lack of calcium, potassium, and magnesium can make the large muscles in the legs hyperirritable," he says.

Calcium, magnesium, and potassium all have an effect on muscle contraction and relaxation. In addition, they help nerve transmission.

Experts say that you can help calm your legs and get some rest by making sure that you're getting enough of all three minerals. Dr. Hauser recommends taking a daily dose of between 800 and 1,000 milligrams of calcium and 500 milligrams of magnesium. Take half this dose in the morning and half at bedtime. Aim for about 3,000 to 5,000 milligrams of potassium by eating a diet rich in fruits and vegetables.

Try 5-HTP for a Good Night's Sleep

Have you ever noticed the little jerking movements that you (or your partner) make just as you're shifting into sleep? Those are outward signs that your brain is closing the gate on muscle movement for the night. If those muscles didn't voluntarily shut down, they'd go on obeying your brain impulses even in the midst of deep sleep. Without that safety switch, if you dreamed of running a marathon, you might end up about 26 miles from where you went to sleep.

For people with restless legs syndrome, that gating mechanism may not be functioning at 100 percent efficiency, says Dr. Lombard. Some movement impulses are getting through, keeping your legs active all night long and leaving you exhausted come morning.

"An interesting supplement called 5-hydroxytryptophan (5-HTP) seems to work well," says Dr. Lombard. Experts believe that 5-HTP is used to make serotonin, a chemical messenger in the brain that can affect sleep quality.

"The rationale behind using 5-HTP for restless legs is that raising serotonin levels will raise the gating effect," says Dr. Lombard. Essentially, it helps to separate mind from body, thus making it easier for your legs to lie still through the night.

Some people with restless legs who try 5-HTP notice a change for the better right away, but you might have to take the supplements for 2 weeks to 1 month before you know whether it will work for you, according to Dr. Lombard.

Start by taking 100 milligrams about 20 minutes before you go to bed, he suggests. You can increase the dose to 200 milligrams if you don't see results after the first few weeks, but don't take any more than that, he advises. Larger doses can cause disturbing dreams and nightmares.

You shouldn't take 5-HTP for longer than 3 months without consulting a doctor. You should also avoid it if you are currently taking antidepressants or have taken them recently. The combined effects could cause a possibly fatal condition called serotonin syndrome. Do not take supplements of 5-HTP if you are pregnant or trying to conceive.

Stabilize Membranes with Horse Chestnut

Preparations of horse chestnut leaves, bark, and seeds are used in Europe for their positive effect on vein health. There's good reason to consider standardized extracts of this herb for the treatment of restless legs, as well, according to Dr. Hauser.

"Horse chestnut is unique in its ability to stabilize vascular membranes," he says. This may give restless legs extra blood flow that can prevent sensations of itchiness or burning.

Give this herbal remedy a try by taking 400 milligrams of standardized extract twice a day, says Dr. Hauser. Generally, people respond within a month, he adds. If your symptoms don't improve in that amount of time, stop taking it and see your doctor for an evaluation.

Horse chestnut is not for everyone. It may interfere with the action of other drugs, especially blood thinners such as warfarin (Coumadin). It may also irritate the gastrointestinal tract. As with other herbs, you should not take it if you are pregnant or breastfeeding.

To use horse chestnut safely, obtain a standardized extract and follow the package directions. A naturopathic doctor or doctor of integrative medicine can help you use this plant safely.

rheumatoid arthritis

If you have rheumatoid arthritis, your body's infection-fighting immune cells decide that you're the enemy. They attack your joints and cause inflammation, with pain, redness, heat, swelling, and tissue damage.

Rheumatoid arthritis (RA) is a chronic inflammatory disease that affects the lining of the joints, mostly in the hands and knees. It's characterized by swelling and redness and can wear down the cartilage between bones. RA is two to three times more common in women than in men. People who develop it tend to have a genetic tendency toward the disease, researchers now know. But not everyone with "RA genes" gets it, so researchers believe some sort of environmental trigger may also set it off.

What those triggers may be is still anyone's guess, and it's likely that there are a number of possible causes, says Jody Noe, ND, a faculty member at the University of Bridgeport College of Naturopathic Medicine and in private practice at Natural Family Health and Integrative Medicine, in Westerly, Rhode Island. Among the possibilities: infectious diseases, such as *Chlamydia pneumoniae,* now recognized as a cause of pneumonia, pharyngitis, bronchitis, and several other chronic inflammation-related diseases.

Other possible causes: leaky gut syndrome, which can lead to autoimmunity as allergens in the GI tract that normally wouldn't get into your bloodstream leak into your body and get attacked by your immune system, and environmental toxins, including mercury fillings, which can trigger an inflammatory cascade.

The inflammation doesn't always confine itself to joints, either, says Andrew Rubman, ND, director of the Southbury Clinic for Traditional Medicine in Connecticut and consultant to the Office of Complementary and Alternative Medicine at the National Institutes of Health. "Other organs, such as the skin, heart, and lungs, can be affected," he says.

Rheumatoid arthritis is usually treated with drugs that suppress your immune system, such as methotrexate, strong anti-inflammatory drugs, and steroid drugs that also knock out inflammation and may suppress your immune system.

Alternative practitioners attack rheumatoid arthritis on several additional fronts, says Dr. Noe. They try to figure out what is making the immune system go awry, and correct that. To do this, they look at GI tract symptoms, toxic chemical exposure, stress, nutritional deficiencies, antioxidant status, and hormone levels, and they correct those as needed.

They also use anti-inflammatory nutrients and herbs. Often, these supplements are prescribed in large doses, so you'll need the advice of a practitioner or doctor before you start taking them.

Some of the recommended supplements, like vitamins D and C, also work to restore proper immunity and to get the adrenal glands functioning better. These glands, located above the kidneys, are powerful little organs that secrete hormones such as epinephrine and steroids, which affect many organ functions and influence the use of energy throughout your body.

If you've been diagnosed with rheumatoid arthritis and want to try these options, be aware that many conventional doctors may not be up on the latest natural remedies. Or they may be very skeptical, and for good reason, as there are many RA products that don't work.

But there are some that do help, as you'll see in the following pages. If you can, find a doctor who specializes in integrative medicine, whether it's an MD, DO, or ND (a naturopathic doctor). Doctors who practice integrative medicine combine conventional and alternative medicine as needed. Seek out one who specializes in autoimmune disorders, including rheumatoid arthritis.

Factor In Friendly Fats

By changing the kinds of fats you eat, you can reduce the amount of inflammation-generating chemicals that your body produces. "Meat and other animal foods provide your body with something called arachidonic acid, which is used to make pro-inflammatory biochemicals," Dr. Noe explains. A diet filled with nuts, seeds, and dark leafy greens will help you cut back on inflammatory fats. And eating cold-water fish like wild salmon, mackerel, herring, and sardines, or taking fish oil supplements, will get you plenty of anti-inflammatory omega-3 fatty acids.

Several studies have shown that fish oil supplements may help reduce morning stiffness with RA. In addition, the omega-3 fatty acids in fish oil help protect against heart disease, which is an added benefit because people with RA are at a higher risk of developing heart disease.

Based on this, supplement with fish oil, Dr. Noe says. The best way to make fish oil work for you is to cut back on pro-inflammatory fats, so it doesn't have to compete with them, and to use other anti-inflammatory aids along with it. That way, using 2 to 3 grams a day will slowly reduce inflammation. It can take months to see the full effects of fish oil supplements, so be patient.

Mind Your D

It's well established now that a deficiency of vitamin D plays a role in the development of autoimmune problems, including rheumatoid arthritis. "This new research is really opening our eyes about the importance of vitamin D for so many systems in the body, including immunity," Dr. Noe says.

A number of population studies have linked low blood levels of vitamin D with an increased risk for rheumatoid arthritis. Women living in northeastern America, for instance, where sun exposure comes with the risk for frostbite during certain months of the year, are more likely to develop rheumatoid arthritis.

Another study showed that once you have RA, your vitamin D status may also play an important role in how bad it gets. The study looked at women with early inflammatory polyarthritis—two or more painful joints for at least 4 weeks. It found that women with higher vitamin D levels were less likely to get worse than women with low D levels. Every 10 ng/ml increase in vitamin D was associated with a 43 percent lower tender joint count, a 25 percent lower C-reactive protein level (a measure of inflammation), and other reduced symptoms, like the number of swollen joints.

So good vitamin D status clearly was associated with less serious RA, over time. But so many women in this group had low vitamin D levels—more than 75 percent had levels lower than 30 ng/ml—that it was hard to even find women with RA with optimal levels.

Vitamin D experts such as John Cannell, MD, director of the Vitamin D Council, are now saying that everyone should take a dose that maintains vitamin D blood levels (25-hydroxy-vitamin D) at 50 to 80 ng/ml, year-round. To attain that level, you may need a high dose of vitamin D_3 (the active form), taken under medical supervision. Once your levels are high

Reining In Radicals with C and E

In our bodies, inflammation is usually a protective response brought on by an infection or injury. If your immune system is in good operating order, it detects any foreign organism that's been able to invade at the site of the wound or infection, and your body begins setting up its defense. The response is designed to wall off the infection or foreign matter from the rest of the body, destroy any organisms involved, and break down any injured tissue, clearing the way for new construction.

The classic signs of inflammation are heat, redness, swelling, and pain. These symptoms are the result of increased blood flow into the affected area. The blood vessels actually change size, making room for immune cells to travel through the bloodstream to the site of the injured or infected tissue. This process also produces a number of chemicals that orchestrate the process and that can cause pain and fatigue.

In this process, free radicals are normally generated, according to Maret G. Traber, PhD, principal investigator at the Linus Pauling Institute and associate professor of nutrition at Oregon State University in Corvallis. Free radicals are molecules that can cause damage to healthy cells by stealing electrons from other molecules in cells. "Immune cells, such as lymphocytes, macrophages, and neutrophils, generate oxygen and hydrogen peroxide as part of the clean-'em-up, move-'em-out process," notes Dr. Traber.

Macrophages are amoeba-like cells that engulf bacteria and foreign matter. Inside the voluminous macrophages are sacs of hydrogen peroxide,

enough, a lower daily dose will maintain them, Dr. Noe says. The suggested starting point is between 1,000 and 2,000 IU a day.

And it's better to take a smaller daily dose than one large dose once a week, as some doctors recommend, Dr. Rubman says. "We believe that large weekly doses of vitamin D can interfere with parathyroid hormone levels," he says. The parathyroid gland controls calcium balance in the body.

Antioxidant Synergy to Ax Inflammation

Any time you have inflammation, there's production of free radicals—unstable molecules that can harm surrounding cells, causing what's called oxidative damage. Some nutrients that may help stop free radicals and prevent that damage include vitamins E and C, beta-carotene, selenium, and zinc.

and when the invaders are trapped in these sacs, they're killed by the interaction with hydrogen peroxide.

As inflammation progresses, some free radicals end up on the wrong side of the battlefield. They may react with the membranes of cells that are essentially innocent bystanders, damaging some of the molecules in those otherwise healthy cells. If the healthy cells' membranes are damaged enough, the cells may be killed or maimed.

If there are antioxidants in the neighborhood during this reaction, less damage may occur. Some antioxidants, such as vitamin E, act as shields. They are incorporated into cell membranes and can give up one of their own electrons, thus neutralizing a free radical and making it settle down rather than hunting for other electrons.

Vitamin C can collaborate in neutralizing free radicals. If vitamin C is available to give vitamin E one of its electrons, vitamin E can put the damper on free radical activity. "It actually travels through the cell membrane, and each molecule of vitamin E can protect about 1,000 molecules in the membrane," Dr. Traber says.

Other antioxidants act in different ways, but the end result is the same: More cells are protected and emerge unscathed despite being under assault from the free radicals that have been unleashed during inflammation.

Several studies have shown that the risk of rheumatoid arthritis is highest among people with the lowest blood levels of these nutrients. Other studies suggest that whether or not people are deficient, these nutrients may help reduce their arthritis symptoms.

In a Belgian study, 15 women with rheumatoid arthritis who took 160 micrograms of selenium or 200 micrograms of selenium-enriched yeast every day for 4 months experienced significant improvement in joint movement and strength. Another study showed that people with rheumatoid arthritis who took 600 IU of vitamin E twice a day had a significant reduction in pain compared with people who took pills with no vitamin E (placebos).

Researchers at the University of Washington in Seattle found that people with rheumatoid arthritis who took 50 milligrams of zinc three times a day for 3 months experienced significant improvement in joint swelling and morning stiffness. It also took them less time to walk certain distances than when they were not taking the zinc.

"Zinc helps your body make an important inflammation-fighting enzyme called superoxide dismutase," says Dr. Noe. She cautions, however, that this doesn't mean that you should take the amounts of zinc that were used in the study. This amount of zinc should not be taken without medical supervision.

Dr. Noe recommends a daily mixture of antioxidant nutrients, including 1,000 to 3,000 milligrams of vitamin C in divided doses, 400 to 1,000 IU of vitamin E, 200 to 400 micrograms of selenium, and 15 to 30 milligrams of zinc picolinate or citrate. Each antioxidant works in a slightly different way, so a mix of lower-dosage antioxidants can really work better than higher doses of just one or two, she says.

You can also take 1 to 2 milligrams a day of copper and 5 to 15 milligrams of manganese, suggests Dr. Noe. Both of these trace minerals help the body make its own antioxidants. Be careful not to take higher doses of these two, however, as they can be toxic in large amounts.

"A good multivitamin/mineral will cover a lot of these nutritional bases," Dr. Noe says. To maximize absorption from a multi, she suggests taking capsules with meals.

Nutrients to Improve Digestion

Some kinds of arthritis have a clear link with inflammatory bowel disease. Those with confirmed links include arthritis of the knees, ankles, and wrists and ankylosing spondylitis (rheumatoid arthritis of the spine).

These links, as well as other clues, have suggested to doctors of alternative medicine that digestive problems can play a role in rheumatoid arthritis. Here's where the leaky gut theory comes in. If incompletely digested food and bacterial fragments are seeping through the intestinal lining and into the bloodstream, so the thinking goes, maybe they're setting off an improper immune response that ends up causing rheumatoid arthritis.

"It's possible to do tests that can confirm if someone is having an immune reaction that could cause rheumatoid arthritis," Dr. Noe says. Your rheumatologist or a naturopathic doctor can order these tests.

In addition, she recommends nutritional supplements that nourish and rebuild the intestinal lining and restore good bacteria in the bowel. Some foods that commonly aggravate leaky gut are wheat gluten, corn, and dairy products.

"I may also recommend enzymes that help break down food for proper digestion if tests suggest that someone's pancreas is not producing enough for normal digestion," Dr. Noe says.

To provide nourishment directly to intestinal cells, she suggests a large number of supplements that are specifically used to treat autoimmune diseases like rheumatoid arthritis and lupus. They include:

- 500 to 750 milligrams of the amino acid glutamine.
- 100 to 300 milligrams of gamma oryzanol, a component of rice bran oil.
- 50 to 100 milligrams of fructooligosaccharides (FOS), taken two or three times a day between meals. (Fructooligosaccharides are naturally occurring sugars that help to promote the growth of friendly bacteria in the intestines.)
- One or two capsules two or three times a day of a supplement containing various forms of lactobacillus and other so-called friendly bacteria— *Lactobacillus acidophilus, L. rhamnosus, L. casei, L. plantarum, Bifidobacterium bifidum, B. longum,* and *B. breve.* The recommended dose is 2 to 5 billion active organisms per capsule.
- 500 to 1,000 milligrams of 10X USP of digestive enzymes. (10X USP is a measure of strength that's listed on the bottle.)
- A mixture of other enzymes derived from plants, including 12,500 to 18,000 USP of protease, 2,675 USP of lipase, 12,000 to 27,000 USP of amylase, and 175 Cu2 of cellulase.

Dr. Noe says that these supplements are safe to take on a continuous basis as long as you get your doctor's approval and remain under supervision. Some of the supplements may only be available through a naturopathic physician or doctor of integrative medicine.

Herbal Anti-Inflammatories

Like the drugs used to reduce inflammation, the herbs and spices used for rheumatoid arthritis target the biochemicals that generate inflammation. They do this in all sorts of different ways, and that's why a mix of them can be more helpful than larger doses of just one, Dr. Noe says.

Curcumin, a component of the yellow Indian spice turmeric, also reduces inflammation, but it's not very well absorbed. So natural care practitioners are using an altered form of curcumin called liposomal curcumin,

A Thunderstorm to Stay Away From

One botanical, thunder god vine, also known as lei gong teng (Latin name: *Tripterygium wilfordii*) has been used in China for health purposes for more than 400 years. A study conducted by the National Institutes of Health's Center for Complementary and Alternative Medicine found that thunder god vine relieved symptoms in patients with RA, including improvements in pain, tender and swollen joints, and physical function. Both oral and topical applications seem to help.

Thunder god vine has a long list of actions that affect the immune system, but the bottom line is that it does indeed inhibit immune cells involved in RA and other autoimmune diseases. The problem, according to the NIH, is that there is no safe, reliable source of thunder god vine in the United States, and that's important because if it is not processed properly, it is poisonous. Even when it is properly processed, it can decrease bone mineral density, impair fertility, and cause birth defects. It should not be taken with other immune-suppressing drugs. Until there is a reliable source of this herb, avoid it, experts say. Even then, it will require close medical supervision to avoid problems.

or Curcumin Phytosome, that is well absorbed. It is available in health food stores and online. Follow the label directions.

Ginger is another anti-inflammatory spice that can fight inflammation. Dr. Rubman recommends 100 to 200 milligrams three times a day of ginger extract standardized to contain 20 percent gingerol and shogaol, the active ingredients. You also have the option of 8 to 10 grams (about 1½ tablespoons) of fresh ginger or 2 to 4 grams (about 1 teaspoon) of dry powdered ginger daily.

Ginger can be especially soothing if your rheumatoid arthritis includes gastrointestinal problems. If you tend to "run hot," as Dr. Rubman puts it—if you tend to sweat a lot or have hot, swollen joints—you're better off avoiding ginger, he says.

sciatica

If all of your nerves were a network of roads, the sciatic nerve would be a busy interstate highway. All of the nerve impulses transmitted to and from the lower half of your body must pass through the sciatic nerve, the largest and longest in the body. From its roots in the spinal cord, the thick conduit branches through the buttocks and down the back of each leg to the foot. Pain that follows this route is called sciatica.

The pain can show up almost anywhere along this route, from your buttocks to your feet. It can vary from tingling to numbness and muscle weakness to searing pains that shoot down your leg.

Certain positions and movements can cause it. Other times, it might seem to be a constant thing. Smokers, people who do a lot of heavy lifting, and people with osteoporosis or arthritis are at highest risk for developing sciatica.

Sciatica can also be the result of bulging or shrinking disks, the cartilage between your spinal vertebrae. It can also be the result of spinal misalignment. Both of these problems pinch or put pressure on the sciatic nerve. In either of these cases, a good chiropractor should be able to provide some relief.

Natural remedies do a few things. They help reduce the inflammation that is invariably generated with chronic sciatica. They help to provide damaged nerves with support for repair. They can plump up those cartilage disks, and they relax spastic muscles.

Check for D-ficiency

One of the symptoms of vitamin D deficiency is unexplained chronic back pain. That means you've had it for at least 3 months and your doctor hasn't found any obvious cause. In one study of 360 patients with back pain, every one of them was found to have inadequate levels of vitamin D. After taking vitamin D supplements for 3 months, symptoms were improved in

95 percent of the patients. All of them with the most severe vitamin D deficiencies experienced back-pain relief once they increased their levels.

And in an extensive review of clinical research, editors at the professional journal *Pain Treatment Topics* concluded that "those with chronic back pain almost always had inadequate levels of vitamin D. When sufficient vitamin D supplementation was provided, their pain either vanished or was at least helped to a significant extent."

Vitamin D is essential for calcium absorption and bone health. Inadequate vitamin D intake can result in a softening of bone surfaces, or osteomalacia, that causes pain. The lower back seems to be particularly vulnerable to this effect, and that's where sciatic pain originates.

Vitamin D shouldn't be seen as a cure for all back pain, but it is worth trying (and much cheaper than a lot of other options), these researchers say. It's best to get your blood levels checked and to take a dosage that maintains your blood level at 50 ng/ml or higher. (For most people, 50 to 80 ng/ml is a good range.) Experts suggest a starting dosage of between 1,000 and 2,000 IU.

Take Magnesium and Calcium, Too

While you're taking extra vitamin D, don't forget calcium and magnesium. "Magnesium is especially important because it takes more energy for a muscle to relax than it does to contract, and magnesium really does help muscles to relax," says Evie Katahdin, ND, a naturopathic doctor specializing in sports medicine at AthletiZen, in Costa Mesa, California. Sciatic pain can be caused by back muscle contractions, or the pain itself can cause them. Either way, you hurt.

Dr. Katahdin advises her patients to take 400 to 600 milligrams of an easily absorbed form of magnesium (such as glycinate, citrate, or malate), orally, at night. "These forms don't get lost in the gastrointestinal tract and usually don't cause any side effects, such as diarrhea, at these dosages," she says. "If it does, you can just back down on the dose a little." As an extra benefit, magnesium can help relax muscles and ease pain so you can sleep better.

Calcium is important, too, for a healthy back and strong muscles, and she likes people to get 1,000 to 1,200 milligrams a day, again, in an absorbable form such as citrate or glycinate.

Try the Osteoarthritis Duo: Glucosamine and Chondroitin

Because sciatica can sometimes be caused by deteriorating spinal disks, which are made of cartilage, some doctors recommend the same supplements used to help preserve joint cartilage in osteoarthritis: glucosamine and chondroitin. These two provide the building blocks needed to maintain and repair cartilage, and they can also be helpful for back problems because your spine does have joints between each vertebrae.

Because the pair works best by preserving the cartilage you have left, don't wait until you're in agonizing pain to start on a supplement program. Take 500 milligrams of glucosamine sulfate and 400 milligrams of chondroitin sulfate twice a day. It can take up to 4 months before you begin to notice benefits. You can take these two supplements indefinitely.

Bring in the Bs

To help muscles repair and relax, and to provide nerves with the energy they need for repair and neurotransmitter production, you also need B vitamins. People don't tend to eat enough B-rich foods, Dr. Katahdin says. "I recommend using a high-dose B-complex in the morning and at noon," she says. During times of acute pain or muscle spasm, she recommends 140 to 280 milligrams of B_6 and 200 to 400 micrograms of B_{12}, she says.

Help Your Body Douse Inflammation

The same list of anti-inflammatories that help many chronic health problems can sometimes help with the pain of sciatica, whether it's being caused by muscle spasms or spinal impingement, naturopathic doctors agree.

On that list is fish oil, which helps your body naturally reduce inflammatory biochemicals. Take 1 to 3 grams a day. "I also like people to be getting about 900 milligrams a day of DHA, which means they need a high-DHA [fish oil] product," Dr. Katahdin says. "Omega-3 fatty acids are highly concentrated in the fatty myelin sheath that wraps around nerve cells and cushions and protects them." To make fish oil work better, it's good to cut back on pro-inflammatory saturated fats and trans fats.

And if you've been taking NSAIDs for back pain, you might want to try some botanicals that ease inflammation without all the stomach-eroding side effects, Dr. Katahdin says. She likes a product called Traumeric, by Ortho Molecular Products, which contains turmeric, ginger, and enzymes that help break up the proteins involved in inflammation. "You use it two or four times a day on an empty stomach while you have pain, and stop using it once the pain is gone," she says.

A Recipe for Relaxation

Sometimes, pain and tingling can be due to muscle spasms in the piriformis muscle, a pear-shaped muscle in the buttocks that surrounds the sciatic nerve. Relaxing this muscle can help relieve pain, says Priscilla Evans, ND, a naturopathic doctor in private practice in Cary, North Carolina.

Naturopaths often use a mixture of soothing herbs such as valerian and passionflower to promote muscle relaxation. Although valerian has become a staple on drugstore shelves, where it is sold as a sleep aid, its powers of reprieve go beyond sleep.

"Valerian is also great for easing tension and for general pain relief," says Dr. Evans. It contains substances known as volatile oils, which work together to make you sleepy and relax your muscles.

Sometimes, your sciatic nerve is in the grip of a spastic muscle, and that no-win tug-of-war is at the root of the pain. Your doctor will need to confirm if a spastic muscle is the source of your pain. If it is, taking 150 milligrams of valerian three times a day may help, says Dr. Evans.

scleroderma

Scleroderma means, literally, "hard skin." It occurs when cells called fibroblasts, concentrated in the skin but also found in other organs, begin to replicate overtime.

The fibroblasts crank out a connective tissue called collagen. "They literally overgrow parts of the body with collagen, the same way these cells would form new tissue to heal a wound," says Richard Silver, MD, head of the rheumatology division at the Medical University of South Carolina in Charleston. Unfortunately, the excess collagen isn't needed for anything. It just messes things up. The end result is fibrosis, thickening, and scarring. It can be limited to patches of skin or involve the intestinal tract, lungs, throat, kidneys—just about any organ in your body.

Moreover, almost everyone with scleroderma also has Raynaud's disease, an extreme sensitivity to cold in their hands and feet that is caused by constricted blood vessels that cut off blood flow to the fingers and toes. (However, you can have Raynaud's disease without having scleroderma.)

No one knows exactly what triggers scleroderma, but "it is considered an autoimmune disorder, meaning that something is wrong with a person's immune system," Dr. Silver says. Certain immune cells secrete chemicals that make the fibroblasts more active than they should be. Your body is actually attacking collagen, a connective tissue that literally holds you together, says Jody Noe, ND, a faculty member at the University of Bridgeport College of Naturopathic Medicine and in private practice at Natural Family Health and Integrative Medicine, in Westerly, Rhode Island.

Genetics and environment both play roles. "Some cases may have been triggered by exposure to organic solvents such as trichloroethylene, a solvent that's used mainly to degrease machinery but can also be found in drinking water," Dr. Silver says. Other possible causes: some sort of infection; food allergies; so-called "leaky gut" syndrome, which is when food particles that would otherwise be contained within the intestines move through the intestinal wall and into the bloodstream, where they become allergens; and other kinds of environmental toxins, such as silica (possibly from leaky breast implants), some drugs, and plastics. Scleroderma has been found in jewelry workers and miners of gold and quartz. People who live near airports also have a higher incidence of this disorder.

Scleroderma is most often treated with drugs that reduce inflammation and muscle spasms, improve blood flow, or reduce high blood pressure if the kidneys are damaged, Dr. Silver says. "Scleroderma can be controlled somewhat, but not cured."

Alternative treatments for scleroderma include ferreting out possible environmental toxins and reducing exposure, and using detoxification programs. Treatment may also include nutritional supplements that help reduce inflammation and improve circulation—the same sorts of things used for other autoimmune diseases, such as rheumatoid arthritis.

Some alternative treatments can also address other possible underlying causes, including digestive problems, says Andrew Rubman, ND, director of the Southbury Clinic for Traditional Medicines in Connecticut and a consultant to the Office of Complementary and Alternative Medicine at the National Institutes of Health.

If you've been diagnosed with scleroderma, work with your doctor if you're taking supplements. Here are some natural remedies that may help.

Antioxidants against Early Damage

Oxidative stress has been found to be significantly increased in people with scleroderma compared to healthy people, says Alan Gaby, MD, author of *Nutritional Medicine*. This suggests that free radical injury plays a role in scleroderma and that antioxidants such as vitamin E might be helpful. Vitamin E might also have antifibrotic effects, in that it helps prevent fibrous scar tissue formation. Some case reports suggest that vitamin E can help various symptoms of scleroderma, including Raynaud's disease, calcium deposits, and hard spots. Dr. Gaby recommends vitamin E in doses of 200 to 1,200 IU a day.

"Vitamins C, A, and zinc are also an important part of the mix," Dr. Rubman adds. "These vitamins are involved in skin production, and zinc helps the body make its own antioxidants, such as superoxide dismutase." It also helps to maintain a healthy lining in the intestinal tract, which is important for anyone with an autoimmune disease, he notes.

Reach for the Right Oils

Getting rid of fats that increase inflammation and increasing your intake of anti-inflammatory fats is an important part of any treatment plan for autoimmune diseases, says Dr. Rubman. Cut back on saturated fats by eating a mostly plant-based diet and take fish oil capsules, starting with 2,000 to 5,000 milligrams a day.

He also recommends another essential fatty acid, gamma-linolenic acid (GLA), in a dose of 2,000 to 5,000 milligrams a day. One source, evening primrose oil, has proven helpful at reducing pain and improving skin texture in people with scleroderma and Raynaud's disease.

"I think the best way to tell whether these oils are having a positive effect is to dose fairly liberally with them initially and see if you perceive a change," he says. "It can take as long as 5 or 6 weeks at these quantities before people notice a difference."

That difference might be a reduction in inflammation that results in less painful, more functional joints. You might also experience fewer muscle spasms, and you may find that your skin is less sensitive to touch and temperature changes, Dr. Rubman says.

An Enzyme-Spice Combination

Naturopathic doctors will sometimes recommend supplements of bromelain, an enzyme derived from pineapple. Some doctors also suggest curcumin, a component of the Indian spice turmeric. "I'll recommend these if a person needs good short-term control over acute inflammation," Dr. Rubman says.

Both bromelain and curcumin act to quiet inflammation. Bromelain has the additional talent of inhibiting the body's production of fibrin, or scar tissue, Dr. Rubman says. Much of its anti-inflammatory action is achieved by activating compounds that break down fibrin. Bromelain also blocks compounds produced by immune cells that increase swelling and cause pain.

Dr. Rubman recommends 1,000 milligrams of bromelain and 500 milligrams of curcumin powder a day during periods of acute inflammation. "If it's going to help, it will work in fairly short order, within a week or so," he says.

In research at the Medical University of South Carolina, scientists found that curcumin causes cell death in scleroderma lung fibroblasts—the cells that produce too much collagen in the lungs, but not in normal fibroblasts. This means that the herb interferes with the "bad" fibroblasts, but not the normal ones.

The researchers concluded that, "curcumin may have therapeutic value in treating scleroderma." They also stated that, "this is especially appealing as a treatment because curcumin is extremely nontoxic and is beneficial for a host of other disorders including many cancers, heart disease, and Alzheimer's disease."

As for how much to take, Bharat Aggarwal, MD, at Anderson Cancer Center at the University of Texas and a leading authority on curcumin, recommends 2 grams a day for a minimum of 3 months to see results. Some forms of curcumin are much more absorbable than others. Lipsomal curcumin and Curcumin Phytosome, both of which are mixed with an emulsifying fat, are very absorbable forms. Several brands of both are available at health foods stores and online.

What about Vitamin D?

Considering how much research has been done on vitamin D in the last 10 years, surprisingly little has focused on how it relates to scleroderma. What is known is that people with scleroderma tend to be quite low in vitamin D. No surprise there, since they tend to avoid the sun.

Research has found that vitamin D deficiency makes the body less tolerant of "self." In other words, low levels of this steroid–hormonelike nutrient may actually induce some of the immune problems associated with autoimmune diseases like lupus, rheumatoid arthritis, multiple sclerosis, scleroderma, and others. In animals, adding vitamin D reverses immunologic abnormalities characteristic of lupus.

One study did look at vitamin D in people with undifferentiated connective tissue diseases (UCTD). It found that people with UCTD whose vitamin D levels were low were more likely to progress to some kind of diagnosable autoimmune disease, such as lupus, scleroderma, Sjögren's Syndrome, or mixed connective tissue disease. In other words, they were more likely to get worse if they had low vitamin D levels.

Everyone with an autoimmune disease should be taking extra vitamin D, Dr. Noe says. "Recommendations for dosages of vitamin D have really increased, and I like to see blood levels of vitamin D (25-hydroxy-vitamin D) at least 50 ng/ml, and even up to 100 ng/ml." To get to that level, some patients have to take high doses, up to 5,000 IU a day. "I'd rather see people take a smaller daily dose than a larger weekly dose," she says. (Some experts think doing one large weekly dose can interfere with parathyroid hormone function. These glands regulate calcium levels in the body.) Start with the 800 IU that's recommended for most people, but if you think you may need more or would like to try it, work with your doctor to get the right dosage.

An Herb That May Help

Gotu kola, an herb with a long history of use in India, China, and Indonesia for wound healing and skin conditions such as leprosy and psoriasis, may help scleroderma. There is not much research, but the little there is shows that gotu kola (*Centella asiatica*) can decrease skin hardness, improve mobility, and decrease pain in people with scleroderma. The herb is also used to improve circulation and reduce swelling in people with diabetes who have impaired microcirculation.

One anti-inflammatory component of the herb, terpenoid extract, seems to improve connective tissue remodeling by increasing fibroblast activity, stimulating collagen synthesis, increasing epithelial turnover, and decreasing capillary permeability. Gotu kola is thought to increase the production of type I collagen in scar formation over type II. Type II collagen is associated with hypertrophic scarring.

In research studies where liver function was monitored, people have safely taken 120 milligrams of gotu kola for 6 months. However, experts suggest you do not take this herb if you have liver damage or are taking a drug that can impair liver function, such as cholesterol-lowering statin drugs. You can buy gotu kola at most health foods stores, but it's a good idea to work with a naturopathic or integrative doctor to make the most of your natural treatments for scleroderma, including gotu kola.

shingles

If you had childhood chickenpox, your parents probably told you that you'd never get it again. That's good news to any kid who has just endured the little blisters, itching, and fever that are all signs of chickenpox.

It's too bad that your parents were wrong.

The same virus that causes chickenpox—the varicella-zoster virus—can continue to live an undercover existence in your nerve cells, and it may emerge later. The second time around you don't get the childhood version of itchy, blotchy chickenpox. Instead, you get the adult version, shingles, which is characterized by searing pain and lesions that can leave a good-size scar.

It's hard to tell why the virus reemerges in some people and not others and it's impossible to tell when it's going to crop up again. Certainly, elderly people get it more often than young people do, and some individuals are more likely to develop shingles when they're under severe stress or when their immune systems have been weakened. Adults may get shingles after an illness. For cancer patients who are undergoing chemotherapy, compromised immune systems may be a factor in bringing on shingles.

What characterizes all of these situations is a weakened immune system in which your body's disease-fighting soldiers, the antibodies, are in short supply.

"The virus looks for the right opportunity when your antibody production is down," says William Warnock, ND, a naturopathic doctor in Shelburne, Vermont. "Stress is one of the biggest causes of reduced antibody production. When people become stressed, they don't eat right, they don't sleep well, and their immune systems just don't function as well."

Typically, during a shingles outbreak, you have tingling and pain around your torso, neck, or face. Lesions, or small blisters, may break out on the skin near the site of the infected nerve. The pain often lasts from 2 to 4 weeks, but in some cases it can last for months. If it does, it's called postherpetic neuralgia.

Fighting the Virus

Once it gets loose, there's no cure for the varicella-zoster virus, but there may be ways to slow it down or limit damage during the outbreak. Medical doctors frequently prescribe an antiviral drug such as acyclovir (Zovirax) or famciclovir (Famvir) to shorten the course of the infection.

In order to hasten healing, treatment should be started within 2 to 3 days of the first appearance of the small blisters. In addition, you may be able to boost your immunity and help fight the virus with some herbs, says Dr. Warnock.

Herbalists believe that astragalus and echinacea are most effective. They work best if you take them as soon as you know you have an outbreak of the virus, says Dr. Warnock. Although you can take an herbal tincture, he recommends taking one 300-milligram capsule of standardized extract three times a day.

If you use capsules of dried echinacea root, he recommends 2,000 milligrams three times a day. Since echinacea is also safe at higher doses, you can take even more than the specified dose if you find it to be effective. "I'd do a high dose for a short period—just a few days. That's when it's most effective," he says.

Support from Astragalus

While echinacea speeds white blood cells to the infection site, you can add astragalus to help with the healing process. This herb provides what is known as deep immune support, working within the bone marrow where immune cells are manufactured, says Anne McClenon, ND, a naturopathic doctor at the Compass Family Health Center in Plymouth, Massachusetts. You can take astragalus in capsule form, following the directions on the label.

"Astragalus provides immune support on a long-term basis. That's important because people who get shingles may have a weakened immune system that needs to be built up again," she says. "I'd recommend taking it for 4 to 6 months."

Some Licorice Aid

Licorice also has strong antiviral properties. During the course of the infection, Dr. Warnock recommends taking 500 milligrams of standardized licorice extract in capsule form three times a day. If you take powdered licorice root in capsules, however, the dose should be 2,000 milligrams three times a day. Continue the treatment for 2 weeks after the lesions have healed, Dr. Warnock says.

Take licorice with caution, and don't take it at all if you are pregnant or nursing or if you have diabetes, high blood pressure, liver disorders, or kidney problems. In general, you shouldn't take high doses of licorice for more than 4 to 6 weeks unless you're under the supervision of a qualified health-care practitioner.

On the High Cs

High doses of vitamin C have been shown to keep the varicella-zoster virus from replicating, according to some studies involving people who were given intravenous injections. There have not been any studies that showed similar effects from taking oral supplements. Dr. Warnock believes, however, that you can help keep the virus from taking hold with a daily dose of 10,000 milligrams of vitamin C until the outbreak disappears. Dr. Warnock recommends five doses of 2,000 milligrams each, taken 3 hours apart. "The dosage goes beyond being a simple immune booster," he says. "The point is to interrupt the virus."

Dr. Warnock thinks vitamin C might prevent the virus from multiplying and spreading along the infected nerve. At the same time, vitamin C may ease inflammation in the nerve and lessen the outbreaks of the lesions, he says.

With a dose this high, you might experience an upset stomach and diarrhea, which is a frequent side effect of excess vitamin C. If so, just reduce the dose until you reach a level that's more tolerable, says Dr. Warnock.

"Also, you need to take this treatment early in the infection," he says. "Once there are millions of virus particles floating around, it becomes a much harder task to keep them from reproducing."

Starve the Virus

Varicella-zoster belongs to a larger family of herpes viruses, all of which share an important characteristic: They multiply with the help of the amino acid arginine and are inhibited by another amino acid called lysine. Lysine may work by blocking the virus's ability to absorb and use arginine.

To keep shingles at bay, doctors advise, you should avoid arginine-rich foods such as chocolate, legumes, and nuts, especially peanuts, and eat more foods that are rich in lysine, such as fish, tofu, eggs, lean beef, and lean pork.

You can also boost your lysine levels by taking a supplement. Dr. Warnock suggests taking 2,000 milligrams of lysine daily until the infection runs its course.

Beat the Pain with a B Vitamin

Shingles is not just painful, it's intensely painful. Because your nerves carry the virus and the virus causes inflammation, having shingles is like having a raw wound inside your nervous system. Even a light touch can give you a jolt, while something as innocuous as a tight shirt can give you a full day of misery.

Vitamin B_{12} seems to maintain the fatty membranes that sheathe and insulate the nerves, says Dr. McClenon. There's also evidence that it reduces the inflammation of the nerve where the virus is causing pain, and it may even shorten the length of the illness.

Some people with shingles take vitamin B_{12} injections, says Dr. McClenon. If the idea of an injection doesn't appeal to you, you can get sublingual B_{12} tablets, which you take by placing them under your tongue. Although some people have difficulty absorbing B_{12}, most people can absorb at least some of the vitamin this way.

"It definitely speeds healing," says Dr. McClenon, "and it may lessen the chances of a person getting the postherpetic neuralgic pain." She suggests taking a 2,000-microgram dose of sublingual B_{12} each day during the course of the infection.

Limit the Lesions

The skin outbreaks and pain of shingles can sometimes be eased with herbal treatments that you can apply directly to the surface of the skin. Among these topical treatments are licorice root extract, capsaicin, and St. John's wort oil.

Licorice root comes in a gel or ointment form that you rub directly on painful skin areas. It seems to interfere with the spread of the virus, says

Dr. Warnock. Licorice gel (Licrogel) is available from your physician or chiropractor. You can also ask your health food store to order a brand called Licroderm.

Although naturopathic doctors find that St. John's wort oil applied to the unbroken skin acts as an anti-inflammatory, it's also used to relieve pain and strengthen nerves, says Dr. McClenon. "Thus, it's a good topical treatment for any kind of nerve pain. I would continue to use it for the residual pain that may linger after the outbreak."

Fight Fire with Fire

Many over-the-counter ointments for shingles contain capsaicin, the substance that makes hot peppers hot. Like St. John's wort, capsaicin cannot be used on open lesions, so use it after they've cleared to relieve the pain of postherpetic neuralgia, says Dr. Warnock. Capsaicin cream is available in a number of different strengths, ranging from 0.025 percent to 0.075 percent.

Capsaicin works by stimulating and then exhausting Substance P, the nerve-related transmitter that sends pain messages from your skin to your brain. After 2 to 3 days of applying capsaicin, you should begin to feel the pain subsiding. The cream itself is irritating to the skin, so start with a tiny amount, and if a high-strength concentration burns too much, just switch to a lower strength, says Dr. Warnock.

Because capsaicin can burn the skin, however, he advises people to use it carefully. "I tell them to apply it four times a day to the affected area," he says. "You should always wear gloves when you apply it, and if you get it somewhere where you don't want it, don't try to wash it off with water. That just reactivates it and makes it worse. Instead, you can lessen the burning by rubbing the area with olive oil."

stress

Daily traffic. Work deadlines. Family squabbles. Rebellious teenagers. Illness. Injury. All of these life experiences add up to big-time stress that can knock you off your feet, spin you around, and keep you dazed. Without some relief, you may feel as if each morning is the beginning of a new melodrama.

Poking fun at stress is one way to help you de-stress. But the truth is that stress is no laughing matter. Whenever you're filled with tension and anxiety, your adrenal glands, located above your kidneys, pump out stress hormones such as adrenaline and cortisol, which give your body that burst of energy it needs to escape danger. Long-term stress causes chronically high levels of stress hormones, which can weaken your immune system, tax your heart and blood vessels, tire you out, and make you more susceptible to illness. Eventually you end up with low cortisol as your adrenal glands poop out.

Fortunately, certain dietary and lifestyle changes can help relieve stress and release tension. For starters, get at least 20 minutes of aerobic exercise three to five times a week to lift your spirits and melt away feelings of pressure and anxiety. Also, don't overlook weight lifting and brisk walking, as they can have similar effects.

Another tip for stress control: Limit your intake of caffeine, alcohol, high-fat foods, and sugar. Caffeine and alcohol can raise the levels of stress hormones in the blood and alter brain chemistry. Caffeine also causes nervousness, anxiety, and irritability. Moreover, when you replace nutritious foods with refined carbohydrates like sugar, you lower the amount of vitamins and minerals in your diet, depleting your body of essential nutrients that protect you from the dangers of stress. You also set yourself up for a roller coaster of high blood sugar, followed by low blood sugar, irritability, and hunger.

Once you have made these changes, you can try a variety of nutritional supplements as added stress protection. Certain vitamins can build up your immune system to prevent stress-related illnesses. Others can boost your energy and lift your mood. Even some herbs can help to calm your nerves, increase stamina, and keep you mentally and physically strong in the midst of turmoil.

Vitamin C: What Happens

Vitamin C gives your immune system the fighting power it needs to prevent many stress-related health problems such as headaches, high blood pressure, diabetes, and heart disease, says Jacob Teitelbaum, MD, medical director of the Fibromyalgia and Fatigue Centers, a nationwide group of clinics, and author of *From Fatigued to Fantastic*. What's more, vitamin C is required to manufacture stress hormones, which can flow excessively if you're stressed for a long time. After a while, your adrenal glands become exhausted from overwork and your body's ability to produce stress hormones declines, Dr. Teitelbaum says. Once this happens, you could experience excessive fatigue, low blood pressure, and low blood sugar. Supplementing with extra vitamin C is one step that you can take to keep your adrenal glands healthy. He recommends at least 500 milligrams a day.

Welcome the B Family

The B-complex vitamins are a treasure trove of stress relief. They can give you more energy, strip away fatigue, produce adrenal gland hormones, and manufacture brain chemicals responsible for keeping you alert and lifting your mood, says Dr. Teitelbaum. "All the B vitamins are important, but the one that really supports your adrenal glands is pantothenic acid, vitamin B_5," he says. "And B_6, folic acid, and B_{12} play important roles in neurotransmitter production." He recommends 50 milligrams of pantothenic acid, which you can take separately along with a balanced B complex supplement that includes 500 to 1,000 micrograms of B_{12}, 800 micrograms of folic acid, 200 micrograms of biotin, and 50 to 75 milligrams of the rest of the Bs.

Using Licorice Safely

Licorice—real licorice root, not the candy—is often recommended by integrative practitioners for support during stressful times. Used carefully, it can be very helpful. But it can also cause high blood pressure, so it is best used with the guidance of a knowledgeable doctor. "Licorice slows the breakdown of the adrenal hormone cortisol in your body, and that keeps it in the system longer so you don't have to make as much of it," Dr. Teitelbaum explains.

An easy way to use licorice is to drink a cup of licorice tea every day. Or you can take about 200 milligrams a day of licorice root extract, he says. Don't use it if you have high blood pressure, and monitor your blood pressure to make sure it doesn't go too high with licorice. (A kind of licorice called DGL, deglycyrrhized licorice, does not help the adrenal glands.)

Ginseng: A Stress-Busting Powerhouse

Ginseng is considered the most notable medicinal herb used to restore vitality, boost energy, reduce fatigue, improve mental and physical performance, and protect the body from the negative effects of stress. With ginseng, your initial reaction to stress is likely to be less intense. It's often referred to as a tonic for the adrenal glands because it tones and maintains their overall health.

You can find different varieties of the herb, including Siberian ginseng, Asian (Panax) ginseng, and American ginseng. Asian ginseng is the most widely used for medicinal purposes. They all have similar properties, although Asian ginseng is more of a stimulant than its Siberian cousin, says Joseph E. Pizzorno Jr., ND, president of Bastyr University in Kenmore, Washington. Thus, if you're acutely stressed or recovering from a long illness, Asian ginseng would be the way to go.

In one study, nurses who had switched from the day shift to the night shift were given either Asian ginseng or an inactive substance (a placebo). Their competence, mood, and general well-being were rated. This study showed that the nurses who took the ginseng were more competent, upbeat, and alert than those who didn't take the herb.

Because potency varies, as does the concentration of active ingredients, you'll need to adjust the amount you take depending on which product you buy. You can take 1,000 to 2,000 milligrams one to three times a day if you choose a high-quality crude Asian ginseng root, says Dr. Pizzorno. If you take an extract standardized to 5 to 7 percent ginsenosides, take 100 milligrams one to three times a day.

If you're taking Siberian ginseng root, says Dr. Pizzorno, you probably should take somewhere between 2,000 and 3,000 milligrams a day in

Food for Your Adrenal Glands

For a nutritional supplement that claims to zap fatigue, boost energy, and help you cope with stress, some people are turning to adrenal gland extracts.

These extracts fall into a category called "glandular supplements" because they come from the glands of animals such as cows and pigs, on the assumption that what helps them will help you. Advocates of these products claim that adrenal gland extracts can put life back into your own adrenal glands, which have become tired from pumping out so much stress hormone during long periods of stress.

At first glance, it seems sensible to assume that an adrenal booster can do some good. Doctors know that unless we have a healthy pair of adrenal glands, we're more prone to infections and stress-related illnesses. When you're under a lot of stress, your glands need all the help they can get.

The results aren't certain, however. It's believed that adrenal extracts can help people who are under a great deal of stress or who have chronic fatigue, but little research has been done to prove their effectiveness. Most naturopathic or integrative doctors who use them first test saliva cortisol levels to make sure a patient actually has low cortisol. Some people's cortisol levels are high, and some have high cortisol at night, which keeps them awake, and low during the day, which makes them tired. "If you've been stressed-out for a long time and, especially, if you have symptoms of 'If I don't eat NOW I am going to kill someone,' chances are you have low cortisol levels," says Jacob Teitelbaum, MD, medical director of the Fibromyalgia and Fatigue Centers and author of *From Fatigued to Fantastic.* He does use adrenal glandulars, and one product he likes is Adrenal Stress-End, by PhytoPharmica. It contains adrenal cortex extract, licorice, and other ingredients.

To find the right dosage, you may need to try products with various potencies and qualities, according to Joseph E. Pizzorno Jr., ND, president of Bastyr University in Kenmore, Washington. "I suggest taking one-third of the recommended dosage on the label and slowly increasing it every 2 days unless you notice any signs of irritability, restlessness, or insomnia," he says. "If you experience any of these symptoms, simply reduce your dosage until the symptoms go away. Over time, you should notice an increase in energy and better resistance to stress." If you don't feel better in 2 to 3 weeks, the supplements are probably not working for you.

divided doses. If you take the extract, take 100 to 200 milligrams of a product that is standardized to 0.8 percent eleutherosides three times a day. Because everyone's response to ginseng is different, start off with the lower dosage and increase it over time, he suggests.

Women taking Asian ginseng may experience breast tenderness. You can simply reduce the dose or discontinue use to make the symptoms go away, says Dr. Pizzorno.

Ginseng has many other potential side effects with long-term use, so limit use to no more than 3 months.

Natural Calmers

For some people, stress and anxiety go hand in hand. If you're one of them, you know that if you can chill out, everything goes more smoothly. "There are plenty of herbal products used for anxiety, but what I think are best to use are valerian, passionflower and Suntheanine, the brand name for a pure form of L-theanine, an amino acid that comes from green tea," Dr. Teitelbaum says.

Valerian is commonly used as a sleep remedy. In a number of studies it has been shown to improve deep sleep, speed of falling asleep, and quality of sleep without next-day sedation. "It's considered a safe choice for mild insomnia, but it is more effective when used continuously rather than as an acute sleep aid," Dr. Teitelbaum says. He recommends 200 to 800 milligrams at bedtime.

Passionflower is calming and can reduce your perception of pain. You can take 90 to 360 milligrams at bedtime.

L-theanine is interesting because it is calming but not sedating, D. Teitelbaum says. Taken during the day, it can promote calm alertness. "It directly stimulates the production of alpha brain waves during the day," he explains. "These brain waves are associated with an awake yet relaxed, almost meditative state." At bedtime, it promotes deep sleep. You can take 50 milligrams two or three times a day, and a larger dose, 100 to 200 milligrams, at bedtime, he says.

sunburn

Sunburn is an inflammation of the skin that results from overexposure to ultraviolet radiation. Get a mild burn, and you might be uncomfortable overnight, but the redness and stinging will dissipate pretty quickly. If you really fry yourself and end up with what's called a second-degree burn, though, your skin will actually blister and ooze.

For a second-degree roasting, see a physician, but for mild sunburn, you can do a number of things to help reduce your day-after discomfort.

When you've been out in the sun too long, the first thing you need is immediate relief from the burning. There are several effective topical treatments for sun exposure, beginning with the old folk remedy of taking an oatmeal bath, says Kathy Foulser, ND, a naturopathic doctor at the Ridgefield Center for Integrative Medicine in Connecticut. Simply pour about $1\frac{1}{2}$ ounces of ground oatmeal, which is sold under brand names like Aveeno, into comfortably warm water and soak for 15 minutes.

Another home-style treatment for sunburn is aloe gel. If you have an aloe plant, break a leaf, squeeze out the gel, and gently rub it into the damaged skin. You can also purchase the gel at drugstores. "The gel is great for cooling and soothing the skin," says Dr. Foulser.

In a study at the University of Texas in Galveston, scientists found that aloe vera inhibited the formation of a substance known as TXA2. This substance is responsible for a lot of the skin damage that results from burns, electrical injuries, and frostbite. By inhibiting TXA2, aloe relieves pain and increases blood supply to the injured area, researchers report.

Oil Your Burn

Because sunburn essentially produces skin inflammation, it's helpful to take herbs with strong anti-inflammatory properties, says Dr. Foulser.

She recommends evening primrose oil, which contains gamma-linolenic acid (GLA). The body transforms GLA into hormonelike compounds called prostaglandins, which have anti-inflammatory effects. When you put more GLA into your system, your body has increased power to reduce inflammation.

The essential fatty acids in this oil provide another benefit: They are good for overall skin health, says Dr. Foulser. She recommends taking six capsules daily of evening primrose oil for long-term use.

"If you want, you can take more, because this oil is quite safe," she adds. Be sure to check the label of the supplement for information on recommended dosages.

Up Your Antioxidants

Whenever your skin burns, cells are damaged. This damage is caused by free radicals, which are free-roaming, unstable molecules that are seeking to stabilize themselves by stealing electrons from healthy cells. As a result of this cell damage, free radicals can cause premature wrinkling, and in the case of repeated sun exposure, even skin cancer. If you take antioxidants, substances that scavenge free radicals in the body, you can speed healing and prevent rapid cell damage.

At your drugstore or health food store, you will find plenty of antioxidant combination products on the shelf. Alternatively, you can choose to take separate supplements of vitamin C, vitamin E, and beta-carotene, all of which have strong antioxidant properties, says Dr. Foulser.

For a mild sunburn, take 50,000 international units (IU) of beta-carotene a day, Dr. Foulser advises. If your sunburn is more severe, you could take 100,000 IU of beta-carotene for a few days and then reduce it to 50,000 IU as the burn heals. Dr. Foulser also suggests taking 800 IU daily of vitamin E, which is known to aid in the repair of damaged skin.

"You should keep this up for a couple of weeks, even after you think the burn has healed," she says. The exceptions are pregnant women and people with liver problems, who should never take high doses of beta-carotene, even for short periods. To be safe, consult a holistic physician before starting this program, Dr. Foulser suggests.

Vitamin E can also be used topically on sun-damaged skin along with other salves and skin conditioners, says Dr. Foulser.

Guarding against Sun Singe

Of course, we all know that a milligram of prevention is worth many pounds of cure when it comes to sunburn. The best way to prevent sunburn is to simply use common sense by avoiding excess exposure and using sunscreen. You can also help your skin by taking some supplements when you know you're going to be exposed to the sun.

Vitamin C has qualities that can help protect skin from sunlight, and it's also well-known for its antioxidant properties, says Leon Hecht, ND, a naturopathic doctor at the North Coast Family Health Center in Portsmouth, New Hampshire.

For people who spend a lot of time in the sun, Dr. Hecht suggests up to 1,000 milligrams of vitamin C three or four times a day. "Vitamin C stimulates repair of sun-damaged skin," he says.

In a controlled study, 10 people took either 2,000 milligrams of vitamin C with 1,000 IU of vitamin E a day or an inactive substance (a placebo). The sunburn reaction after 8 days of treatment revealed that the skin of people in the treatment group showed less damage than that of those in the placebo group.

Dr. Hecht also states that vitamins C and E used in topical sunscreens prove effective, as well. "Early studies show that it is prudent to add vitamins C and E to your sunscreen to protect against ultraviolet phototoxic injury to your skin," he says. Sunscreens with these vitamins already added can be found in drugstores.

You can also prepare your skin to withstand the harmful effects of ultraviolet rays by taking a beta-carotene supplement, says Dr. Hecht. He recommends taking 100,000 IU of beta-carotene for a month or two before you plan to expose yourself to intense sunlight—before the first beach day, for instance, or before a midwinter skiing vacation. This preventive works particularly well for light-skinned people, says Dr. Hecht. You should talk to your doctor, though, before taking this amount.

"It pigments the skin a little bit and just gives you a kind of base. It's no substitute for protecting yourself from the sun, but it does help prevent some burning," he says.

taste and smell loss

"Take time to stop and smell the roses," goes the saying.

That's very good advice, but it's impossible to follow if you're losing your sense of smell.

If you don't smell things as well as you once did, there could be many explanations. Advancing age can be a contributing factor, possibly because infection has taken its toll or because you've sniffed too many noxious fumes over the years. Moreover, you shouldn't be surprised if you temporarily lose your sense of smell because you've had an infection such as a bad cold.

Head injury is another possible cause, if the delicate nerves leading from your nose to your brain are damaged. Also, certain prescription drugs can rob you of some ability to enjoy the fragrance of flowers, perfume, or freshly baked apple pie.

As smell slips away, your sense of taste may suffer, too. The two senses are so closely related that people who complain of not being able to smell often say that they also have trouble tasting.

Depending on the cause, disturbances in your senses of taste and smell are sometimes permanent. In other cases, though, you might regain these senses after a while, says Charles P. Kimmelman, MD, associate professor of otolaryngology at Weill Medical College of Cornell University in New York City and attending physician at Manhattan Eye, Ear, and Throat Hospital. If smell loss is linked to a head cold, for instance, you can expect your nose to work normally after you've shaken off the cold.

When the problems last longer, talk to your doctor. "Disturbances of the taste and smell senses are best treated by a physician," says Barbara Silbert, DC, ND, a chiropractor and naturopathic doctor in Bethel, Vermont. She adds, however, that people who are deficient in zinc often have taste and smell problems, and in those cases, supplementing with zinc is an excellent remedy to the problem.

Taste for Heavy Metal

Not having enough zinc can make smelling and tasting things such as a festive holiday meal a real challenge. Here's why: The cells in your taste buds and nose that help you to smell depend on zinc. In fact, cells in the salivary glands make a zinc-dependent protein called gustin that is secreted into your saliva. An important contributor to your sense of taste, gustin helps develop cells that can distinguish among different flavors.

Although zinc deficiencies are pretty rare in the United States, it's worth asking your doctor to test for a deficiency if you are experiencing taste and smell loss. Many things can lead to a deficiency, including poor eating habits, alcoholism, certain drugs, kidney disease, and the stress of surgery or serious burns.

"If I discover a zinc deficiency, I typically recommend 25 milligrams of zinc picolinate twice a day to start," says Dr. Silbert. Of course, you can also eat more of the foods that contain zinc. Your best bet is seafood, such as cooked oysters and crab. Meats such as lean beef and lean pork also provide zinc, but they're not really recommended because they are high in saturated fat. Other sources include eggs, whole grains, nuts, and yogurt. If you plan to take more than 20 milligrams of zinc a day, it's best to do so under your doctor's care.

tinnitus

Imagine having the whoosh of a vacuum cleaner, the roar of the breaking surf, or even the innocent chirping of a cricket inside your head. You can't turn it off, walk away, or stomp on it. Earplugs won't help. It's there when you wake up, when you're trying to fall asleep, and when you're talking or trying to watch TV.

That's tinnitus in a nutshell: It's ringing in the ears. While this condition can be caused by a buildup of earwax or by allergies, it is often due to damage to the nerve cells in the ears.

Exposure to loud noises can cause ear damage, and some medicines can contribute to it. Alcohol abuse can also lead to tinnitus, as can an overdose of caffeine. Or it could be the result of direct damage to some portion of the ear, such as a blockage in the tiny arteries that feed blood to the ears, hardening of the tiny bones in the inner ear, or viral infections that damage the inner ear. Even high blood pressure can be a contributing factor.

With so many possible causes, you and your doctor should try to figure out what's causing your tinnitus, says William H. Slattery III, MD, director of clinical studies at the House Ear Institute in Los Angeles. Once that's established, some natural remedies may be helpful for improving blood circulation to the ear, if that's your problem, or protecting the nerves of your ear from further damage. Here's what some experts recommend.

Magnesium Shields against Noise Damage

An essential mineral, magnesium, can help protect your ears from noise-induced damage, Dr. Slattery says. "I would recommend that everyone, especially those who already have some hearing loss, make sure they are getting adequate amounts of magnesium."

When magnesium-deficient laboratory animals were exposed to noise, their inner ears were damaged far more than the ears of animals that had adequate magnesium. When magnesium is in short supply and there's a lot of exposure to noise, the inner-ear cells can become exhausted. That in turn can lead to cell damage or destruction.

Low magnesium levels can also cause blood vessels to constrict, affecting the tiny arteries leading to your inner ear. When the arteries constrict even farther in reaction to loud noises, the result is tinnitus.

Israeli researchers found that soldiers who got an additional 167 milligrams of supplemental magnesium daily during 2 months of basic training had less inner ear damage than those getting inactive substances (placebos). Extra magnesium from supplements can also protect against long-term noise exposure.

If you're often in a noisy environment, make sure you're getting the Daily Value of magnesium, which is 400 milligrams from food and supplements, Dr. Slattery says. Most people get less than this amount from food, with men averaging about 329 milligrams and women 207 milligrams a day. Make sure that your multivitamin/mineral supplement has enough magnesium to make up the difference, he advises.

Try N-Acetylcysteine

N-acetylcysteine (NAC) can reduce cochlear and hair cell damage in the ear and can therefore help prevent hearing loss associated with drug treatments such as cisplatin, or hearing loss associated with prolonged exposure to loud noise or exposure to sudden loud pulses of noise, such as that caused by gunfire. How so? This amino acid helps your body make the powerful natural antioxidant glutathione. While glutathione cannot cross the cell membrane, NAC can, and once it gets there it is eventually converted into glutathione. Once inside your cells, the glutathione can help repair free radical damage that causes hearing loss. A normal dose of NAC is 600 to 1,800 milligrams a day, in divided doses. If you've been exposed to a sudden, damaging noise, call your doctor to talk about a different dose.

Add In Alpha-Lipoic Acid

This versatile antioxidant does a couple of things: It regenerates other protective antioxidants, such as vitamins C and E, and glutathione; it can get into places some other antioxidants can't, like the brain and nerve cells; it helps symptoms of peripheral neuropathy; and it may even help prevent brain damage caused by neurotoxins. All of this may help alpha-lipoic acid to show promise in experimental models to prevent aminoglycoside-induced cochlear damage. (Aminoglycosides are found in some antibiotics, like neomycin, streptomycin, and others.) It also appears to help protect hearing loss from neurotoxins such as lead, arsenic, cadmium, mercury, and hexachlorobenzene, a fungicide that can accumulate in your body. Doctors typically recommend that you take 600 to 1,200 milligrams of alpha-lipoic acid a day, in divided doses.

The Enzyme to Use

Coenzyme Q_{10} is often recommended for conditions where cells are having trouble making the energy they need to function properly. It does improve energy output and can help overcome damage to nerve cells, including cells in the ears, from neurotoxins. While there is no direct evidence that it can help tinnitus, it is added to some tinnitus nutritional formulas based on its general effects on nerve cells. A usual dose is 150 to 300 milligrams a day. Start with the lower dose for a few weeks, then move up to 300 milligrams if you don't feel any benefit.

Go after Ginkgo

If there's a blockage in the tiny arteries that go to your ears, the herb ginkgo may help your tinnitus symptoms, says Jennifer Brett, ND, a naturopathic doctor at the Wilton Naturopathic Center in Stratford, Connecticut.

"Ginkgo works a number of ways to improve blood flow, especially in tiny blood vessels," says Dr. Brett. It also acts as an antioxidant, which means that it helps to protect your cells from all kinds of damage, including damage from drugs like quinine (Quinamm), furosemide (Lasix), and some antibiotics, such as streptomycin and gentamicin (Garamycin). Ginkgo also stabilizes cell membranes. With more stable membranes, your nerve cells conduct signals more efficiently, so it's quite possible that the nerves in your ears will work better even if they're damaged.

Ginkgo also enhances the use of oxygen by cells. Even if blood flow is restricted so that a cell isn't getting all the oxygen it needs, the cell may function better if you're taking ginkgo. "In my experience, ginkgo improves symptoms in about half the people who try it," says Dr. Brett. Even if you've had tinnitus for more than 3 years, ginkgo can be effective, although it seems to be more helpful in people who haven't had tinnitus that long.

Take 40 to 80 milligrams of ginkgo extract three times a day. Dr. Brett recommends a concentration of 24 percent ginkgoflavonglycosides, a product that is available in many health food stores.

"Try it for about 6 weeks and see if you notice an improvement in your symptoms," she says. If you do, continue taking it.

Bet on the Bs

Your body needs vitamin B_{12} to manufacture myelin, the fatty sheath that wraps around nerve fibers, insulating them and allowing them to conduct their electrical impulses normally. That's apparently important for ears as well as the rest of your body.

The same Israeli researchers who found that magnesium helped protect ears also found that 47 percent of a group of 113 army personnel with tinnitus had a B_{12} deficiency. All of the people low in B_{12} received injections of 1,000 micrograms weekly for about 4 months. At the end of that time, all of them reported some improvement in their tinnitus, including a decrease in loudness.

If your tinnitus is accompanied by memory problems, depression, or difficulty walking, talk to your doctor about having your blood levels of B_{12} or zinc checked. It's possible that you may not be absorbing the vitamin or mineral properly, and you may need injections.

vaginitis

If you're a woman who's never had a bout of vaginitis, you're lucky—but the odds are good that you'll have to deal with it at some point in your life. It's all part of being a woman.

Vaginitis is an umbrella term for inflammation, irritation, and redness of the vulva and vagina. The most common form is bacterial vaginosis, an infection characterized by a yellowish, fishy-smelling discharge. Yeast infection is another form, which reveals itself with a white, cottage cheese–like discharge, intense itching, and burning.

Trichomoniasis is yet another type, an inflammation triggered by a single-celled organism that's transmitted sexually and causes itching, burning, and a frothy green or yellowish, foul-smelling discharge. Due to hormone level changes, women are more likely to be plagued by vaginitis before menstruation, during pregnancy, or after menopause, when thinning vaginal walls caused by decreasing estrogen become more susceptible to infection. This same lack of estrogen also causes vaginal dryness, which can lead to irritation, inflammation, and a higher risk of developing a bacterial infection.

Whatever the cause or the symptoms, vaginitis needs attention. If left untreated, trichomoniasis can put you at risk for other sexually transmitted diseases, and untreated bacterial vaginosis may lead to urinary tract infections and pelvic inflammatory disease, which can cause infertility. Be sure to see your doctor without delay if you have any of these symptoms. After a proper diagnosis, your doctor can help you decide if supplements are right for you.

If you're plagued by chronic yeast infections that are causing vaginitis, you can make some dietary changes that could help prevent recurrences. Try to eliminate sugar and milk and other dairy products from your diet, naturopathic doctors advise. You should also avoid foods that contain mold and yeast, including alcoholic beverages, cheeses, dried fruit, melons, mushrooms, and peanuts.

There's a clear rationale behind the ban on these foods, naturopathic doctors believe. *Candida albicans,* the fungus that causes yeast infections, thrives on sugar, and because milk is high in lactose—also a sugar—it may contribute to a yeast infection.

While you're dodging those foods, naturopathic doctors say that you can also take a number of nutritional supplements that have been known to clear up more than one stubborn case of vaginitis. Vitamins and minerals can reduce the severity of symptoms and boost your immune system at the same time. Supplementing with probiotics, a mix of friendly bacteria that muscle out the bad ones in your intestines and vagina, can create a more stable and healthy environment in your vaginal area. Certain herbs, such as black cohosh and dong quai, which help balance female hormones, can restore the vaginal moisture that some women lose when they experience hormonal changes during menopause. Other herbs laced with powerful immune-stimulating properties, such as garlic, can destroy fungi and bacteria on contact.

Fight Back with Vitamins C and E

Whether your bout with vaginitis is caused by bacteria, yeast, or hormonal changes, supplementing with a powerful arsenal of vitamins and minerals may help shorten the duration and lessen the severity of the infection, says Pamela Jeanne, ND, a naturopathic doctor and owner of Mount Hood Holistic Health in Gresham, Oregon.

Among these stars are vitamins C and E. Taken together, they can help reduce the pain and inflammation associated with vaginitis, says Dr. Jeanne. Vitamin C kicks your immune system into high gear, strengthening your body's ability to fight off the infection. Vitamin C helps reduce the inflammation and strengthens the capillary walls and mucous membranes lining your vagina so they can ward off infection, says Dr. Jeanne. "Make sure the vitamin C you take contains bioflavonoids or rose hips," she says. "Bioflavonoids prevent the infected vaginal cells from releasing immune system chemicals called histamines, which cause the inflammation."

Take 2,000 milligrams of vitamin C daily to maintain a healthy vagina, Dr. Jeanne suggests. If you suffer from chronic vaginal infections, take 3,000 to 4,000 milligrams a day over a 2-week period.

Vitamin E should be the number one nutrient for women during and after menopause, says Dr. Jeanne. Estrogen levels drop and remain low once menopause is under way, leading to the irritation, inflammation, and other vaginal problems related to low estrogen. Dr. Jeanne believes that vitamin E can lower this risk by strengthening the cell membranes lining your vagina. The stronger the membranes, the less likely it is that bacteria will invade them and wreak havoc.

With your doctor's consent, you can take 400 to 800 IU of vitamin E daily, says Dr. Jeanne. Some women also find it soothing to prick or cut open a capsule of vitamin E oil and apply it directly to inflamed tissues.

Strike a Balance with Friendly Bacteria

If you get repeated yeast infections, the yeast may have moved beyond your vagina and into your intestinal system, says Jennifer Nevels, ND, who specializes in women's health at East Valley Naturopathic Doctors in Mesa, Arizona. To get the yeast out of your entire body, switch to an anti-yeast diet—cut out sugars, refined carbs, alcohol, and yeast-containing foods such as breads. Also, start taking natural supplements with probiotics, which are friendly bacteria that keep yeast in check. *Lactobacillus acidophilus* is one of these, but it's best to take a mix that contains both *Bifidobacterium bifidum* and *L. acidophilus*. A good product will list the number of colony-forming units (CFU) it contains, and you're looking for at least 10 billion. Some probiotics also contain prebiotics— "food" in the form of fiber that the bacteria feed on. This can help you to establish colony-forming units in your intestines and is especially helpful if you are on a low-fiber diet or have to take antibiotics, Dr. Nevels says.

Herbs to Wipe Out Yeast and Bacteria

To clear up bacterial infections and control yeast, consider taking some garlic or echinacea. Whether you take them together or separately, naturopaths believe that these herbs can muster up a tough defense against bacterial offenders. They also help to restore the natural flora to the vagina, reinforcing the efforts of good bacteria to defend you from the bad and the ugly.

Garlic strengthens the immune system so that your body can fight off the infection on its own, plus it has both antifungal and antibacterial properties, says Tori Hudson, ND, professor at the National College of Naturopathic Medicine in Portland, Oregon, and author of *Women's Encyclopedia of Natural Medicine*.

When garlic comes on the scene, invading bacteria and overgrowing yeast don't stand a chance. The number one ingredient in garlic that kills bacteria and stunts the growth of yeast is allicin, and experts believe this is one of the plant kingdom's most potent antibiotics.

Echinacea also deserves a mention. This powerful immune system stimulant has antiviral powers, as well. It increases levels of a body chemical called properdin, which activates the part of the immune system responsible for destroying bacteria and viruses. Taking echinacea orally in combination with a topical antifungal cream applied to the infected area can help prevent recurrent vaginal yeast infections.

During an acute infection, take one or two capsules of garlic daily for 3 to 14 days, or until the infection clears up, says Dr. Hudson. Take two capsules daily for 4 weeks or longer if your infection is chronic. Products that contain at least 4,000 micrograms of allicin may be the most effective, she says.

Take 300 milligrams of echinacea three times a day for at least one week, says Dr. Jeanne. When symptoms subside, drop the dosage to 300 milligrams twice a day. Dr. Jeanne says that this dose can be taken for 4 to 6 weeks, but after that it's best to stop for a while.

Herbs for Vaginal Dryness

Most women in their twenties and thirties probably take their abundant supply of estrogen for granted. It's only when the supply runs low as they get older that they begin to notice the effects of a shortfall.

During and after menopause, women produce less estrogen, which is one of the "basics" that's needed to prevent vaginal problems. "Estrogen feeds the vaginal tissue and promotes circulation and natural lubrication, which protects the vagina from bacteria," says Liz Collins, ND, a naturopathic doctor and co-owner of the Natural Childbirth and Family Clinic in Portland, Oregon.

Herbs can replenish some of the estrogen that's lost during the menopausal and postmenopausal years and give you the moisture and protection you need. Naturopathic doctors recommend herbs like horopito, dong quai, and black cohosh. (If you're pregnant, talk with your doctor before using any of these herbs, topically or orally.)

Horopito (*Pseudowintera colorata*), a relative newcomer to the herbal market, is from New Zealand. It contains a compound called polygodial, which helps kill bacteria and fungus and relieves pain. It also seems to be a vasodilator, which means it improves blood flow to an area, which can help it heal faster. And horopito contains two powerful antioxidant flavonoids, quercitin and taxifolin. Both of these help stop itching and allergic reactions. One product Dr. Nevels likes to use for vaginitis is Kolorex Intimate Care Cream, with horopito extract, tea tree oils, apricot kernel oil, aloe vera, and natural source vitamin E. "Women just love it," she says. "It's very soothing and healing."

Try a Woman's Tonic

Dong quai is a Chinese herb with a centuries-old reputation as a woman's tonic. Herbalists say that it relieves vaginal dryness associated with menopause and menstrual problems. Sometimes promoted as the "female ginseng," this herb is a general tonic for the female reproductive system.

Many women find great relief from using dong quai, which is sometimes called dang gui, tang kwei, or Chinese angelica. It also helps lower blood pressure and relieve headaches and arthritis, and it has been shown to stimulate immunity, says Dr. Jeanne.

Take 300 milligrams of dong quai two or three times a day along with licorice for 1 to 2 months for chronic or recurring infections, says Dr. Jeanne. You shouldn't take it while you're menstruating, however, since it can increase blood loss. It also contains substances that can cause a rash or severe sunburn if you're exposed to sunlight.

varicose veins

Varicose veins aren't just a cosmetic problem. They can make your legs swell or make them feel heavy and tired. They can also aggravate muscle cramps.

When you have varicose veins, it means that the blood returning to your heart is extremely sluggish. Within the veins, valvelike mechanisms that help maintain upward blood flow aren't doing their job any more. It may get to the point where blood is simply pooling in the veins rather than moving along as it should.

Blood vessel damage can set the stage for thrombosis, or clotting, so be sure to see your doctor for a proper diagnosis. If your veins present a real danger to your health, your doctor may recommend sclerotherapy, a procedure that shuts them off, says Decker Weiss, NMD, director of the Weiss Center for Naturopathic Excellence in Scottsdale, Arizona, and author of *The Weiss Method: A Natural Program for Reversing Heart Disease and Preventing Heart Attacks*. While that may seem drastic, Dr. Weiss points out that sclerotherapy could relieve discomfort. "The veins aren't helping you in any way," he says. "They are just creating pain."

Most doctors' nutritional recommendations for varicose veins are limited to "Lose weight and eat more fiber." That's good advice, but some naturopathic doctors also recommend nutrients that help to strengthen blood vessel walls or reduce the likelihood of blood clots that could block the veins. Just be sure to talk to your own doctor before you start taking supplements for this condition.

Take Fiber for Vein Strain

Straining to have a bowel movement puts a lot of pressure on the veins of your lower body, and over time, it can promote the development of varicose veins in your legs, Dr. Weiss says. "I've had patients who, once they have their constipation problems under control, see their varicose veins improve, especially the hemorrhoid type."

To prevent constipation, it's best to eat foods that contain a mixture of fiber, such as beans, fruits and vegetables, and whole grains. If you also need to take a fiber supplement, find one that contains both soluble and insoluble fibers, Dr. Weiss advises. Whatever kind of fiber you're getting, also make sure you drink at least eight glasses of water and other fluids every day.

Bromelain Breaks Up Bumps

Bromelain, an enzyme that's extracted from green pineapple, can help prevent the development of the hard and lumpy skin found around varicose veins, says Joseph E. Pizzorno Jr., ND, president of Bastyr University in Kenmore, Washington.

People with varicose veins have a decreased ability to break down fibrin, one of the compounds involved in the formation of blood clots and tissue scarring. In healthy veins, a substance called plasminogen activator helps break down fibrin, but veins that are varicose have decreased levels of this substance.

Bromelain acts similarly to plasminogen activator to help break down fibrin, so it's particularly helpful for varicose veins, says Dr. Pizzorno. It can also help people who have a tendency to develop phlebitis, or blood clots in leg veins.

Dr. Pizzorno recommends taking 500 to 750 milligrams of bromelain on an empty stomach two or three times a day. If you take it with meals, it simply works as a digestive enzyme and is used up in your intestines rather than passed along to your bloodstream.

Bioflavonoids Keep Veins Strong

Even if you seem destined to get varicose veins, the powerful antioxidant and anti-inflammatory properties of bioflavonoids might help make the walls of your veins stronger, says Stephen T. Sinatra, MD, an integrative cardiologist in private practice in Manchester, Connecticut, and author of *Reverse Heart Disease Now.*

"Bioflavonoids can help protect the structural integrity of the vascular walls and help prevent free radical stress inside the vessel," he says.

The "Compression Stocking" Herb

Which would you rather do to treat your varicose veins: wear surgical compression stockings that make you feel like you're encased in elastic or take an herbal tincture of horse chestnut seed extract?

In a study, people with varicose veins were divided into two groups. One group took an extract of horse chestnut that provided 50 milligrams a day of escin, one of the active ingredients. The other group used compression stockings, which are commonly recommended by doctors as a way to relieve the discomfort of varicose veins. After 12 weeks, researchers found that both groups had an almost identical reduction of swelling in their legs.

Horse chestnut contains compounds called bioflavonoids. When you take this herb, the bioflavonoids seem to move into the bulging varicose veins, says Decker Weiss, NMD, director of the Weiss Center for Naturopathic Excellence in Scottsdale, Arizona, and author of *The Weiss Method: A Natural Program for Reversing Heart Disease and Preventing Heart Attacks.* "I'd recommend it as a first-line treatment, along with correcting constipation," he says.

Horse chestnut seed extract—the supplement form that's used—has anti-edema properties, which means that it helps prevent the buildup of

Two bioflavonoids that seem to promote vascular health are grape seed and Pycnogenol, commonly called oligomeric proanthocyanidins, or OPCs. In one study, OPCs demonstrated powerful antioxidant activity by being able to trap the free-roaming, unstable molecules that can do so much cell damage. In fact, the antioxidant ability of OPCs was found to be many times greater than that of vitamin C and vitamin E.

If you have varicose veins, you should take 200 to 300 milligrams of grape seed extract or Pycnogenol a day with meals for at least 6 months, says Dr. Sinatra. If your discomfort improves, you can continue taking the supplement indefinitely.

Get Your C and B

Vitamin C is needed to help your body manufacture two important connective tissues, collagen and elastin. "Both of these tissues help to keep vein walls strong and flexible," says Dr. Pizzorno. Vitamin C may be especially important if you bruise easily or have broken capillaries, fluids. It also helps prevent inflammation, and it can decrease fluid leakage from capillaries by reducing the number and size of the small pores in the capillary walls.

Horse chestnut also improves the tone of blood vessels so veins become more elastic. With this boost in elasticity, they can contract more strongly and relax better, Dr. Weiss says.

How much you'll need to take depends on what kind of horse chestnut you buy. If you get a standardized extract of horse chestnut seed, use an amount that provides you with a daily dose of 50 milligrams of escin, Dr. Weiss says. Reduce the dosage after symptoms improve, he advises.

"I haven't had many problems with it, and I've had people on it for 7 or 8 months at a time," says Dr. Weiss. There have been some reports of side effects such as itching, nausea, and stomach discomfort. If you experience these side effects, simply stop taking horse chestnut until the symptoms go away. If you are pregnant, don't take this herb without your doctor's okay. Horse chestnut may also interfere with the action of other drugs, especially blood thinners such as warfarin (Coumadin), so check with your doctor to rule out drug interactions.

which may show up on your skin as tiny spider veins, he says. He recommends 500 to 3,000 milligrams of vitamin C daily.

Some doctors also recommend a combination of B vitamins, especially to people who have a history of blood clots. It's particularly important to make sure that you're getting sufficient amounts of folic acid, B_{12}, and B_6, Dr. Weiss says.

"I recommend B vitamins to all my patients with heart or circulatory problems as part of a high-potency multivitamin," says Dr. Weiss. If people have absorption problems, he will suggest B_{12} injections. Otherwise, you can take B-vitamin supplements in pill or capsule form.

Bring on the Es, Too

Vitamin E can also help, Dr. Pizzorno says. "Vitamin E helps keep platelets, blood components involved in clotting, from sticking together and from adhering to the sides of blood vessel walls," he says.

Research shows that reducing platelet stickiness with vitamin E may help people who are at particularly high risk for blood-clotting problems, such as those with type 1 (insulin-dependent) diabetes.

Taking 200 to 600 international units of vitamin E a day should be sufficient, Dr. Pizzorno says. If you've had bleeding problems, however, or are taking prescription anticoagulants to help prevent clotting, get your doctor's okay before you take vitamin E.

Go for Gotu Kola

The herb gotu kola is particularly good for varicose veins and also has a reputation as an antiaging herb, says Roberta Bourgon, ND, a naturopathic doctor at the Wellness Center in Billings, Montana. This herb seems to be able to strengthen the sheath of tissue that wraps around veins, reduce formation of clogging scar tissue, and improve blood flow through affected limbs.

"It's really more of a preventive measure than a cure," says Dr. Bourgon. "If you know you're prone to varicose veins, this can help you slow down or perhaps prevent the problem."

Even if it doesn't help the varicosity itself, gotu kola often improves the symptoms of varicose veins, including pain, numbness, and leg cramps, Dr. Bourgon says. Try taking 60 to 120 milligrams a day in capsules.

water retention

Fluid retention, or edema, is an excess of water in the body's tissues. It occurs when fluid that normally circulates in blood vessels and lymph ducts is diverted into the tiny channels between cells, called interstitial spaces. This makes the tissue swell.

Fluid accumulates for two primary reasons, says David B. Young, PhD, professor of physiology and biophysics at the University of Mississippi in Jackson. First, increased blood pressure in your veins causes increased pressure in the tiny capillaries that form a network throughout your tissues. This causes fluid to filter out of the capillaries and into the tissues.

"Increased blood pressure in the veins is usually caused by heart failure, often to the right side of the heart," Dr. Young says. "During the later stages of pregnancy, a woman may also experience swollen ankles because the baby is pressing against veins in her abdomen, hindering blood flow back from the legs and increasing pressure."

You don't have to be carrying a baby to have edema, however. Just standing for a long period of time can also increase blood pressure in veins. That's why your feet may be swollen at the end of the day.

Anything that changes the permeability of the capillaries can also cause swelling. Allergic reactions, such as a reaction to a bee sting, are one common cause. Also, if you have an injury that causes the capillaries to leak, that will create swelling.

No doubt you've heard that an ice pack or cold pack will reduce the swelling. There's much more than wishful thinking behind that advice. "Ice is so effective at reducing swelling because it constricts blood vessels, helping to reduce the flow of fluid from capillaries to tissue," Dr. Young says.

While leakage from capillaries is one clear cause of swelling, it's less clear why women often have fluid retention premenstrually for a few days each month. No one knows exactly why that happens, Dr. Young says. "It's a huge question, and certainly hormonal changes are involved, but nobody has a clue as to exactly how to explain it."

An Herb That Gets the Bloat Out

Many herbs act as diuretics—that is, they help your kidneys to remove water from your body. One of the best at getting the bloat out is dandelion.

In an animal study, dandelion leaf removed fluid from the body as well as furosemide (Lasix), a powerful diuretic often used for congestive heart failure. Dandelion leaf also supplies potassium, which other diuretics tend to drain out of your body.

For temporary bloating such as that which may occur premenstrually, you can drink 2 to 4 cups of dandelion leaf tea per day. Although teas work better as diuretics, you can also take one or two capsules of dried dandelion leaf.

(You'll also find alcohol-based tinctures of dandelion on store shelves, but because they're not as effective as teas or capsules, you'd have to take an extremely high dose, and that means too much alcohol.)

If you have fluid retention due to heart problems, you'll want to work with your doctor. You may be able to slowly increase your dosage of dandelion and decrease your dosage of pharmaceutical diuretics. If you have gallbladder disease, however, do not use dandelion preparations without medical approval.

Normally, a healthy body eventually recovers from swelling on its own. If you put your feet up for an hour or get a night's rest, your feet shrink to normal size. If you put a cold pack on a sprained ankle, the swelling goes down. Once hormones shift and menstruation starts, most women find that bloating quickly disappears. Additionally, there are ways that you can help your body to recover or to not be so prone to fluid retention. Here's how.

The Potassium Connection

Your body uses a balance of dissolved minerals to help regulate fluids. Two of the most important minerals in this regard are sodium and potassium, Dr. Young says. For optimal fluid regulation, your body needs to have a proper balance of both.

Unfortunately, most people get too much sodium and barely enough potassium. This can raise your blood pressure and your potential for fluid retention, Dr. Young says.

He suggests that you double your potassium intake to about 5,000 milligrams a day by consuming potassium-rich foods such as fruits and vegetables. It is possible to get potassium from supplements, but by law, over-the-counter supplements contain only 99 milligrams per tablet, because large doses have the potential to cause stomach irritation. For tablets that contain more potassium, you'll need a doctor's prescription. As for sodium, "your body needs very little and is very good at conserving it, so the less, the better," Dr. Young says.

Try B$_6$ for Hormone-Related Bloating

Vitamin B$_6$ plays a role in the body's use of hormones associated with fluid retention in women, including estrogen and progesterone, says Marilynn Pratt, MD, a doctor in Playa del Rey, California, who specializes in women's health. "By helping the liver to metabolize, or break down, these hormones, B$_6$ may help the body remove excess amounts that may be present during the premenstrual period," Dr. Pratt says.

In one study, 500 milligrams a day of vitamin B$_6$ relieved the breast tenderness, headaches, and weight gain associated with water retention in 215 women.

If you'd like to try B$_6$ for hormone-related fluid retention, take 50 milligrams four times a day for the 5 days before your period begins, Dr. Pratt suggests. In addition, take a supplement containing the rest of the B vitamins. "These nutrients interact and tend to work better as a team than individually," she says. Look for a supplement that contains a total of about 50 milligrams of most of the other B vitamins.

Vitamin B$_6$ can cause nerve damage in large doses if you take it for a number of weeks without a break, so generally, it's best not to take more than 100 milligrams on a daily basis, Dr. Pratt says.

wrinkles

We don't like wrinkled sheets. We don't like wrinkled apples. And we sure don't like wrinkled skin.

What is it about wrinkles? They suggest two things that we'd rather not think about—age and overuse. Of course, when it comes to wrinkles caused by aging, we have to accept a certain number as an inevitable part of the process. But your skin can defy the passage of years if you take certain precautions.

If you smoke, drink alcohol, eat poorly, and spend a lot of time in the sun, you can expect your face to become as lined and craggy as any weathered mountain. If, however, you take better care of your overall health, protect your skin from the sun, and feed it the proper nutrients and vitamins, you'll still age, but you will look younger than your years.

"You can definitely take better care of your skin, and that can make a difference in the number of wrinkles you eventually get," says Hope Fay, ND, a naturopathic doctor in Seattle. "The number one advice is: Don't stay in direct sun for long periods."

Undoing the Damage

When your skin is exposed to the sun, cells are damaged. These damaged cells give off free radicals—unstable molecules that cause cell damage.

By taking antioxidants, medicines that scavenge free radicals in the body, you can prevent further cell damage and protect your skin, says Dr. Fay. Three of the most common antioxidant vitamins are vitamin C, vitamin E, and beta-carotene.

If you've gotten a sunburn, Dr. Fay recommends taking 400 to 800 IU of vitamin E per day. "Vitamin E is really good for preventing free radical damage to the skin," she explains.

Vitamin C may be even more powerful because not only is it an antioxidant, it's also an essential developer of connective tissue. It aids in the formation of collagen, a protein in all connective tissues, including skin. Collagen binds cells together somewhat like mortar binds brick. It maintains the integrity and firmness of the skin, and firmer skin means fewer wrinkles.

You can get vitamin C from citrus juices, red bell peppers, and broccoli, says Michael Gazsi, ND, a naturopathic doctor in Danbury, Connecticut. "If your goal is healthy connective tissues and skin, taking 500 milligrams of vitamin C each day may help," he adds.

Selenium for Skin

Like the antioxidant vitamins, the trace mineral selenium is very effective at consuming free radicals caused by sun damage. You have to be careful when taking a selenium supplement, however, Dr. Gazsi warns. "I'd start with a multivitamin that contains some selenium—usually less than 100 micrograms," he says. "Then you can work your way up to a higher dosage." The maximum he recommends is 200 micrograms.

The dose that's right for you may depend on how much selenium you have in your diet, he adds. Selenium is found in the soil and makes its way into our bodies through plants and animals. Regions in the Great Lakes and Atlantic Seaboard have little selenium in the soil, while vast swatches of the Great Plains and Midwest have rather high amounts. If you live in one of the high-selenium areas and eat lots of local produce, you probably get enough selenium from your diet.

Hormone Helpers

Although we all get wrinkles as we age, sometimes they seem to come on more suddenly after pregnancy, menopause, or emotional stress. These triggering events may upset the balance of hormones in the body. Proper regulation and production of these chemical messengers are essential to maintaining soft, elastic skin.

To prevent hormone imbalances, you can begin by eating more legumes and soy products such as tofu, says Dr. Gazsi. These foods contain phytoestrogens, plant compounds that mimic the biological activities of female hormones.

Other important building blocks for hormone production are essential fatty acids, which are also generally good for the health of the skin, says Dr. Gazsi.

Upping Your Fatty Acids

Fatty acids aren't manufactured by the body but must be obtained from food sources like eggs, nuts, vegetables, butter, and whole milk. Some people who have poor, unbalanced diets don't get enough fatty acids for healthy skin, says Dr. Gazsi, and "unhealthy skin can lead to permanent wrinkles."

Whether your diet is deficient or not, you can help your skin fight off the effects of aging and sun exposure by taking a supplement of either flaxseed oil or evening primrose oil, both of which are sources of essential fatty acids, says Dr. Gazsi. He recommends four capsules per day of evening primrose oil or 2 tablespoons of flaxseed oil. "I'd probably start with the flaxseed oil and see how it works," he says. "It may take several months, however. Skin responds pretty slowly."

yeast infections

Few people would sign up to do battle with microscopic plant life, especially if they knew that the plant life would use guerrilla tactics at every opportunity.

Unfortunately, most women are destined to fight this battle. An estimated 75 percent of women get at least one yeast infection during their lives. To deal with a yeast infection, many women head for the local drugstore and buy an over-the-counter treatment such as miconazole nitrate (Monistat). But if the treatment you choose addresses only vaginal symptoms, you're getting at only half of the problem, says Lorilee Schoenbeck, ND, in private practice at the Vermont Women's Center in Burlington and coauthor of *Menopause: Bridging the Gap Between Natural and Conventional Medicine.*

When it comes to chronic or recurring infections, the heart of the problem is often the intestines, rather than the vaginal area, according to many naturopaths. *Candida albicans,* the organism that most frequently causes yeast infections, can sometimes become overgrown in your intestines. Yeast that exits the gastrointestinal tract can migrate into the vagina. That area can become infected repeatedly, says Dr. Schoenbeck. (See Vaginitis on page 605.)

Yeast infections can also mimic urinary tract infections or sexually transmitted diseases, so it's important to get an accurate diagnosis from a medical practitioner before beginning treatment. Also, you should definitely consult with your doctor if this is your first experience with symptoms of a yeast infection or if you are pregnant and have an underlying condition such as diabetes. Your doctor can determine whether you have a yeast infection.

Fortunately, there are many things that you can do to ward off yeast infections in the first place. To start with, limit the amount of sweets you eat, suggests Dr. Schoenbeck. Candida breeds even more profusely when you ingest a lot of sugar.

Another preventive measure is spelled d-r-y. Candida loves a warm, moist environment. Panty hose, tight jeans, wet bathing suits, and sweaty exercise clothes all provide the yeast with an ideal set of moist conditions. If you get damp clothes off as fast as you can and change into something dry and airy, you just might discourage the little diehards. Also, wear only pure cotton underwear and change it daily, says Dr. Schoenbeck.

Apart from these precautions, fighting off a chronic yeast infection usually requires a combined approach. While over-the-counter creams may knock out the occasional yeast infection, chronic or recurring ones may need more help. With the correct diet, herbs, and a good topical treatment regimen, most women can expect to begin winning the battle against chronic or recurring infections in about a month, says Dr. Schoenbeck. As for supplements, consider them potent allies in this battle. Some can help clear up a minor infection, and others can actually help ward off a yeast invasion.

Probiotics—The Right Stuff

Because the vaginal itching, redness, and pain can drive you absolutely nuts, you have to take care of the immediate outbreak first, says Dr. Schoenbeck. Probiotics—friendly bacteria found throughout your body—help keep candida in check.

When levels of your good bacteria are down (like when you take antibiotics), candida starts growing like wild. In the process of killing off infectious bacteria, antibiotics inadvertently kill off the good bugs as well, giving candida an extra chance to flourish. One easy way to get more probiotics is to eat live-culture yogurt, but probiotics also come in supplement form. Look for a supplement that contains a mix of *Lactobacillus* and *L. bifidus* bacteria and guarantees at least 10 billion colony-forming units (CFU).

Probiotics can help reestablish normal intestinal health, says Dr. Schoenbeck. Take the capsules only when you have an active yeast infection or are having a problem with recurring infections.

Taking oral doses of probiotics for just 2 to 4 weeks can help decrease candida in both your vagina and your intestines, she says. That makes you less prone to repeat infections.

Turning to Herbs

"Garlic is one of the best things to take for yeast infections," says naturopathic doctor Tori Hudson, ND, professor at the National College of

Naturopathic Medicine in Portland, Oregon, and author of *Women's Encyclopedia of Natural Medicine*. It is both antifungal and immunity-boosting, she says.

In a laboratory study, researchers gave some animals with yeast infections a solution of aged garlic extract and others a plain saltwater solution with no active ingredients. After 2 days, the animals that received the garlic extract showed no signs of yeast infection. The animals in the other group still had infections.

In humans, two garlic capsules a day are enough to protect against yeast, according to Dr. Hudson. It's best to take enteric-coated capsules because the coating prevents the active ingredients in garlic from breaking down in the stomach. Look for garlic capsules with 4,000 milligrams of allicin, which is the antifungal agent found in garlic, she says.

Herbs such as Oregon grape root extract, tea tree oil extract, and lavender extract all help reduce the amount of candida growing in the intestines. "There are supplements that contain all of these extracts, but they are hard to find. I'd ask an alternative practitioner to prescribe one," Dr. Schoenbeck says. She recommends taking two tablets three times a day. After a month, see your practitioner to be sure the infection is gone.

Echinacea is beneficial, too. A German study found that women taking antifungal medicine plus echinacea extract had only a 10 percent recurrence of yeast infections. In the study, this group was compared to women who took only antifungal medicine. Nearly 60 percent of that group had recurrent infections.

Another great antiyeast herb is goldenseal, says Dr. Schoenbeck. Like Oregon grape, goldenseal contains berberine, a chemical that has antibiotic properties and works particularly well against yeast. You can buy echinacea and goldenseal separately or in combination capsules. Whichever you choose, take them daily as directed on the product you buy. If the capsules contain 450 milligrams of an echinacea and goldenseal combination, a typical dose would be two or three capsules daily with water. Do not use goldenseal if you are pregnant, however.

index

Underscored page references indicate boxed text.

A

Acerola berries, 15
Acetyl-L-carnitine
  for Alzheimer's disease, 316
  for angina, 326
  for chronic fatigue syndrome, 369
  for diabetes, 391
  for infertility, male, 470
  for memory loss, age-related, 64, 316
Acetylcholine, 301, 319
Acid reflux, 438
Acyclovir (Zovirax), 414, 587
Adaptogen herbs, 36–37, 220–21. *See also specific type*
Adenosine triphosphate (ATP)
  alpha lipoic acid and, 55
  coenzyme Q_{10} and, 520
  creatine and, 143–44
  magnesium and, 244–45
  riboflavin and, 287
Adrenal gland extracts, <u>594</u>
Adrenal glands
  chronic fatigue syndrome and, 368
  DGL and, 593
  DHEA and, 496
  gotu kola and, 226–27
  hormones, 114
  licorice root and, 497
  menopause and, 506
  pantothenic acid and, 267
Adrenal Stress-End, 368, <u>594</u>
Age-related macular degeneration (AMD),
    500–503
  beta-carotene for, 502
  B vitamins for, 502–3
  carotenoids for, 502
  dry form, 500
  fish oil for, 503
  lutein for, 272, 502
  vitamin C and, 502–33

vitamin E and, 502–3
wet form, 500
zeaxanthin for, 272
zinc for, 502
Aging
  coenzyme Q_{10} and, 134, 136
  digestion and, 174
  dowager's hump and, 122
  macular degeneration related to, 500–503
  memory loss related to, 313–19
  minerals and, 20
  nutritional needs and, 8, 18–20
  oxidative damage and, 164
  preventing/treating effects of
    DHEA, 157–58
    ginkgo, 212–13
    gotu kola, 229
    vitamin C, <u>113</u>
  riboflavin and, 19
  selenium and, 19–20
  supplements and, 18–20
  taste and smell loss and, 599
  thiamin and, 19
  vitamin B_6 and, 19
  vitamin B_{12} and, 19
  vitamin C and, 19–20
AIDS. *See* HIV and AIDS
Ajoenes, 205
ALA. *See* Alpha-linolenic acid; Alpha lipoic acid
Alanine, 63, 562
Alcohol
  addiction, 75, 301, 323
  cirrhosis from, 58
  headaches and, 428
  impotence and, 460
  insomnia and, 471
  multiple sclerosis and, 516
  stress and, 591
  withdrawal from, 301
  wrinkles and, 618